ETHICS & AIDS IN AFRICA

THE CHALLENGE TO OUR THINKING

Editors: Anton A. van Niekerk, Loretta M. Kopelman

Left Coast Press Inc.

WALNUT CREEK, CALIFORNIA

We dedicate this volume to the persons with HIV/AIDS and hope this discussion of the moral issues of their disease helps them and those who love them.

Left Coast Press Inc.

Published outside Africa by
Left Coast Press, Inc.
1630 N. Main Street #400
Walnut Creek, CA 94596
www.LCoastPress.com

First published in Africa by David Philip Publishers, an imprint of New Africa Books (pty) Ltd, 99 Garfield Road, Claremont 7700, South Africa, www.newafricabooks.co.za

Hardback ISBN 1-59874-070-9
Paperback ISBN 1-59874-071-7
Library of Congress Control Number 2006924267

Printed in the United States of America

This book is printed on New Leaf EcoBook 50, containing 100% recycled, 50% post-consumer waste, processed chlorine free; remaining content is elemental chlorine free. EcoBook 50 is acid-free and meets the minimum requirements of ANSI/astm D5634-01 (Permanence of Paper). ∞™

05 06 07 08 5 4 3 2 1

Editing by Celia Fleming
Proofreading by Glynne Newlands
Layout and design by AN dtp Services
Cover design by Nic Jooste

FOREWORD

For 25 long years, we have grappled with humankind's worst pandemic since the plague cut down one-third of Europe's population nearly seven centuries ago. We have struggled to grasp the virology of AIDS, its demography, its impact on human physiology, its social and economic consequences, its responsiveness to medical treatment. But most of all we have struggled with the moral and ethical implications of so much suffering and death, first in North America and Western Europe, and now in Africa, where the epidemic's fiercest toll is being exacted.

AIDS is an economic and social challenge. But more than this, it is a moral test. For underlying the practical challenges of leadership, organisation and decision-making — themselves so critical when so many lives are at stake — are the ethical tests of our own thinking. How do we conceive an epidemic that was first diagnosed amongst the morally still-marginalised gay men of North America and Western Europe, and that now strikes hardest at the materially marginalised populations of the world's poorest continent? How do we conceive a world that has effective means to treat most people with AIDS, but in which the life-saving benefit of antiretroviral medication is still denied to most of those with the greatest need?

These challenging questions have already tested South Africa's and Africa's leadership, and that of the Western world, whose societies are more fabulously powerful and wealthy than any in human history. But they challenge us also. For in Central and Southern Africa, AIDS is not someone else's problem: it is our own. And our response to AIDS — in our own lives and households and workplaces and communities and organisations — will help determine the calibre of our future societies.

These are the questions that powerfully inform the contributions to this important collection of essays that Anton van Niekerk and Loretta Kopelman have compiled. In it, distinguished authors, including those at the forefront of the debates that most bear on life and death in the African epidemic of AIDS, discuss its central ethical issues. What are our means of knowledge in the epidemic? How do we know whether the epidemic is real (for, astonishingly, this question is still asked, and asked with aggression and righteousness by those who dispute the existence of AIDS, or its viral, mostly sexually transmitted causes)? What imperative response does the availability of life-saving medications demand of us? And how do we assess our own judgment of those who have HIV and AIDS?

Not only are these questions asked in the pages that follow, but also the contributing authors provide clarity and new moral direction in answering them. As far as I know, this is the first collection of essays dedicated to ethics and AIDS and Africa. Its appearance is most welcome. The power and clarity of its contributions is even more welcome. For far from hiding in abstraction or generalities, the authors contributing to Prof. Van Niekerk's and Prof. Kopelman's book take bold and lucid stances. Their writing adds to our understanding of the epidemic and provides suggestions for how societies should respond to this crisis. That response necessarily requires moral leadership, and this is a bold book that provides it.

Edwin Cameron
Supreme Court of Appeal
February 2005

TABLE OF CONTENTS

LIST OF CONTRIBUTORS

Richard E. Ashcroft is Reader in Biomedical Ethics and Head of the Medical Ethics Unit at Imperial College, London.

Tony Barnett is ESRC Professorial Research Fellow at the Development Studies Institute, London School of Economics, and founder of LSEAIDS.

Solomon R. Benatar is Professor of Medicine, Director of the Bioethics Unit at the University of Cape Town and Visiting Professor of Medicine and Public Health Sciences, University of Toronto, Canada.

Gavin George is a Researcher at the Health Economics and HIV/AIDS Research Division of the University of KwaZulu-Natal.

Loretta M. Kopelman is Professor and Chair of the Department of Medical Humanities at the Brody School of Medicine, East Carolina University, USA.

Keymanthri Moodley is Associate Professor of Family Medicine and Head of the Tygerberg Division of the Unit for Bioethics in the Centre for Applied Ethics, University of Stellenbosch.

Nicoli Nattrass is Professor of Economics and Director of the AIDS and Society Research Unit in the Centre for Social Science Research at the University of Cape Town.

David B. Resnik is a Bioethicist at the National Institute of Environmental Health Sciences, National Institutes of Health, Washington D.C., USA.

Udo Schüklenk is Professor of Ethics and Public Policy and Head of the Centre for Ethics and Public Policy at Glasgow Caledonian University in the UK.

Catherine Slack is a Clinical Psychologist and Project Co-ordinator of the HIV/AIDS Vaccines Ethics Group (HAVEG) at the University of KwaZulu-Natal.

Melissa Stobie is Senior Lecturer in the School of Philosophy and Ethics at the University of KwaZulu-Natal.

Ann Strode is a Senior Lecturer in the Faculty of Law at the University of KwaZulu-Natal.

Godfrey Tangwa is Associate Professor of Philosophy and Head of the Department of Philosophy at the University of Yaounde 1, Cameroon.

Anton A. van Niekerk is Professor of Philosophy, Director of the Centre for Applied Ethics and Head of the Unit for Bioethics at the University of Stellenbosch.

Alan Whiteside is Professor of Economics and Director of the Health Economics and HIV/AIDS Research Division at the University of KwaZulu-Natal.

INTRODUCTION

A little more than 20 years ago, The Centers for Disease Control in Atlanta, USA, first reported in its *Morbidity and Mortality Weekly Report* that a few men had died of a deadly form of pneumonia. Since that 5 June 1981 publication, 23 million people have been documented as dying from what is now identified as acquired immune deficiency syndrome (AIDS). More than half, over 17 million of these people, are Africans. Currently, 39.4 million persons live with the human immunodeficiency virus (HIV) and 25.4 million (64 percent) of them reside in sub-Saharan Africa (Whiteside 2005). In Africa, the disease is mainly transmitted through heterosexual sex; whereas, in the developed world, contaminated needles of intravenous drug abusers and homosexual male sex are also major contributors to its persistent spread.

The most disturbing fact about HIV/AIDS is that, although there has been significant improvement in the management of the disease, largely brought about by the introduction of highly active antiretroviral therapies (HAART), and although progress is seemingly being made with the development of effective and safe AIDS vaccines, there is, as yet, no cure for or vaccine against this disease. HIV/AIDS has therefore become the overwhelming reality in the seemingly pervasive predicament of the African continent. Never in the history of pandemics have we seen such a persistent increase in the number of people infected over such a prolonged period of time. Epidemics are usually characterised by sharp rises in infection rates, followed by similarly sharp declines once appropriate management measures are taken. This was, for example, seen in the case of the recent SARS epidemic in the East and Canada. HIV/AIDS defies this 'law of epidemics' since its inception, in part, because of its long incubation period. It has therefore become a global catastrophe, and poses the major challenge to both health care and social stability on the African continent.

Nowhere is the catastrophic impact of HIV/AIDS more apparent than in the region of Southern Africa. Botswana and Swaziland have infection rates in excess of 40 percent of its population – a figure that, a few years ago, was widely regarded as inconceivable as far as epidemics go. South Africa has, in absolute numbers, the highest rate of infection in the world. More than five million South Africans are currently HIV positive. In 2004 alone, more than 311 000 people died of HIV/AIDS-related diseases in South Africa (i.e. almost 900 per day) (Benatar 2005b).

The catastrophic nature of the pandemic is well illustrated by the fact that, in the absence of effective interventions (none of which seem forthcoming), it is expected that 40 to 50 percent of South Africa's workforce will die in the next ten years. In this coming year, there will already be 800 000 orphans under the age of 15 in South Africa (Benatar 2005b). UNICEF estimates that by 2010 an estimated 20 million children in Africa will have lost one or both parents to HIV/AIDS (Whiteside 2005). One should ask: what happens – economically and socially – to societies in which this occurs?

Much has been written about the medical, demographic, economic, political and social-psychological dimensions of the pandemic. This book, however, is the first comprehensive volume about the *ethical* dimensions and problems associated with the pandemic, and particularly so in Africa. Ethics is the discipline that deals systematically with the nature of obligation, including with the issues, judgments, theories and possible answers pertaining to the question: when are our actions right or wrong, and what things are good or bad? The HIV/AIDS pandemic has revealed a remarkable array of ethical problems that occur in the effort to identify HIV-positive people and to treat patients suffering from AIDS appropriately, and, eventually, to vaccinate the population against the disease, should a vaccine eventually be successfully developed – something that is not foreseen to occur within the current decade.

However, as will be argued in some of the contributions that follow, the ethical problems related to HIV/AIDS transcend the sphere of the day-to-day clinical practice of administering medical care to patients by health care workers. It is becoming increasingly clear that the phenomenon of HIV/AIDS reveals dramatic problems in the global interactions between countries and institutions in the developed and developing worlds. As such, HIV/AIDS has, almost more than any other health care phenomenon in recent times, revealed the necessity of the development of what can nowadays indeed be called a 'global bioethics'. The contributions to this book deal with both these dimensions of the problem.

In what follows, we shall briefly introduce the main arguments and insights of the chapters that follow:

- **Chapter 1** ('AIDS in Africa: facts, figures and the extent of the problem') is by Alan Whiteside, South Africa's leading AIDS demographer. In this chapter, the exact extent of the problem in Africa will be discussed, with emphasis on what is to be expected if current trends of (in)action regarding treatment continue, and what the effect of interventions might be. The latest and most reliable figures about the pandemic are provided, as well as remarks about the significance of apparent discrepancies that occur between data from different sources. Whiteside goes on to discuss the 'dramatic and far reaching' consequences of the pandemic, particularly their impact on the economy and on the social welfare of orphaned children, which is generally foreseen to be catastrophic in Africa. Some appropriate responses are explored in conclusion.

- In **Chapter 2**, Alan Whiteside, Tony Barnett, Gavin George and Anton A. van Niekerk ('Through a glass, darkly: data and uncertainty in the AIDS debate') discuss the problem of unreliable statistics about the AIDS epidemic and how the moral controversies surrounding AIDS can be related to unreliable data about the pandemic. The limitations of the use of antenatal clinic surveys, which provide the bulk of our information, are discussed. While it can be claimed that there are problems with the reliability of the data from antenatal clinics, this by no means suggests that the available figures are over-inflated. On the contrary, given the fact that access to antenatal clinics is quite limited in the deep rural areas of Africa, it is safer to assume that our available figures on the pandemic are too conservative. The authors then turn to the evidence of impact of the epidemic, showing how the long incubation period for HIV infections to turn to AIDS, and for AIDS to translate into deaths has profound consequences, including orphaning, increasing poverty and changing population structures. Furthermore, it means that once the HIV prevalence has peaked, AIDS impact will take years to work through; this epidemic is a 'long-wave' event. They argue that insufficient and/or unreliable data have allowed leaderships, particularly in Africa, to deny the scope and scale of the problem and that this is unacceptable. However, it is incumbent on these leaders to accept the moral responsibility for choices and the consequences of their work, and this includes funding and supporting those who gather, interpret and use the data.

Chapter 3 ('Rolling out antiretroviral treatment in South Africa: economic and ethical challenges') is by Nicoli Nattrass, an economist from the University of Cape Town who is well known for her recent book *The moral economy of AIDS in South Africa* (Nattrass 2004). In this chapter, she develops three moral-economic arguments that are all related to the issue of whether treatment with HAART is, from both a social and economic perspective, a viable option for (South) Africa at present. First, she argues, in response to some policy makers, why a rollout of HAART is likely to contribute to fewer new HIV infections. She also disputes the counterclaim that a HAART rollout will lead to less responsible lifestyles and thus increased infections. Her second argument deals specifically with the issue of cost-effectiveness. She argues: 'Once HIV-related costs are included in the calculation, the cost per HIV infection averted is lower in a treatment plus prevention intervention scenario than it is in a prevention-only scenario'. Her conclusion is that the constraints on funding a large-scale, comprehensive intervention in the current pandemic in Africa are politically and not economically driven. It is, contrary to what many policy makers seemingly accept, economically feasible to fund such a comprehensive treatment programme with HAART. Finally, Nattrass turns to an ethical issue specifically generated by the spending of tax money on AIDS. This is the phenomenon that many people living with AIDS in South Africa are increasingly becoming dependent on disability grants provided to them by the government. Given the insufficiency of other poverty relief measures in a developing country such as South Africa, these grants are apparently becoming an incentive to either contract HIV or to fudge information when ability to go off the grant is restored. Nattrass develops an impressive argument why this phenomenon ought to provide an additional reason for considering the introduction of a Basic Income Grant for South Africa (Nattrass 2005).

- In **Chapter 4** ('Moral and social complexities of AIDS in Africa') we move from these demographic and economic issues to other moral and socio-political complexities of the HIV/AIDS pandemic in Africa. Anton van Niekerk discusses some of these, as well as the importance of finding responses that empower people living with HIV/AIDS in Africa. Complexities include poverty, denial, poor leadership, illiteracy, women's vulnerability and the disenchantment of intimacy as people worry about whether their partners will give them a deadly disease. Seeking long-term and comprehensive solutions to its moral, social and political problems could exacerbate the sense of hopelessness and helplessness that is engulfing the region as so many become orphans, get sick or die. Rather than wait for comprehensive solutions and warning against the disempowering consequences of tendencies to politicise the discourse about AIDS in Africa, he argues that we should focus upon what needs to be done immediately to respond to HIV/AIDS.

- In **Chapter 5** ('The HIV/AIDS pandemic: a sign of instability in a complex global system'), Solomon R. Benatar deals with the HIV/AIDS pandemic as a 'sign of instability in a complex global system'. He argues that Van Niekerk's view that we should not wait for comprehensive solutions before acting should be supplemented by conceding the role of global politics, especially the exploitation, discrimination and imperialism by first world countries of sub-Saharan Africa. For the sake of world stability and common decency, more affluent countries should realign their development aid priorities and help Africans create a better quality of life by responding to their poverty, hunger and diseases. He acknowledges that since colonial independence, some problems have resulted from 'poor governance, corruption, internal exploitation, nepotism, tribalism, authoritarianism, military rule and over-population through patriarchal attitudes and disempowerment of women, [but urges that] these shortcomings must be seen in the context of powerful external disruptive forces acting over several centuries to impede progress in Africa'. According to Benatar, 'a biomedical approach cannot, in isolation, sufficiently improve the health of populations. To achieve the latter will require understanding and addressing the powerful social forces that allow pandemics to emerge and spread in order to ensure that real development and empowered independence can take the place of perpetual philanthropy. Broadening the discourse on ethics to include public health ethics and the ethics of international relations could contribute to reducing the impact of the pandemic and to preventing the emergence of new infectious diseases in the future' (Benatar 2005a).

- In **Chapter 6**, ('Principles of global distributive justice and the HIV/AIDS pandemic: moving beyond Rawls and Buchanan'), Anton A. van Niekerk draws on some of Benatar's insights to develop the perspective of a global bioethics by specifically contributing to the debate between Allen Buchanan and John Rawls about the appropriateness and contents of principles of global distributive justice (PGDJ), as these are specifically called for in view of the HIV/AIDS pandemic. He briefly reviews the main tenets of Rawls's theory of justice, particularly as it concerns health care. In this respect, he draws on the work of Norman Daniels who has applied Rawls's theory to the issue of the provision of just health care. Secondly, he argues for the necessity of a global approach to biomedical ethics in view of the need for a more equitable provision of health care between developed and developing worlds. Thirdly, he discusses the main tenets of Rawls's *The Law of Peoples*, the book in which Rawls extrapolated the implications of his theory of justice to the sphere of just international law. Allen Buchanan's criticisms of this Rawlsian enterprise are then critically reviewed. Finally, Van Niekerk evaluates this debate, arguing that, although he largely (but not wholly) agrees with Buchanan's identification of the shortcomings in Rawls's *The Law of Peoples*, two additional principles of global distributive justice (PGDJ) ought to be added to the two formulated by Buchanan with which the author agrees. One of these additional principles shows the importance for special measures in cases of catastrophic occurrences such as the current HIV/AIDS pandemic. The other emerges from another problem the author has with Buchanan's analysis: his tendency, when formulating PGDJ, to concentrate the burden of responsibility implied by these principles entirely to the wealthy societies. Van Niekerk argues that this principle involves the responsibility of poor societies to not only be on the receiving end of aid and to bask in continuous entitlements, but to also exert responsible policies that create sustainable conditions for the meaningful redistribution of global wealth and health. This is again illustrated with reference to issues in the current debate about the global response to the AIDS pandemic.

- **Chapters 7 to 13** deal with more specific ethical issues provoked by the HIV/AIDS pandemic: the cost of drugs (Chapters 7 and 8), mother-to-child transmission (Chapter 9), ethical issues related to the development of AIDS vaccines (Chapters 10, 11 and 12) and the issue of whether HIV/AIDS can rightly be seen as 'punishment' (Chapter 13). In Chapter 7 ('Access to Affordable Medication in the Developing World: social responsibility vs. profit'), David Resnik deals with the issue of access to affordable medication in the developing world, and specifically the question as to how concerns about the profits of large multinational pharmaceutical companies weigh up against concerns of their (alleged) social responsibility. The gist of his argument is that 'large, global pharmaceutical companies have a moral obligation to develop affordable drugs for the developing world and to make these drugs accessible, and that developing nations should cooperate with these companies in achieving these goals'. His view is that 'although pharmaceutical companies and developing nations are often in conflict they must work together to develop drugs for the developing world' (Resnik 2005). He emphasises that his view does not stem from a naïve defence of the pharmaceutical industry; pharmaceutical companies have social responsibilities that they often do not take seriously. His defence of intellectual property rights for pharmaceutical companies 'stems from a pragmatic approach to the justification of intellectual property, not from an ideological commitment to big business' (Resnik 2005).

- **Chapter 8** ('Affordable access to essential medication in developing countries: conflicts between ethical and economic imperatives') by Udo Schüklenk and Richard Ashcroft offers an alternative perspective to the views expressed by Resnik. They argue that given the public health crises, compulsory licensing of essential AIDS medications is justifiable on consequentialist grounds. Alternatives such as discounted pricing and donation schemes by drug manufacturers are, they argue, both morally and pragmatically inferior.
- In **Chapter 9** ('Mother-to-child transmission of HIV/AIDS in Africa: ethical problems and perspectives'), by Anton van Niekerk, the subject is mother-to-child transmission (MTCT) of HIV/AIDS in Africa and its concomitant ethical issues. The author first deals with the relevant facts about MTCT. This is followed by a discussion of two ethical problems, viz. the issue of the morality of placebo-controlled trials for drugs to prevent MTCT in Africa, and the issue of the lack of political leadership and responsibility to implement proven programmes that will combat MTCT. In conclusion, the author discusses a number of insights that these disputes yield for our understanding of our powers over disease in the contemporary world, the implications of these issues for our understanding of scientific methodology in medicine, the dangers of politicising a health problem such as HIV/AIDS, the need for renewed reflection on the global disparities in the provision of health care, and the need for imaginative and responsible political leadership and co-operation between the developed countries, Africa and the pharmaceutical corporations to address and combat a catastrophe of unprecedented global proportions.
- In **Chapters 10 to 12** the issue is ethical problems related to the development of AIDS vaccines in Africa. In Chapter 10 ('HIV vaccine trial participation in South Africa – an ethical assessment'), Keymanthri Moodley discusses tensions when first world countries sponsor research in sub-Saharan Africa. In order to study HIV/AIDS, especially in rural African regions, interpretations tailored to specific communities may be needed of such key notions in research ethics as informed consent, fair treatment of subjects and risk assessment. These societies, she argues, employ a moderate form of communitarianism referred to as 'Ubuntu' or 'communalism' that could help these

people understand research as an altruistic endeavour benefiting communities as a result of risks taken by individuals. The first world individualistic focus may fail to emphasise such forms of communalism, thereby thwarting the sort of approach likely to gain approval and co-operation for research needed in Africa today.

- In **Chapter 11** ('The HIV/AIDS pandemic, African traditional values and the search for a vaccine in Africa'), Godfrey B. Tangwa also argues for the importance of traditional African values and how they should be enlisted to fight the HIV/AIDS pandemic. These values emphasise empathy and providing for people in genuine need, irrespective of their ability to pay. This contrasts with the more libertarian, market-driven, profit-oriented practices of important sectors of first world countries. Not only should these traditional African values be respected, he argues, but they could also teach others how to deal with those in need.
- In **Chapter 12** ('The dilemma of enrolling children in HIV vaccine research in South Africa: what is in 'the child's best interest'?), Melissa Stobie, Ann Strode and Cathy Slack examine whether and how to involve children in the research for HIV vaccines. Many children are infected with HIV in (South) Africa, and are entitled to benefit from the development of a vaccine. How, then, are we to think of the thorny issue of the 'child's best interest' in a situation where they will inevitably be put at risk if they participate in research to develop vaccines? The authors of this chapter argue that the 'best interest principle', so often invoked as the guiding ethical principle in moral issues regarding children, may, ironically, 'work to the long-term detriment of children if interpreted too strictly on individual grounds. This is especially so in South Africa, where the prevalence and rate of HIV infection mean that the only way to effectively stem the epidemic would be to vaccinate children against HIV infection'. Vaccinations of children, however, can only occur safely if children are included in the vaccine trials – a move which, in turn, may not be in their individual 'best interests'. The authors thus 'explore the ethical and legal framework in South Africa, and evaluate it in terms of the best interests standard'. In doing so, they 'try constantly to bear in mind not just the best interests of the individual child, but also of children as a class'. They conclude by 'suggesting some tools research ethics committees may need to use in order to determine whether the best interests of children are being respected' (Stobie et al. 2005).
- In the final chapter, **Chapter 13** ('If HIV/AIDS is punishment, who is bad?'), Loretta M. Kopelman takes as her starting point the fact that HIV/AIDS strikes with the greatest frequency in sub-Saharan Africa, a region uniquely lacking resources to deal with this epidemic. To keep millions more people from dying, wealthy countries and people must provide more help. Yet deeply ingrained biases may distance the sick from those who could provide

> far more aid. One such prejudice is viewing disease as punishment for sin. This 'punishment theory of disease' ascribes moral blame to those who get sick or those with special relations to them. Religious versions hold that God or other divine beings punish to castigate, encourage virtue, warn, rehabilitate or maintain some cosmic order. Its various religious and secular forms are untenable; they lack cogency, risk blaming people unjustly, and jeopardise compassionate care for people. These views are not only irrational but also dangerous because they influence policies and cost lives and lead people to deny the reality of the danger. We need to cooperate and respond as befits this global public-health disaster and not engage in the misguided and bad faith activity of dividing the world into the blameworthy and blameless.

The authors of this book agree that for compassionate as well as pragmatic reasons, there must be both a national and a global effort to find a solution to the HIV/AIDS pandemic. Each author discusses some of the fault lines and upheavals that this plague has exposed and the radical changes that this pandemic is likely to leave in its wake. They conclude that good solutions must be cooperative ventures amongst countries within and outside of sub-Saharan Africa, with wealthy countries making more generous contributions to help fight the world's worst plague.

This book is the outcome of a project initiated by the editors in 2002 when they were invited to edit a special edition of the *Journal of Medicine and Philosophy* (volume 27, no. 2, April 2002) on the ethical problems related to AIDS in Africa. All the articles published in that volume are republished in this book. We would like to express our sincere gratitude to the Editor-in-Chief of the *Journal of Medicine and Philosophy* (JMP), Dr H. Tristram Engelhardt, not only for the original invitation, but also and in particular for granting permission to republish edited varieties of the seven articles originally included in the JMP edition, i.e. the (considerably changed) Introduction as well as Chapters 4, 5, 8, 10, 11 and 13 of this volume.

Chapter 2 was originally published in *Developing World Bioethics*, an extended version of Chapter 6 in the *South African Journal of Philosophy* and Chapter 9 in *Jahrbuch für Wissenshaft and Ethik*. We thank the publishers for permission to republish. The other chapters (1, 3, 7 and 12) were written specifically for this volume, subject to peer review similar to all the other material included. We would specifically like to thank these authors – Alan Whiteside, Nicoli Nattrass, David Resnik, Melissa Stobie, Ann Strode and Cathy Slack – for their excellent work in this regard. Our thanks, naturally, also extend to Tony Barnett, Gavin George, Solly Benatar, Udo Schüklenk, Richard Ashcroft, Keymanthri Moodley and Godfrey Tangwa for their contributions.

We appreciate New Africa Books and their representative, Jeanne Hromnik, for taking on this project and rendering outstanding professional service. Anton van Niekerk particularly wishes to thank his assistant Liezl Dick for rendering invaluable help with the preparation of the manuscript; and Loretta Kopelman wishes to thank Evangelyn Okereke, and Lisa Bagnell for their help in preparing these manuscripts. Loretta Kopelman and Anton van Niekerk wish to give special thanks to Debra Duncan for her diligent proofreading and for helping to compile the index.

Finally, we express our sincerest gratitude to Justice Edwin Cameron of the Supreme Court of Appeal in South Africa for his very generous Foreword. His stature as one of South Africa's foremost advocates of accelerated action to curb the pandemic lends significant credibility to this project.

Anton A. van Niekerk
Centre for Applied Ethics, University of Stellenbosch, South Africa

Loretta M. Kopelman
The Brody School of Medicine at East Carolina University, North Carolina, USA

February 2005.

References

Benatar, S.R. (2005a).The HIV/AIDS pandemic: a sign of instability in a complex global system, Chapter 5 of this volume.

Benatar, S.R. (2005b). The lost potential of our health system. *The Cape Times*, 14 January 2005, p. 14.

Kopelman, L.M. (2005). If HIV/AIDS is punishment, who is bad? Chapter 13 of this volume.

Nattrass, N. (2004). *The moral economy of AIDS in South Africa*. Cambridge: Cambridge University Press.

Nattrass, N. (2005). Rolling out antiretroviral treatment in South Africa: economic and ethical challenges. Chapter 3 of this volume.

Resnik, D. (2005). Access to affordable medication in the developing world: social responsibility vs. profit. Chapter 7 of this volume.

Stobie, M., Strode, A. & Slack C. (2005). The dilemma of enrolling children in HIV vaccine research in South Africa: what is in 'the child's best interest?' Chapter 12 of this volume.

Whiteside, A. (2005). AIDS in Africa: facts, figures and the extent of the problem. Chapter 1 of this volume.

Chapter 1

AIDS in Africa: facts, figures and the extent of the problem

Although there are some discrepancies in statistics, the figures given here by **Alan Whiteside**[1] *prove that Africa has been hardest hit by the AIDS epidemic. The impact is, and will be, devastating across many sectors, and an immediate and appropriate response is necessary.*

Every year UNAIDS releases new data on the extent of the epidemic across the world. The trend is inexorably upwards. At the end of 2004 there were an estimated 39.4 million [35.9 million–44.3 million] people living with the virus. Of these, 4.9 million [4.3 million–5.4 million] people were infected in 2004. An estimated 3.1 million [2.8 million–3.5 million] people died of the disease in the past year (UNAIDS and WHO 2004).

Sub-Saharan Africa is the worst affected continent, with 25.4 million [23.4 million–28.4 million] people living with HIV at the end of 2004, an increase of one million since 2002. About two thirds (64 percent) of all people living with HIV are in sub-Saharan Africa, as are more than three quarters (76 percent) of all women living with HIV. There is not 'one' epidemic in Africa. There are differences in the size and trajectory of the disease – Southern Africa has by far the worst epidemic, while in North Africa there is no significant HIV infection.

This chapter will:

- look at the recent debate on how data are collected;
- discuss the African epidemics;
- examine the figures to understand future impact, especially with regard to demographic, development and economic consequences;
- point to the moral issues.

Data debates: an update

Where do data come from? How can UNAIDS say that there are between 23.4 and 28.4 million people infected in Africa – how certain are they about this? As with so many other fields, we need to understand the limitations of data and data collection. This is well described in the chapter 'Through a glass darkly, data and uncertainty in the AIDS debate', an article first published in *Developing World Bioethics*, 3(1), May 2003: 49–76 by Alan Whiteside, Tony Barnett, Gavin

George and Anton A van Niekerk and included in this collection as Chapter 2. This chapter does not revisit that discussion, but rather updates it.

Scientists (and social scientists) recognise the imperfections of the data we have. However, this is not the case for others. Indeed for South Africans, one of the depressing features of 2004 was the renewed questioning of data by ill-informed people who 'discovered' the fact that we do not 'know' and therefore assume that all data must be wrong.

The 18 December 2003 issue of the British magazine *The Spectator* ran an article by South African journalist Rian Malan under the headline 'Africa isn't dying of AIDS' (Malan 2003). This article was picked up by the British and South African press and read widely. Malan was given additional credibility by being quoted extensively – although not on the issue of AIDS – by President Thabo Mbeki in his state of the nation address on 6 February 2004. Two days later Mbeki used Malan's arguments in a TV interview to argue that AIDS is not as serious a problem as we think.

Malan made two key arguments: the first, that while AIDS is a serious issue for Africa, the size of the problem and its long-term effects on society and the economy have been exaggerated; the second suggested that there is something of a cover-up of the true (and more limited) extent of the epidemic as it would not suit the AIDS industry for whom this disease provides employment. There were a number of responses to Malan, one co-authored by myself (Barnett, Prins & Whiteside 2004). Rather than rehash the debates, in the next section this chapter will review the latest data and assess what it means for Africa, and will return to the data issue in the last section.

Before we do this, let us spend a few minutes looking at where data come from. When 'Through a glass darkly' (Chapter 2) was written, almost all of the information on HIV prevalence came from antenatal clinics (ANC). The reason was that this is a sexually active, convenient population from whom blood was drawn anyway. Sampling an entire population is expensive and difficult, especially when the test requires blood. It had been done in a few locations and the results of these surveys suggested that ANC data over-estimated prevalence in younger women and underestimated it in older women. It was also believed that although more women would be infected at younger ages, the increased prevalence among older men would even this out.

It has become apparent that in sub-Saharan Africa HIV/AIDS is affecting women and girls in increasing numbers.

With time it has become apparent that in sub-Saharan Africa HIV/AIDS is affecting women and girls in increasing numbers. While globally, just under half of all people living with HIV are female, women and girls make up almost 57 percent of all people infected with HIV in sub-Saharan Africa. In the younger age groups (15 to 24 years), 76 percent of those infected are female.

But there are also new data sources. There have been a number of population-based surveys. In South Africa we have two new surveys – the Nelson Mandela/

HSRC population study in 2002 (Nelson Mandela/Human Sciences Research Council 2002) and the 2004 Reproductive Health Research Unit (RHRU) survey of 15- to 24-year-olds (Pettifor et al. 2004). In countries to the north, HIV prevalence is being surveyed as part of some of the Demographic and Health Surveys. This has been done in Kenya and Ghana (where preliminary results are available), and Burkina Faso. There are a number of other studies ongoing and these will report in 2005.[2]

What these studies show varies. In South Africa, the HSRC survey found a prevalence rate of 17.7 percent among women aged 15 to 49, while the 2001 antenatal survey figure for the same age group was 24.8 percent. However, among pregnant women the prevalence was 24 percent in the HSRC survey – albeit in a very small population. The South African ANC survey shows the prevalence rising steadily. HIV prevalence amongst pregnant women in 2002 was 26.5 percent rising to 27.9 percent in the 2003 – and most recent – survey. According to the RHRU survey HIV prevalence among 15- to 24-year-old South Africans was 10.2 percent. This was 15.5 percent among women and 4.8 percent among men. Prevalence among 21-year-old women was over 30 percent.

Are these differences in South African prevalence levels significant? According to the RHRU report: 'The HIV findings from this study are similar to those found in the 2002 Nelson Mandela/HSRC survey and the 2002 Antenatal Clinic Survey. Differences are most likely the result of sampling from different populations. Given the paucity of comparative data it is not possible to gauge definitive trends from these findings' (Pettifor et al. 2004). Referring to the 2003 ANC survey results, the Department of Health writes: 'These findings show that South African HIV prevalence rates remain high and the epidemic is still in the stabilisation phase and has not yet begun to decline' (South Africa, Department of Health 2003).

The reality facing South Africa is that we have a serious epidemic and there is as yet no sign of a downturn.

The reality facing South Africa is that we have a serious epidemic and while there may be some debate about the exact numbers, there are many people infected (see Table 1), prevalence remains high, and there is as yet no sign of a downturn. Knowing what we do of how AIDS cases lag behind the HIV curve (see Chapter 2), we can also predict that the number of people falling ill and dying will rise, the number of orphans will grow, and the impact of the disease has yet to be fully felt.

In the case of the Kenyan DHS survey, the results were significantly lower than those obtained from antenatal surveys. As a result they were seized on, by the press, to suggest that national HIV prevalence had been overestimated. The UNAIDS figure was that 9.4 percent of all Kenyans were living with HIV/AIDS, the DHS estimated that 6.7 percent of Kenyans were infected (Kenya Central Bureau of Statistics, 2004). The inference was that the 'AIDS industry' has been caught out. As the full results have not been released we cannot make detailed comments, but UNAIDS notes that when the results are broken down by gender, the HIV prevalence of 8.7 percent among women is in the same range as the 9.4 percent prevalence estimated by UNAIDS and WHO.

A hard look at the population surveys shows that they too are not without problems. In both Kenya and South Africa there were high refusal rates – people who would not be interviewed, provide specimens or who were not contactable. In South Africa in the HSRC survey of the 13 518 individuals who were selected and contacted for the survey, 73.7 percent persons agreed to be interviewed, and 65.4 percent agreed to give a specimen for an HIV test. In Kenya, 70 percent of eligible people agreed to give blood samples. Epidemiologists are concerned when participation rates fall below 80 percent.

An additional problem is the lax way in which numbers are thrown around by both the press and many AIDS activists. For example, Swaziland currently has the highest HIV prevalence rate among ANC attenders in the world. The 2002 survey found prevalence of 38.6 percent among those tested (Swaziland Ministry of Health and Social Welfare 2002). But this is then presented as though 38 percent of adults are infected, or even as though 38 percent of Swazis have HIV. The result is either complete confusion or black despair – or both.

Sub-Saharan African epidemics

So how bad is the epidemic in Africa? The first and perhaps most important point is to recognise that there is not *an* African epidemic – there are many epidemics. In the continent-wide review below, I primarily draw on the UNAIDS Global Epidemic updates. The data are dependent on information from the countries and these are of very variable quality. No international agency goes out and conducts its own surveys! In some cases this means that data are very old or of dubious quality. For example, there are no estimates of national HIV prevalence in Liberia. The last HIV prevalence survey was in 1993 and was confined to urban areas.

In North Africa and parts of the Sahel there is little evidence of an AIDS epidemic. Some countries do not report any cases and where there are data, the prevalence rate is below 0.25 percent amongst adults. There have been some signs of outbreaks amongst drug users, although sexual intercourse remains the dominant form of transmission. High levels of stigma and discrimination may mean the epidemic is hidden in these countries but the reality is that it has not taken hold in these areas. There are issues around levels of conflict, poverty and unemployment, which needed to be monitored.

In eastern Africa the epidemic has been turned round in Uganda. Prevalence fell from about 25 percent of pregnant women in the early 1990s to the current five to six percent. There is some debate about the accuracy of these figures but the reality is that there have been significant declines in HIV prevalence. There are also encouraging signs from Kenya where data from antenatal clinics show median HIV prevalence falling from 13.6 percent (12.2–27.1 percent) in 1997–

1998 to 9.4 percent (6.6–14.3 percent) in 2002 and then staying largely unchanged in 2003[3]. In Ethiopia the epidemic is most severe in urban areas including in the capital, Addis Ababa. However, HIV prevalence among pregnant women in the capital has been falling. By 2003, HIV prevalence in the city had fallen to 11 percent, less than half the level (24 percent) it had reached in the mid-1990s (UNAIDS and WHO 2004: 25-29).

In the rest of the region the evidence is that HIV prevalence is stable overall – but even in individual countries there is not one epidemic. In Tanzania, for example, the national HIV prevalence is stable, but it has fallen in the Mbeya region and risen in the Rukwa region. It has to be remembered that even with declines in HIV prevalence this turns into horrific numbers of people infected: over 2 million Ethiopians and 2.3 million Kenyans.

Although varying in scale and intensity, the epidemics in West Africa appear to have stabilised in most countries.

The 2002 UNAIDS Update suggested that in west and central Africa, the relatively low adult HIV prevalence rates in countries such as Senegal (under 1 percent) and Mali (1.7 percent) are shadowed by more ominous patterns of growth. HIV prevalence is estimated to exceed five percent in eight other countries of west and central Africa, including Cameroon (11.8 percent), Central African Republic (12.9 percent), Côte d'Ivoire (9.7 percent) and Nigeria (5.8 percent) – sobering reminders that no country or region is shielded from the epidemic. The sharp rise in HIV prevalence among pregnant women in Cameroon (more than doubling to over 11 percent among those aged 20 to 24 between 1998 and 2000), shows how suddenly the epidemic can surge (UNAIDS and WHO 2002: 21).

The 2004 update notes:

> Although varying in scale and intensity, the epidemics in West Africa appear to have stabilised in most countries. Median HIV prevalence measured among women in 112 antenatal clinics in the sub-region remained at an average three to four percent between 1997 and 2002. Overall, HIV prevalence is lowest in the Sahel countries and highest in Burkina Faso, Côte d'Ivoire and Nigeria – the latter having the third largest number of people living with HIV in the world (after South Africa and India).

In Nigeria the 2003 HIV Sentinel Survey put national HIV prevalence at five percent, a rise from the 1.8 percent found in 1991 but roughly level with the 5.4 percent recorded in 1999. However, there are strong regional differences: prevalence ranges from a low of 2.3 percent in the South West to a high of seven percent in the North Central regions. At state level, the variations are even greater: in Benue it was 9.3 percent and in Cross River 12 percent. This suggests that several distinct epidemics are underway.

Côte d'Ivoire reports the highest HIV prevalence in West Africa. In Togo, Ghana and Benin, HIV prevalence is stable. In Central Africa, Cameroon and the Central African Republic are worse affected; HIV prevalence has stabilised at around ten percent. In Congo and the Democratic Republic of the Congo, data suggests prevalence of about five percent.

The UN system finds it difficult to comment on the quality of the data with which they are presented. It is my view that in some situations we simply do not know what is going on. For example, there is little data from states in conflict such as the Democratic Republic of the Congo or Sudan. In others there was (and in some cases, is) not a functioning government to collect, collate and disseminate information: Liberia, Sierra Leone and Somalia. In some instances HIV/AIDS is not high on the agenda. Finally, there are those examples such as Nigeria where data are simply not credible due to inefficiency and government failure or where data are politically sensitive and may actually be manipulated, as may be the case in Zimbabwe.

The one place from which we have generally good data is the epicentre of the epidemic: Southern Africa. The expectations in the early 1990s were that HIV prevalence would not exceed 25 percent in any country. The countries of Southern Africa have confounded this. In June 2002, the UNAIDS Global Report said:

> Circulating in Southern Africa (where the epidemic is the most severe in the world) has been the hope that the epidemic may have reached its 'natural limit' beyond which it would not grow. Thus it has been assumed that the very high prevalence rates in some countries have reached a plateau. If a natural HIV prevalence limit does exist in these countries, it is considerably higher than previously thought (UNAIDS 2002).

The update released six months later was even more plaintive:

> The worst of the epidemic clearly has not yet passed, even in Southern Africa where rampant epidemics are under way. In four Southern African countries, national adult HIV prevalence has risen higher than thought possible, exceeding 30 percent: Botswana (38.8 percent), Lesotho (31 percent), Swaziland (33.4 percent) and Zimbabwe (33.7 percent).

In Southern Africa we have the best data, the best projections and the worst epidemic.

In the 2004 Epidemic Update, the best UNAIDS could say of this region was that in a number of countries, notably Namibia and Swaziland, comparisons of prevalence levels at selected antenatal clinics have shown no evidence of a decline. In other parts of the region HIV infections in pregnant women appear to be stabilising at lower levels – around 18 percent in Malawi (2003), 16 percent in Zambia (2003), and 25 percent in Zimbabwe (2003) – but there is little evidence of an impending decline (UNAIDS and WHO 2004: 24).

The Southern African epidemic

I will now turn to look at Southern Africa in more detail. It is this part of Africa where we have the best data, the best projections and the worst epidemic. The progress of the epidemic over the past 14 years (since data were first collected) using antenatal clinic data is shown on Figure 1 for the five southernmost countries. In South Africa, HIV prevalence rose from about 0.5 percent in 1990 to over 27.9 percent in 2002. Botswana and Swaziland both began collection data in 1992. In Botswana the first survey showed a prevalence rate of about 18 percent; this rose to close to 40 percent by 2000 and has remained at these levels. By contrast in Swaziland, 1994 prevalence was just four percent but by 2002 it had reached 38.6 percent - currently the highest in the world. In Lesotho the 1991 survey was even lower - about three percent but according to the 2003 ANC survey, it is now approaching 30 percent. The odd country out is Namibia. Here the 1991 survey found a predictable three percent but since then, although there has been a steady increase in prevalence, it is lower than that found in the rest of the region.

Figure 1: Antenatal seroprevalence in selected Southern African countries[4]

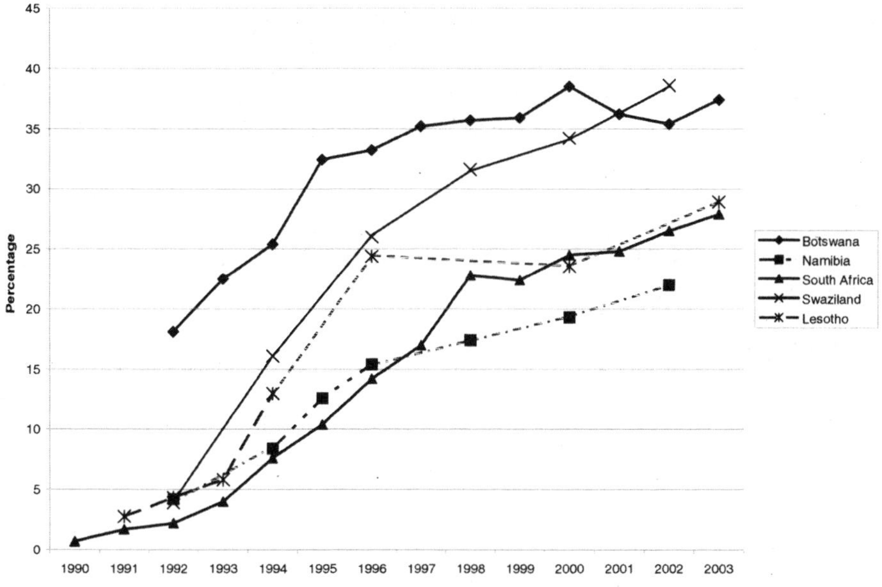

Of great interest is what is happening in the younger population - the 15 to 19 age group and the 20- to 24-year-olds. If HIV prevalence is being controlled, it is here that we would expect to see declining prevalence rates. This is the age group that is becoming sexually active and where, if interventions are making a difference, we have the most chance of seeing it reflected in the data we collect. These data are shown for our Southern African countries in Figure 2. The picture is mixed but the reality is that the best we can say at the moment is - as UNAIDS notes - the epidemic has stabilised!

Figure 2: Antenatal seroprevalence in selected African countries (15–19 yrs)[5]

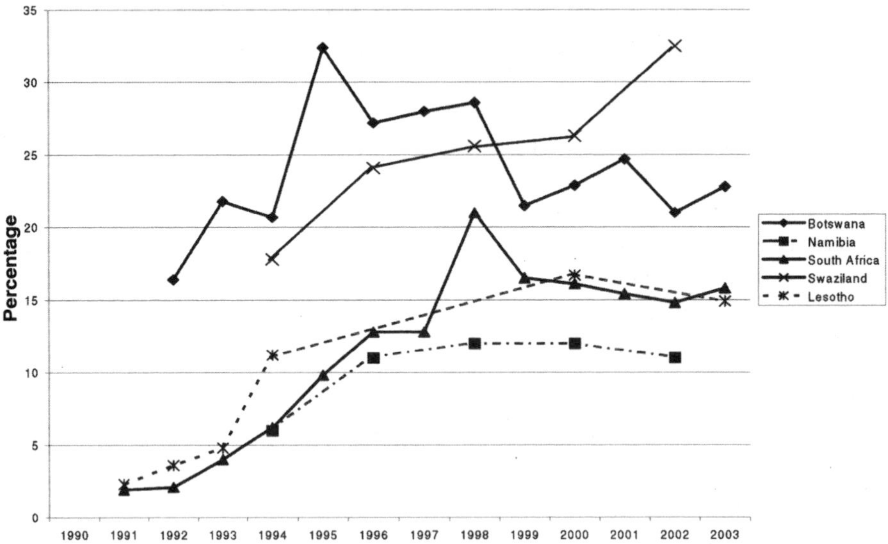

We take a closer look at the South African data in Table 1, which shows the number of infected South Africans as calculated by the Department of Health. This table gives figures for men, women and babies. The government estimates that between 5 155 000 and 6 123 000 South Africans are infected, a difference of nearly a million between the low and high estimates. These are infections that have already occurred and we will have to deal with the consequences as these people fall ill and die.

Table 1: Estimated infected South Africans 2003

	Low	High	Median
Women	2 831 658	3 369 822	3 100 864
Men	2 233 442	2 650 178	2 441 485
Babies	89 897	102 552	96 228
Total	5 154 997	6 122 552	5 638 577

Note: Derived from the Department of Health, *National HIV and Syphilis Antenatal Sero-Prevalence Survey in South Africa 2003*, Government of South Africa 2003, tables 5a, 5b and 5c.

The consequences of HIV/AIDS

What will happen if the epidemic continues unchecked? The hard truth that most simply do not grasp is that even if there were no new infections from 2005, we are still going to see the impact of the disease. The reason for this can be seen in Chapter 2, Figure 1. The reality is that the HIV epidemic curves – across much of the continent and certainly in Southern Africa – have risen, and in the absence of affordable, effective and deliverable treatment we are certain to face the AIDS epidemic and AIDS impact curves.

The effects of AIDS will be dramatic and far-reaching:

- There is no cure and treatment is inaccessible for the majority of infected Africans, due to both the cost and lack of health care staff.
- Impact is felt through the illness (morbidity) and deaths (mortality).
- Most of those who die will be young adults who have completed education, started families and begun working careers.
- HIV/AIDS is a long wave event as compared to other epidemics.
- The true toll cannot be estimated until the full evolution of the epidemic has been seen. The social and economic impacts, in particular HIV/AIDS-related poverty, will get worse over the coming decades.

Demographic consequences are increased mortality and decreased fertility. Mortality rises among infected adults and those infants infected through mother-to-child transmission and adults. A summary of the key demographic impacts of this disease is shown in Table 2.

Table 2: Summary of estimated and projected impact of HIV/AIDS on mortality indicators 2003

Indicator	**53 countries where HIV/ AIDS impact included in 2002 UN estimates**[1]			**7 countries with prevalence > than 20 percent**		
	1995–2000	2010–2015	2020–2025	1995–2000	2010–2015	2020–2025
Number of deaths (millions)						
Without AIDS	159	174	193	3	3	4
With AIDS	170	207	231	5	10	9
percent difference	7	19	20	71	193	142
Life expectancy at birth (years)						
Without AIDS	63.9	68.4	70.8	62.3	67	69.6
With AIDS	62.4	64.2	65.9	50.2	37.6	41
percent difference	2.4	6.1	6.9	19.3	43.9	41.1
Child mortality rate (per 1000)						
Without AIDS	93.9	68.8	56.1	80.2	56.9	44.8
With AIDS	98.8	75.8	62.3	108.8	100.2	84.3
percent difference	5.3	10	11.1	35.7	76.2	88.4

Note: These countries are listed in the report and include the USA, Russian Federation, India and China. There are no data given just for African countries.
Source: United Nations Secretariat, Population Division, 2003.

UNICEF estimates that by 2010 an estimated 20 million children in Africa will have lost one or both parents to HIV/AIDS.

Infected women are less likely to fall pregnant and carry a child to term, and premature mortality means there will be fewer women of childbearing age. This has an impact on fertility. For Uganda the number of births was reduced by approximately 700 000, corresponding with almost 5.9 percent of all births that would have occurred during the last two decades (Lewis, Ronsmans, Ezeh, Gregson 2004). Only in the very worst affected countries (Botswana and Swaziland) might the population decrease. But it is certain there will be a change in the population structure as young adults die.

The increase in 'orphaning' is a demographic impact but it also has social and economic consequences. UNICEF estimates that by 2010 an estimated 20 million children in Africa will have lost one or both parents to HIV/AIDS. For over 80 percent of orphans in the worst affected countries, the cause will be HIV/AIDS. These children face severe stress, they are less likely to attend school, more likely to be exploited and experience premature mortality, and they also have a more pessimistic outlook on life (UNICEF 2003).

The economic impact of the disease varies by country and level. A survey of 700 households with at least one person already sick with AIDS in South Africa gives a clear indication of the impoverishing nature of the epidemic (Steinberg et al 2004). The survey found:

- two thirds reported loss of income as a consequence of HIV/AIDS;
- half reported not having enough food and that their children were going hungry; and
- almost a quarter of all children under age 15 had already lost at least one parent.

Will AIDS cause national economies to grow more slowly? This is not clear, but the most optimistic projections are that economic growth will be slowed in all affected countries. It was believed that AIDS had reduced Africa's economic growth by just under one percent in the 1990s.

The earlier comparisons of 'with AIDS' and 'without AIDS' treated the disease as an 'exogenous' influence that was added to models derived on the presumption that the workforce is HIV-free. Yet in reality HIV/AIDS is an 'endogenous' influence, requiring feedback loops to appreciate accumulative impacts. In late July 2003 the World Bank released a study on the long-run economic costs of AIDS to South Africa presenting a very different view (Bell, Devarajan, Gersbach 2003). This warned that previous models greatly underestimated the potential macro-economic impact of HIV/AIDS and 'if nothing is done to combat the epidemic, however, a complete economic collapse will occur within three generations'. The authors argue that the long-run economic costs of AIDS are almost certain to be very much higher than that predicted to date and may even be devastating. They emphasise the importance of *human capital* and how it is transmitted across generations, making an 'overlapping generations' model more appropriate in understanding how AIDS will impact people. According to the authors, AIDS will retard economic growth:

- by destroying human capital, particularly of young adults;
- by weakening and wrecking mechanisms that generate human capital and investment in people, through loss of income and the death of parents; and
- by giving rise to a new generation with little education and knowledge, therefore less able to raise their own children and invest in their education.

While this most recent economic model was applied to South Africa as an example, it is important to appreciate the new way of looking at potential economic impacts that can be applied in other contexts. 'Endogenous growth models' are recognised as providing a more accurate assessment of the effects of epidemiological crises such as HIV/AIDS on developing countries (Drouhin, Touze & Ventelou 2003: 383–412). Importantly, such models consider persisting effects on development. They identify productivity variables that act as catalysts to development, and further consider the impact of HIV/AIDS on these variables.

Macroeconomic models estimate impact often without considering policy changes and the possibility of newly emerging interventions. Looking again at the conclusions of the World Bank paper, economic growth will be maintained (albeit slower) if there is optimal spending on combating HIV/AIDS, continuing economies of scale to service provision and benefit pooling. Governments therefore face a challenge in proving macroeconomic predictions wrong, by finding a balance of interventions that will contribute towards mitigating economic impacts.

If macroeconomic growth is slowed or the economy contracts, this will have significant implications for poverty, government revenue and spending on service delivery. Sectors such as health and social services will be hardest hit because not only do they face the impact of the disease on their staff and other resources, but they are also required to provide additional care and support.

In development terms AIDS has an adverse effect. Here we can see an impact through international data sets. The most generally accepted measure of human development is the UNDP's Human Development Index (HDI), which looks beyond simple economic measures. It is constructed from three indices: life expectancy, a proxy indicator for longevity; educational attainment which is measured by literacy and enrolment rates; and standard of living which is measured by real GDP per capita. The measure that will be affected first is life expectancy consequent on increased infant and child mortality and premature deaths among adults.

In Table 3 we look at the UNDP's Human Development Reports tracking how life expectancy has fallen with the consequent decline in HDI and changing of the ranking of countries. This updates Table 5 in Chapter 2. We have to ask how countries will cope with these dramatic falls in life expectancy.

Table 3: Life expectancy and place in the HDI (UN 2004, 2001, 1999, 1996)

	1996 Report (1993 data)		1999 Report (1997 data)		2001 Report (1999 data)		2004 Report (2002 data)	
	Life Expect.	**HDI (Rank)**	**Life Expect.**	**HDI (Rank)**	**Life Expect.**	**HDI (Rank)**	**Life Expect.**	**HDI (Rank)**
Botswana	65.	0.741 (71)	47.4	0.678 (97)	41.9	0.577 (114)	41.4	0.589 (128)
Nigeria	50.6	0.400 (137)	50.1	0.391 (142)	51.5	0.455 (136)	51.6	0.466 (151)
South Africa	63.2	0.649 (100)	54.7	0.717 (89)	53.9	0.701 (94)	48.8	0.666 (119)
Swaziland	57.8	0.586 (110)	60.2	0.597 (115)	47	0.583 (113)	35.7	0.491 (137)
Zimbabwe	53.4	0.534 (124)	44.1	0.507 (130)	42.9	0.554 (117)	33.9	0.491 (147)

Responding to the epidemic

The question is how should we respond to the disease, and how should the discussion on data (above) inform this response? Obviously the first prize is to prevent the virus spreading. Most Africans become infected through sex with an infected person. There are various measures that can be put in place to reduce the risk. These include abstinence and fidelity, much promoted by the USA under the conservative republican administration. Male circumcision, the use of condoms and the treatment of other sexually transmitted infections greatly reduce the chance of transmission.

We have to ask how countries will cope with these dramatic falls in life expectancy.

The Copenhagen Consensus 2004 project shows how seriously we need to take AIDS as an issue. For this project a panel of eight economic experts set priorities for confronting ten great global challenges by answering the question: 'What would be the best ways of advancing global welfare, and particularly the welfare of developing countries, supposing that an additional $50 billion of resources were at governments' disposal?' Highest priority was assigned to measures to prevent the spread of HIV/AIDS, with the conclusion that costs are substantial (estimated $27 billion), but small in relation to what stands to be gained by averting nearly 30 million new infections by 2010 (Copenhagen Consensus 2004).

The problem with these interventions is that they do not address the underlying reasons as to why people put themselves at risk, and in the case of abstinence and fidelity makes the axiomatic assumption that these are sought after qualities.

We need to understand that behaviours are determined by the social, economic, political and cultural milieu in which people live and operate. This is particularly important in Southern Africa. In terms of the United Nations Development Programme's GDP per capita (purchasing power parity) figures, South Africa, Botswana and Namibia are the second, third and fourth richest countries in sub-Saharan Africa (only beaten by oil-rich Equatorial Guinea). It is therefore apparent that wealth alone is not a protector against infection.

The second largest group of HIV-positive Africans are children infected through mother-to-child transmission (MTCT). In the absence of interventions an infected woman has about a 30 percent chance of passing the infection to the child. Infection may occur prior to birth, during the birth process or during breastfeeding. Prevention during birth is relatively easy through provision of a single dose of certain antiretroviral drugs to the mother during labour and to the infant after delivery. Providing formula feed as an alternative to breastfeeding is rather more complicated. It requires safe water and that a bottle-feeding mother not be stigmatised. Table 1 in this chapter shows that in South Africa between 89 900 and 102 500 babies were infected in 2004. Appropriate and inexpensive treatment could reduce this by at least two thirds. It is striking that we can still present these figures and not reflect on the fact that these infections do not have to happen.

The data gives us an idea of the number needing treatment across the continent, and of how woefully inadequate our response has been.

Finally, the data gives us an idea of the number needing treatment across the continent, and of how woefully inadequate our response has been.

AIDS is the major issue facing most of Africa at the beginning of this century. But it is not the only issue. Unfortunately, it has the effect of amplifying other social, economic and political problems. Responding to HIV/AIDS is not just an ethical issue; it will affect the survival of many people. This is not a time to quibble over the exact numbers but rather to move forward.

Endnotes

[1] The time taken by the author to write this article was supported by a Department of International Development (UK) Knowledge Programme. All interpretations are the author's.

[2] http://www.measuredhs.com/aboutsurveys/survey_status.cfm.

[3] This is antenatal data rather than the DHS data discussed above. If the DHS is right then this confirms that ANC data and gives ground for optimism.

[4] This figure was compiled in HEARD from data collected from National AIDS Control programmes.

[5] This figure was compiled in HEARD from data collected from National AIDS Control programmes.

References

Barnett, T., Prins, G. & Whiteside, A. (2004). AIDS denial costs lives. *Spectator*, 25th September.

Bell, C., Devarajan, S. & Gersbach, H. (2003). *The Long-run Economic Costs of AIDS: Theory and an Application to South Africa*. Washington: The World Bank.

Copenhagen Consensus. (2004). *Copenhagen Consensus: The results*. [Online] Available: http://www.copenhagenconsensus.com/.

Drouhin, N., Touze, V. & Ventelou, B. AIDS and economic growth in Africa: a critical assessment of the 'base-case scenario' approach. In: Moatti, J.P., Coriat, B., Souteyrand, Y., Barnett, T., Dumoulin, J. & Flori, Y.A. (eds) (2003). *Economics of AIDS and Access to HIV/AIDS Care in Developing Countries. Issues and Challenges*. Paris: ANRS.

Kenya Central Bureau of Statistics (2004). Demographic and Health Survey Highlights [Online]. Available: http://www.cbs.go.ke/kdhs2003_highlights.html.

Lewis, J.J.C., Ronsmans, C., Ezeh, A. & Gregson, S. (2004). The population impact of HIV on fertility in sub-Saharan Africa. In: B. Ties & Z. Basia, 'Demographic and socio-economic impact of AIDS: Empirical Evidence' *AIDS, 18, Supplement, 2nd June.*

Malan, R. (2004). Africa isn't dying of AIDS. *Spectator,* 18th December.

Measure DHS (2004). Demographic and Health Surveys. [Online] Available: http://www.measuredhs.com/aboutsurveys/survey_status.cfm.

Nelson Mandela/Human Sciences Research Council (2002). *South African National HIV Prevalence, Behavioural Risks and Mass Media Household Survey 2002*. Cape Town.

Pettifor, A.E., Rees, H.V., Steffenson, A., Hlongwa-Madikizela, L., MacPhail, C., Vermaak, K. & Kleinschmidt, I. (2004). *HIV and sexual behaviour among young South Africans: a national survey of 15–24 year olds*. Johannesburg: Reproductive Health Research Unit, University of Witwatersrand.

South Africa. Department of Health (2003). *National HIV and Syphilis Antenatal Sero-Prevalence Survey in South Africa 2003*. Pretoria.

Steinberg, M., Johnson, S., Schierhout,G., Ndegwa, D., Hall, K., Russell, B. & Morgan, J. (2002). *Hitting Home: How Households Cope with the Impact of the HIV/AIDS epidemic. A survey of household affected by HIV/AIDS in South Africa*. Health Systems Trust and The Kaiser Family Foundation.

Swaziland. Ministry of Health and Social Welfare. National AIDS/STDs Programme. (2002). *Eighth HIV Sentinel Seroprevalence Report 2002*. Mbabane: Government Printer.

UNAIDS (2004). *Global AIDS Epidemic*. Geneva: UNAIDS.

UNAIDS (2002). *Report on the global HIV/AIDS Epidemic*. Geneva: UNAIDS.

UNAIDS & WHO (2004). *Global AIDS Epidemic*. Geneva: UNAIDS.

UNAIDS & WHO (2002). *AIDS Epidemic Update*. Geneva: UNAIDS.

UNICEF (2003). *Africa's Orphaned Generation*. New York: UNICEF.

United Nations (2004). *Human Development Report*. New York: Oxford University Press.

United Nations (2001). *Human Development Report*. New York: Oxford University Press.

United Nations (1999). *Human Development Report*. New York: Oxford University Press.

United Nations (1996). *Human Development Report*. New York: Oxford University Press.

United Nations Secretariat, Population Division, Department of Economic and Social Affairs. (2003). *The Impact of AIDS*. ESA/P/WP.185 2nd September 2003.

Chapter 2

Through a glass, darkly[1]*: data and uncertainty in the AIDS debate*

Is the insufficiency of data on the AIDS epidemic a sufficient reason for inaction? **Alan Whiteside, Tony Barnett, Gavin George** *and* **Anton A. van Niekerk** *acknowledge and discuss the problems surrounding AIDS data, but argue that incomplete figures are not enough for governments to hide behind when their moral responsibility towards the pandemic is in question.*

There can be no doubt that AIDS is truly a global epidemic although it is Southern Africa that bears the brunt of the epidemic, as the figures presented in the previous chapter make evident. In their 2002 'Report on the global HIV/AIDS epidemic', UNAIDS estimated that 40 million people globally were living with HIV and a further 20 million had died. The majority of new infections occur in young adults, with young women particularly vulnerable. It is estimated that one-third of those who have contracted HIV/AIDS are aged between 15 and 24. It is truly a global epidemic.

At the time of writing, the fastest growing epidemic is in Eastern Europe, fuelled by drug use. At the end of 2001, it was estimated that in that area one million people were living with HIV, with 25 percent of those infections occurring in the 2001 calendar year. Asia and the Pacific have an estimated 7.1 million people living with HIV/AIDS. The Middle East and North America are experiencing a slow but marked spread with 440 000 people now living with HIV/AIDS. In Latin America and the Caribbean there are an estimated 1.8 million adults and children infected with HIV.

Sub-Saharan Africa suffers most. Just over 70 percent of those infected with HIV are found here. AIDS deaths in 2001 alone totalled 2.3 million. UNAIDS estimates that with the 3.5 million new HIV infections in sub-Saharan Africa in the past year, 28.5 million Africans now live with the virus. Even here the picture is by no means uniform. There are variations between regions and countries, and between provinces and districts within countries.

In this chapter we will examine some of the available data on the epidemic and discuss how data are presented and the implications of this. To illustrate our discussion we will use data from five African countries: Botswana, Nigeria, South Africa, Swaziland and Zimbabwe. We will then go on to look at the impact of AIDS, and assess what actual evidence there is for this. We will show that we rely on very few data points to estimate the scale and scope of the epidemic and these data must be treated with caution. We shall argue that the unreliability of data is not only a contingent curiosity of the current international debate about AIDS, but indeed a problem with significant moral dimensions and ramifications.

Although there is a problem with sufficient data about the AIDS pandemic, this is not an excuse for continued denial and obfuscation.

We must stress that we are not questioning the 'HIV causes AIDS' hypothesis. We believe there is an AIDS epidemic in Africa, and it will have far-reaching consequences. We believe that HIV causes AIDS. We argue AIDS is the most serious threat facing Africa at present; it will reverse the limited development gains of the past two decades and will push parts of the continent into political and economic crisis.

However, we show that *seeing* and *believing* this requires imagination and judgement. So, although there is a problem with sufficient data about the AIDS pandemic (as this article will show), this is not an excuse for continued denial and obfuscation, as occur in the statements and policies of some African countries, South Africa in particular. The problems with the data are no indication that the crisis of AIDS in Africa is not extremely serious. To the contrary, we shall argue that the problems with the data require, on ethical grounds, that a much more imaginative effort to acquire and corroborate sufficient data is called for – an effort which policy makers in developing countries ought to fully support.

The moral dimension of the phenomenon of unreliable data

The reliability of data has become one of the most controversial issues in the debate about AIDS in Africa. The denial that has characterised so much of the response from the political leadership[2] in South Africa and other African countries to the AIDS pandemic is, in an important sense, the outcome of both the explicit and implicit challenge of the reliability of data on the pandemic.

There are two moral problems that must be pointed out in this regard. The *first* is that scientists have a moral responsibility to provide the most reliable data possible. Science is not only an intellectual enterprise. It is also a practice that is not value-free, and it has a moral dimension. Accuracy and reliability are fundamental values that accompany the practice of science. The moment the perception is created that regard for truth and accuracy is devalued, science is bound to lose both credibility and support in our society. In addition, it must be noted that so much of the policy decisions of modern societies rely on accurate scientific knowledge. Responsible policy formation in modern societies without the continual input of reliable scientific knowledge has become almost inconceivable.

This is also and particularly true of the formation of a responsible policy to manage HIV/AIDS, which brings us to the *second* moral problem that must be pointed out, viz. the responsibility of leadership in disease-riddled societies to rise to their task of responsible disease management. Responding to reasonably reliable scientific data, the government of Uganda has, for example, launched a comprehensive, co-ordinated national strategy over the past few years, and has, in the process, attained considerable success. The HIV prevalence in pregnant women in the urban areas of Uganda has, for example, consistently come down over the past eight years from a peak of 29.5 percent in 1992 to 11.25 percent in 2000 (UNAIDS 2001).

The fact, however, is that such a national strategy is sorely lacking in most African countries. There are probably many reasons for this phenomenon, but one of them undoubtedly is denial based on the questioning of reliable data on the pandemic. This article will show that data about the AIDS pandemic are far from completely reliable. This fact oils the fire of denial in Africa. The irony is that inaccuracy of data, as will be shown, is hardly a reason for complacency based on the perception that scientists over-estimate the seriousness of the crisis. In fact, as will be shown, inaccuracy of data more often implies an under-estimation of the crisis!

Denial is the main reason why so many millions suffer – in many instances unnecessarily.

Denial is the main reason why so many millions suffer – in many instances (e.g. where programmes could have been launched to prevent vertical transmission from mother to child) unnecessarily. As the numbers of the infected grow, the drain on Africa's meagre resources increases and the social catastrophe widens in scope. There is therefore both an urgent moral duty on scientists to try and minimise the margin of error as regards AIDS statistics, but also on the national leadership in societies where the AIDS epidemic is out of control (as is the case in most of Africa) to act responsibly on the basis of this data. This problem is a clear indication of how science and morality are seamlessly linked and ought to be conjointly theorised and practised.

Understanding the epidemic

Epidemics usually follow an 'S' curve as shown in Figure 1. They start slowly and gradually and if a critical mass of infected people is reached, then the growth of new infections accelerates. The epidemic then spreads through the population until all those who are susceptible to infection and are exposed have been infected. In the final phase of an epidemic – where the 'S' flattens off at the top – people are either getting better or deaths outnumber new cases so that the total number alive and infected passes its peak and begins to decline.

What sets HIV and AIDS apart from other epidemics is there are two curves, as shown in Figure 1. The HIV curve precedes that of AIDS by about seven to ten years, reflecting the incubation period between infection and onset of illness. This is why HIV is such a lethal epidemic compared to, say, cholera. In the

Figure 1: The two epidemic curves

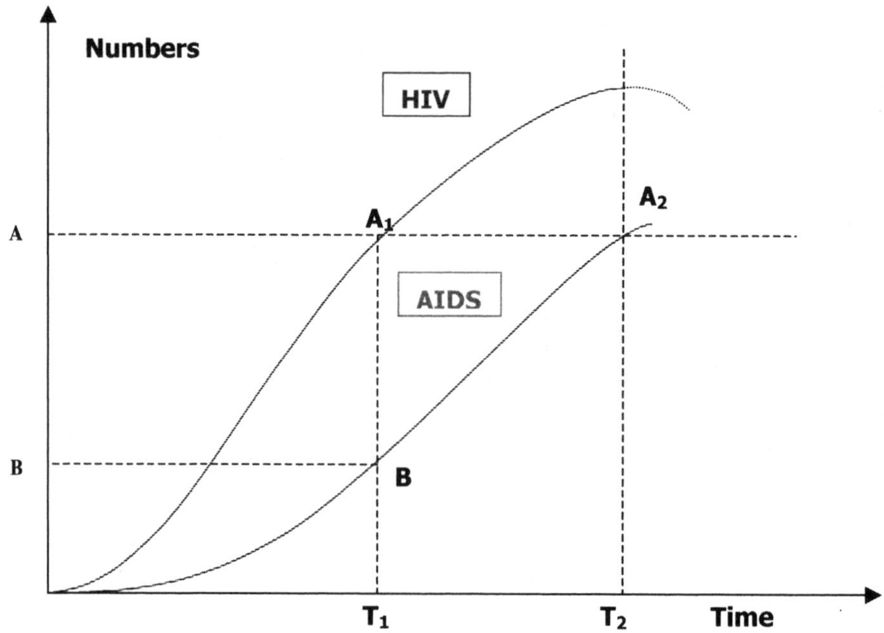

latter case, victims of the disease die quickly which puts the general population and public health professionals on their guard. They take precautions to halt the spread. In the case of HIV, however, the epidemic is silently creeping through the population and it is only later – when the HIV pool has risen to a considerable level – that the true impact of the epidemic is felt in terms of AIDS deaths. By then, the epidemic is in full swing and the only way people leave the pool of infections is by dying, since there is no cure yet. Figure 1 illustrates this point clearly. The vertical axis represents numbers and the horizontal axis time. At T1, when the level of HIV is at A1, the number of AIDS cases will be very much lower at B1. The AIDS cases will only reach A2 (i.e. the same level as A1) at T2. A considerable amount of time will have elapsed and HIV will have risen even higher though it may be levelling off.

Incidence and prevalence

Incidence and prevalence are two important concepts to grasp when looking at HIV/AIDS data. *Incidence* is the number of new infections over a given period of time. The *incidence rate* is the number per specified unit of population (this can be per 1 000, per 10 000 or per million for rare diseases). *Prevalence* is the absolute number of people infected. The *prevalence rate* is the percentage of the population which exhibits the disease at a particular time (or averaged over a period of time). The incidence and prevalence are key statistics for tracking the course of an epidemic. With HIV, prevalence rates are given as a percentage of a specific segment of the population, e.g. children below the age of five, adults aged between 15 and 65, antenatal clinic attenders, blood donors, men with STDs, or the 'at risk' population which is generally taken to mean 15- to 49-year-olds who are sexually active. HIV is unique in that it is the only disease where prevalence is given as a percentage rather than a rate.

Unfortunately, we do not have HIV incidence figures because we don't know when people were actually infected – but only the date on which we *discover* they are infected. The data, which would be most helpful in measuring the spread of the epidemic and impact of prevention efforts, are simply not available. Moreover, high incidence may occur even when prevalence has levelled off because newly infected people are replacing those dying.

Data sources

HIV data

Epidemiological data are drawn from official sources. The HIV data are taken from surveys of specific groups. In the early years of the epidemic they included blood donors, STD clinic attenders, people with TB and women attending antenatal clinics. Until recently, the only way to test for HIV was through blood. This meant that whatever population was used for surveys, blood samples had to be taken, which immediately created a bias as it was expensive. New methods of testing using saliva have been developed in the last few years but have not yet been extensively used.

Our most consistent data come from antenatal clinic surveys. The reason for this was that epidemiologists needed a sample which was broadly representative of the general population, and which they could draw on at regular intervals, usually every year or two. Antenatal clinic attenders provide a good sample because they are adults and sexually active, and blood is routinely taken from women attending these clinics for a number of standard tests. Most ANC surveys are done on an anonymous, unlinked basis – women cannot be linked to the samples. This means that informed consent is not necessarily required.

It is the ANC prevalence data that are quoted most frequently. UNAIDS produces an estimated adult prevalence rate (the percentage of adults between 15 to 49 infected). The UNAIDS data provide the most easily accessible public domain information. In addition to the national data, they provide reports for each country and as Table 1 shows, figures are given for urban and rural areas. (See the epidemiological fact sheets on the UNAIDS website: www.unaids.org.) UNAIDS bases its data on the HIV database maintained by the United States Bureau of Census where data from different sources, including national reports, scientific publications and international conferences are compiled.

Table 1: HIV prevalence amongst pregnant women in selected countries in percent

Country	Area	1989	1990	1991	1992	1993	1994	1995	1996	1997	1998	1999	2000	2001
Botswana	Major Urban Areas		6.0	8.0	19.3	26.8	27.8	34.1	37.8	38.5	43.0	39.9	43.9	44.9
	Outside Major Urban Areas		4.1		10.1	17.8	19.4	29.9	31.6	33.7	30.0	31.7	35.4	34.8
Nigeria	Major Urban Areas	1.0		3.2	0.7		4.0	1				4		4.2
	Outside Major Urban Areas	0.0	0.2		0.5		2.9	2.3				4.3		5.3
South Africa	Major Urban Areas		0.6	0.9	1.8	3.0	6.0	9.0	11.8	14.9	19.2	21	24.3	
	Outside Major Urban Areas		0.4	1.2	1.1	2.2	6.7	8.3	15.8	18.1	21.3	23	22.9	
Swaziland	Major Urban Areas				4.3	21.9	15.5	19.1	26.3		30.3		32.3	
	Outside Major Urban Areas				4.1		16.7		26.5		31.5		34.5	
Zimbabwe	Major Urban Areas	10.0	18.7	17.1		25.8	36.1	31.0	30.4	30			31.1	
	Outside Major Urban Areas		16	18.5	0.0	21.3	24.3	39.5	41.6	28.7	31	22.3	33.2	

Source: UNAIDS – Epidemiological Fact Sheets by country, 2002 Update.

Fortunately, in most cases there are more complete data sets and we give the data for Botswana, South Africa, Swaziland and Zimbabwe below. We have been unable to locate additional data for Nigeria.

The data for Botswana, shown on Table 2, are given by site of clinic. Until recently there was no attempt to calculate the national average. This meant Botswana could not be compared to other countries.

Table 2: Botswana's HIV prevalence by site

	1992	1993	1994	1995	1996	1997	1998	1999	2000	2001
Francistown	23.7	34.2	29.7	39.6	43.1	42.9	43.0	42.7	44.4	44.9
Gaborone	14.9	19.2	27.8	28.7	31.4	34.0	39.1	37.1	36.2	39.1
Ghantsi		9.5		18.9			22.3		26.4	26.4
Kanye (Southern)			16.0		21.8		24.67		40.7	34.0
Molepolole (Kweneng East)		13.7		18.9			37.2		30.4	32.4
Selebi Phikwe			27.0		33.1		49.89		50.3	55.8
Tutume			23.1		30.0		37.45		35.4	50.9

Source: Botswana 2000 and 2001 (crude prevalence rates for pregnant women attending the above sites) HIV Sero-Prevalence Sentinel Survey amongst pregnant woman and men with sexually transmitted diseases.

Data from South Africa are shown on Table 3 by province. What is significant here is the national trend. In 1998 it was estimated 22.8 percent of those surveyed were infected, in 1999 22.4 percent, in 2000 24.6 percent and in 2001 24.8 percent. Simple mathematics in calculating the weighted average indicates the 1999 national figure must have been miscalculated. This was remarked on in the South African Medical Journal in 2000. Four independent researchers, Dorrington, Bradshaw, Bourne and Abdool Karim argued that the officially stated decline in HIV prevalence from 1998 to 1999 (from 22.8 to 22.4 percent) was incorrect (Dorrington et al. 2000). An examination of the 1999 results showed that prevalence fell only in Mpumalanga, a province with a mere seven percent of South Africa's population. Otherwise rates of infection showed little or no change in three provinces and rose in the remaining five.

Dorrington et al. (2000) concluded, using population weighted methods, that national prevalence should not have fallen. Rather a small increase was to be expected. Government officials and a respondent from the South African Medical Research Council argued that the data were accurate, and castigated Dorrington et al. for their pessimism, failure to approach the Department of Health before writing with 'whatever suggestions they might have', and not 'joining in an active partnership against HIV/AIDS' (South African Medical Journal November 2000).

Table 3: South African HIV prevalence by province

	1994	1995	1996	1997	1998	1999	2000	2001
KwaZulu-Natal	14.4	18.2	19.9	26.8	32.5	32.5	36.2	33.5
Mpumalanga	12.1	18.3	15.8	22.6	30	27.3	29.7	29.2
Free State	9.2	11	17.5	19.6	22.8	27.9	27.9	30.1
North-West Province	6.7	8.3	25.1	18.1	21.3	23	22.9	25.2
Gauteng	6.4	12	15.5	17.1	22.5	23.9	29.4	29.8
Eastern Cape	4.5	6	8.1	12.6	15.9	18	20.2	21.7
Northern Cape	1.83	5.3	6.6	8.6	9.9	10.1	11.2	15.9
Limpopo	3	4.9	7.9	8.2	11.5	11.4	13.2	14.5
Western Cape	1.2	1.7	3.09	6.3	5.2	7.1	8.7	8.6
South Africa	7.6	10.4	14.2	16	22.8	22.4	24.5	24.8

Source: National HIV and Syphilis Sero-Prevalence Survey of Women attending Public Antenatal Clinics in South Africa 2000 and 2001.

However, survey results can be wrong as well as miscalculated. The official Swazi data are given in Table 4 on page 22. This shows data for every second year. What is not generally known is that the second survey, carried out in 1993, recorded ANC prevalence of 21.9 percent. It was evident that either the first or second survey results were wrong but it was not until the third and fourth surveys had been carried out that we could see which was the rogue data – that from 1993. Unfortunately these data (which were excluded from all subsequent official documentation) were used by one of the authors of this paper in preparing a report on the potential impact of AIDS in Swaziland (Whiteside & Wood 1994).

Table 4: Swaziland: HIV prevalence in ANC clients 1992–2000

		1992	1994	1996	1998	2000
Sample Size		726	2,343	2,468	1,659	2,316
National HIV prevalence, percent (CI 95 percent)		**3.9** (2.5; 5.3)	**16.1** (14.5; 17.5)	**26.0** (24.2; 27.8)	**31.6** (29.3; 33.9)	**34.2** (32.3; 36.2)
Age Groups (yrs)	< 20	–	18.4	24.7	25.2	25.9
	20–24	–	18.8	33.1	38.4	42.5
	25–29	–	14.3	28.0	38.0	40.7
	30–39	–	10.3	23.7	23.7	25.4
Women aged 15-24yrs		–	**18.4**	**29.8**	**32.9**	**35.4**

Source: 7th HIV Sentinel Sero-surveillance Report Year 2000.

Data also have political sensitivity. In the case of Zimbabwe, a good survey was carried out among women attending ANC clinics in late 2000 (Health Information and Surveillance Unit, Department of Disease Prevention and Control, National Survey of HIV and Syphilis). The report was not made available until early 2002 and even now it has not been publicly released and is hard to obtain. The report shows HIV prevalence of 35 percent compared to 29 percent in 1997, the date of the last survey. This document is as important for what it does not say as what it does. There is little attempt to compare with earlier data, thus we learn that 27.8 percent of women aged 15 to 19 were HIV positive in 2000, but have no idea of the infection level by age in earlier years. It is stated that: 'The HIV/AIDS epidemic in Zimbabwe is severe', but there is no attempt to provide figures (apart from the 35 percent). Why is this? In part it must be because the data show prevention efforts have not worked and there are political problems of having an epidemic of this scale.

The problem with ANC data is that there are biases: younger women will be over-represented as they are more sexually active and likely to fall pregnant; and HIV-positive women will be under-represented as HIV infection reduces fertility. An obvious drawback to the present method of sampling is that it applies solely to women attending the state antenatal clinics. It does not cover those who do not visit government facilities because they are too poor or do not have access to such services. In Southern Africa this group is probably small, but in Nigeria it may be large. It also does not pick up better-off women who attend private doctors – an issue in South Africa and Botswana with their well-developed private health sector.

Nonetheless, once the raw data from the state antenatal clinics are available, it is possible to estimate the percentage of all women, men and adults who are infected, as well as the percentage of children who will be born HIV positive. This is done using a model which adjusts for: the degree to which antenatal clinic attendance figures are unrepresentative due to the adverse impact of HIV on fertility of women; the fact that there are young and old members of both sexes who are not (or not as) sexually active; the lower prevalence in men; and the number of children expected to be infected through mother-to-child transmission. The raw data can then be turned into more representative numbers using various computer models, some of which are in the public domain and accessible through the Internet.[3]

Aside from the obvious problems with HIV data and their representativeness, they are subject to misinterpretation and political spin. The data from Zimbabwe are just one example. The significance of 1998/99 South African data has been alluded to above. Sometimes, of course, the interpretation is simply wrong. To return to the Swaziland data, the 1998 survey found that 31.6 percent of women attending the clinics at the time of the survey were infected (Swaziland Sentinel Report 1998: 21). The antenatal surveillance report then estimated that HIV prevalence among the *adult* Swazi population, those aged between 15 and 49, was 23 percent. However it gave the number of infected people in the country as 293 100. The total population in Swaziland in 1997 was about 978 200. This would give an adult prevalence of nearly 60 percent – assuming half the population was adult. Clearly the interpretation of the data left something to be desired.

AIDS case data

In the early years of the epidemic, AIDS case data were what hit the headlines. But in Africa, most AIDS cases are not officially recorded. In many countries, one of the principal stumbling blocks to cases being reported is that most people are not seen by the formal medical services. Even if they are, cases may not be recorded. There are a number of reasons for this: reporting may be very slow; it takes time for data to flow into a central point and be collated; data may be inaccurate because of the unwillingness of medical staff to report cases due to the stigma associated with AIDS or medical aid societies and insurance companies paying out more for other diseases; AIDS may not be the condition diagnosed (instead the patient may be recorded as having TB or meningitis), and health professionals may feel that it is pointless to report cases as there are always problems with collecting and collating the data.

Impact

This epidemic is only 20 years old. The curve of HIV infection is followed by the curve of AIDS illness and death. Impact flows from the excess illness and deaths in a society caused by this disease. In the countries we are using as examples, HIV prevalence rates appear to still be rising. This means that the full extent of the HIV epidemic is not apparent and it will take even longer for the AIDS cases to emerge. The full impact of this disease is going to take decades to become apparent. AIDS is a long-wave, intergenerational disaster. For example, orphaned female children have a higher likelihood of infection, thus potentially perpetuating the epidemic for a further generation. They are also more likely to be withdrawn from school. This means their children will have higher mortality rates as female education is correlated with infant and child mortality rates. Thus AIDS impacts over three generations.

We have a fairly clear idea of the current scale of the HIV epidemic in some countries, as our examples of Botswana, South Africa and Swaziland show. From this we can make reasonable assessments of potential morbidity and mortality using modelling techniques. Demographic impacts can be estimated but others are speculative.

What do we know about impact?

There are a few literature reviews, some region specific (Loewenson & Whiteside 1997) and some global (Chong Szu Fuei 1999, Barnett & Whiteside 2000). What is particularly significant, and evident from these reviews, is how little original research there has been! The reviews tend to refer to the same studies again and again. Indeed, there is a general problem that reports of 'impact' are sometimes no more than recycled anecdotes, a game of 'Chinese whispers'.

As might be expected (and this is no criticism of researchers who are operating with limited funds and time), impact studies usually focus on one geographical area, one company or one community. The problem is that these results are then applied without discrimination to whole populations or nations. An example is the study done for the Zimbabwe Farmers Union in one communal and small farm area. This found that any adult death had an adverse effect on output, but that in the case of AIDS, this effect was worse. An adult death resulted in a 45 percent decline in marketed output of maize, but where the cause of death was identified as AIDS, there was a 61 percent loss (Kwaramba 1998). The study is good, with 56 key informants and a survey of 544 households, and is well analysed and clearly written up. The problem is that others then applied the findings simplistically to the whole country.

On the basis of this one study in one area, another 'study' reported that there would be a decline in agricultural output not just in Zimbabwe as a whole, but more generally across Africa, and that this could be ascribed to AIDS. This tendency is particularly worrying from an ethical perspective. If one adopts a utilitarian approach to ethical decision-making, as will mostly be done in this article, concerns about the greater good for the most people involved are paramount. This kind of approach, however, requires much responsibility when making claims about the position and/or needs of 'the majority'. Simple and indefensible extrapolations of findings to larger groups of people as has been described are indefensible from both a scientific and ethical perspective.

Impact is hard to see but inevitable, and by the time it is visible it will be too late to take many of the actions that are needed. However, the one exception is in regard to the demographic effects of the epidemic.

The demographic impact of AIDS

Unusual levels of death alter population dynamics. Demography looks at populations and their dynamics. It is concerned with the numbers, growth rates and structure of populations. It measures and predicts size and growth rates, structure by gender and age, and key indicators like birth, death and fertility rates, life expectancy and infant and child mortality.

Demographers derive raw data from two main sources[4]: the census and vital registration statistics. Most countries conduct censuses every ten years. A census is 'the total process of collecting, compiling, evaluating and publishing or otherwise disseminating demographic, economic and social data pertaining at a specific time to all persons in a country or a well delimitated part of a country' (Petersen & Petersen 1985). The United Nations sets out what should be collected – and this includes data on age, sex, place of birth, citizenship, household and family structure, marital status, number of children and child deaths, literacy and educational qualifications, urban and rural domicile and economic status.

Vital registration is information about births, deaths and marriages. In many countries it is compulsory to register these events. But in poorer countries, these data may not be recorded or collected. An exception is South Africa and we will draw on these data later.

There are three main problems in looking at demographic impact. The first concerns the difference between an event and a process. The impact of AIDS is felt as a process: a person begins to feel unwell and so, perhaps, does not grow as much food, the family has less to sell and can't afford to send children to school. When the person dies, household composition changes. The demographer records the death and its effect on household composition and dependency ratios. But the impact of the events leading up to the death and flowing from it are unrecorded. Demography is one of the most 'counting' of the social sciences (Greenhalgh 1996), and because of this, it may insulate its exponents and readers of its reports from the underlying human processes.

Secondly, demographic indicators look at nations, provinces or areas. The impact of the disease may be very concentrated – cases will tend to cluster in households and among specific groups. A large-scale perspective, which concerns itself with averages, will not pick up small-scale impacts. This will only happen if the data are reanalysed in ways specific to the exploration of impact issues.

The third problem concerns the frequency with which demographic changes are measured. A census is carried out every ten years and analysis and reporting of the results may take several years. In the absence of vital registration, trends and changes have to be calculated on the basis of the census data alone.[5] International compilations of data rely on national statistical agencies, central banks and so on. The impact of a new and evolving disease will not be picked up and reflected in most national official data and has even less chance of appearing in international data sets.

Mortality

The most direct demographic consequence of AIDS is an increase in mortality (Carel & Schwartlander). In the absence of effective treatment, the period from infection to illness is between seven and ten years (Stover & Way 1998). UNAIDS states: 'Someone who has just been infected with HIV can expect to live nine years on average before falling seriously ill and to survive up to a year beyond that, even in the absence of antiretroviral therapy' (UNAIDS 2000). Even with recent price decreases and the withdrawal from litigation in South Africa by the multinational pharmaceutical corporations, available antiretroviral therapy is unlikely to make a difference to life expectancy in the poor world. These drugs are too expensive and need a fairly sophisticated delivery infrastructure. This is not to say that access is impossible. Elites in many countries are accessing some form of treatment. For others, there is a lottery of buying drugs when they can afford them and stopping when they can't. As prices fall, the number of people accessing treatment will increase. However, even at $350 per year for the drugs – the price offered by the Indian company CIPLA to NGOs in Africa in early 2001 – the cost of providing ARV treatment remains beyond the reach of most. The bleak conclusion is that demographic impacts are seemingly unstoppable.

The bleak conclusion is that demographic impacts are seemingly unstoppable.

In countries where HIV is primarily spread through sexual transmission, the peak age of infection is 20 to 40 years and the peak ages of AIDS death are seven to ten years later. Thus, AIDS increases mortality in adult age groups that would otherwise typically have the *lowest* mortality rates. Mother-to-child transmission, which is estimated to occur in about 30 percent of births to infected mothers (in the absence of interventions), accounts for increased infant and child mortality.

What evidence is there that the AIDS epidemic is causing increased mortality?

To know the answer, we need to measure mortality accurately. A metanalysis found mortality rates in African adults and children had risen in the mid-1990s (Timæus 1998). However, the data were limited, reporting slow and therefore mortality reflected the state of the HIV epidemic a decade previously. For most poor countries, we are never going to have really up-to-date information about the demographics of HIV/AIDS. We will always be working with history.

Data are, however, available for some specific sites and cohorts. AIDS has been identified as the major cause of deaths of adults aged 15 to 44 in Abidjan, Côte d'Ivoire, and of adults aged 15 to 59 in Tanzania (Adetunji 1997, Boerma et al. 1997). More recent information on excess mortality for sub-national locations comes from Uganda. In Rakai, a team of researchers followed a cohort of 19 983 adults aged 15 to 59 at ten-monthly intervals over four surveys. HIV prevalence in this cohort was 16.1 percent. Mortality in HIV-positive people was 132.6 per 1 000 person years, while in HIV-negative people, it was only 6.7 (Sewankambo et al. 2000). In other words, HIV-positive people were 18 times more likely to die than their peers who were not infected.

South African mortality data

There is one location in which the system of vital registration is good enough to estimate mortality, and this is South Africa. Mortality data have been collected for years in South Africa. Until recently these were not processed or released. One of the few good things to come out of the messy debate over the causes (and even existence of AIDS) that dominated South Africa in 2000 and 2001 was analysis and release of these data. One of the contentions of the 'dissident' group of scientists was there was no evidence of increased mortality in South Africa. The Medical Research Council and Actuarial Society of South Africa collected and analysed mortality data from the Department of Home Affairs' Population register. They estimated that coverage of adult deaths (over age 14) improved from 54 percent in 1990 to 89 percent in the 12-month period to the end of June 2000. The government is clearly succeeding in establishing a system to give accurate information on adult deaths.

The South African government is clearly succeeding in establishing a system to give accurate information on adult deaths.

After much delay the MRC report was finally released in November 2001 (Dorrington et al. 2001). This shows that there is a changing pattern of adult mortality, as is shown for men and women respectively on Figure 2. Mortality of young adult women has increased rapidly in the last few years with the mortality rate in the 25- to 29-year age range in 1999/2000 being some 3.5 times higher than in 1985. Mortality of young men starts from a higher base, but it too has increased. In the 30- to 39-year age range in 1999/2000 it was nearly twice the 1985 rate (Dorrington et al. 2002).

Figure 2: Estimated increase in adult death rates relative to the 1985 death rates

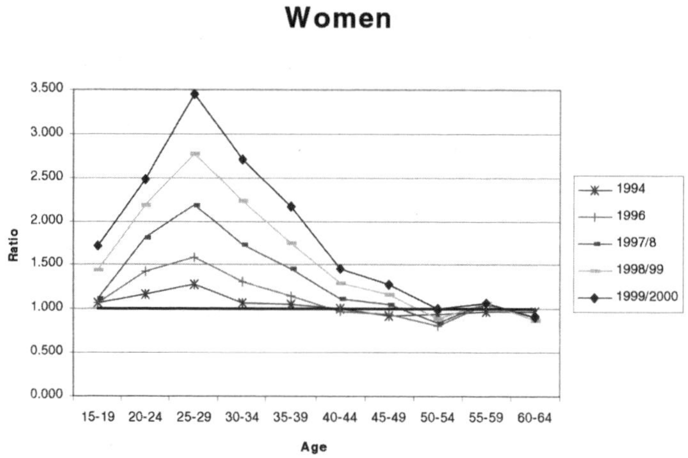

Source: The impact of HIV/AIDS on adult mortality in South Africa, MRC technical report.

The South African data prove conclusively that there is increased mortality in the country. In the absence of any other plausible explanation, AIDS is implicated. In 2000, of the adult deaths aged 15 to 49, some 40 percent were due to HIV/AIDS. It is estimated that AIDS accounted for about 25 percent of all deaths, making it the single biggest cause of death. Most worrying is that, without treatment, the number of AIDS deaths can be expected to grow in the next ten years to more than twice the number of deaths due to all other causes.

The fact that these data prove conclusively that South African mortality rates are rising sharply because of AIDS ought to be more than an ample incentive for the South African government to explore all possible and ethically justifiable interventions to try and curb the pandemic. We have earlier noted the possibilities in terms of a cure, a vaccine and ARV treatments for mother-to-child transmissions – the issue which currently consumes the news and public debate in South Africa. The one area that remains is the issue of motivating people to change their sexual behaviour. It is in this respect that, in particular, the South African government is currently seriously undermining its moral responsibility. Whereas, on the one hand, it is widely known that policy interventions are generally not guaranteed to change people's behaviour, *morally* speaking that cannot serve as an excuse *to refrain from trying*, as is currently happening in South Africa.

South Africans have, up till now, not once heard their President, their Minister of Health, or any other cabinet minister publicly denounce the irresponsible sexual practices that are the main cause of the pandemic. No official appeal or call has been made by such leaders that people should refrain from promiscuity, or use condoms and keep their sexual relations closed. This call ought to be made for reasons of national survival or economics. To refrain from such an appeal, given the extent of the pandemic in South Africa and the undeniable increase in mortality, as shown above, is immoral negligence on the part of the South African government, and posterity will judge them harshly for it.

The Swazi mortality notices

Given the problems with official data an obvious question is: are there alternative data sources? These are important if policy makers and politicians are to be convinced of the seriousness of the epidemic. In addition, if such data can be found, this will allow these people to acknowledge the reality of what they may well know through anecdote. We carried out a study in Swaziland [which had an ANC prevalence of 34.2 percent in 2000 (Swaziland Sentinel Report 2000)] using death notices from the local paper (Whiteside et al. 2001).

Figure 3: Modelled and reported deaths: Swaziland

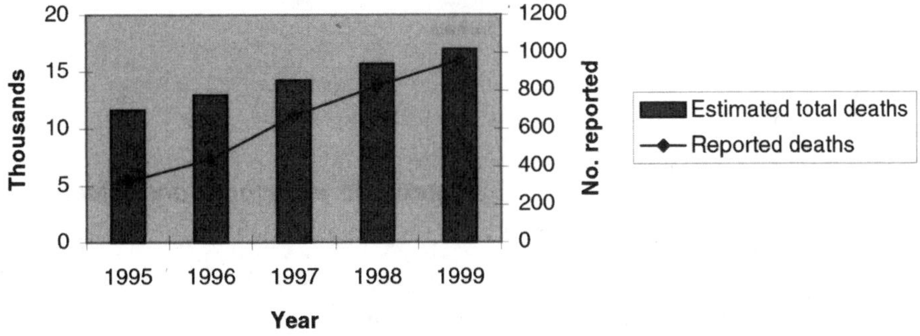

Many people place bereavement notices in the local press. Increasingly, these notices include a photograph and some biographical details. The study reviewed death notices in the *Swazi Times* from 1st July 1994 to 30th June 1999. The total number of deaths rose substantially during the period and tracked the trajectory of deaths predicted from models (The Futures Group, personal communication from John Stover). This is shown in Figure 3. When the data are analysed by age (Figure 4), it is apparent that the majority of deaths are in the 26- to 40-year-olds. This is also the age group with the largest increase. While this method of analysis has biases, it has the advantage of being consistent and illustrating the magnitude of an existing problem.

Figure 4: Reported deaths by age: Swaziland

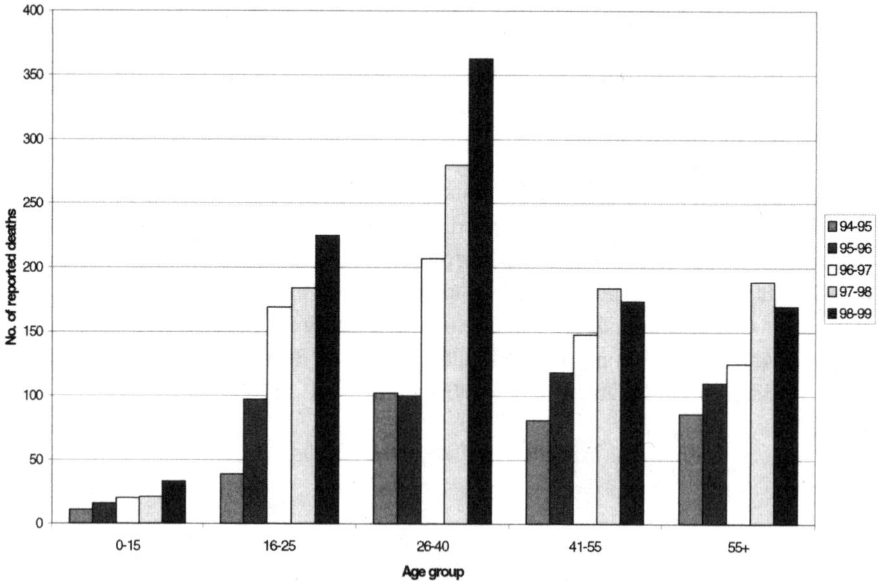

Source: Whiteside et al. 2000.

Measuring AIDS impact on human progress: life expectancy and infant and child mortality data

In the last part of this article we ask what evidence of impact is available from international data sets. The main sources of internationally comparative data are the multilateral agencies such as the World Bank and United Nations Development Programme. The most basic and popular measures of human progress and development are life expectancy and infant and child mortality. In Japan the life expectancy of a citizen born in 1999 was 80.8 years. By contrast, a Sierra Leonine born in the same year had a life expectancy of just 38.3 years. For every 1 000 Japanese babies born in that year, four would die before their first birthday; in Sierra Leone, 182 babies would not survive to age one (UNDP 2001). Without any other information, it is clear where most people would prefer to live.

These indicators in turn feed into the UNDP's Human Development Index or HDI which was introduced in 1990 to look beyond financial measures to assess development and progress toward it. It is constructed from three indices: life expectancy which is a proxy indicator for longevity; educational attainment which is measured by literacy and enrolment rates; and standard of living which is measured by real GDP per capita.

So what information do we have about the impact of AIDS on life expectancy and infant and child mortality? The UNDP's Human Development Report and World Bank's World Development Report produce data purporting to show what has happened up to the present. However, although the multilateral agencies should start from the same epidemic data, their results and interpretation are different. In some cases the difference is significant. For example, UNDP puts Botswana's 1998 child mortality at 48 per thousand, the World Bank at 105. It is not clear whether and/or how AIDS impact is considered in these official figures. UNDP did not put AIDS into its population calculations before its 1997 report and up to 1999 did not do so for all countries.[6] The impact of AIDS on life expectancy, HDI and ranking for our selected countries is shown in Table 5.

Table 5: Life expectancy and place in the HDI (UN HDP, 1996, 97, 99, 2001)

	1996 Report (1993 data)		1997 Report (1994 data)		1999 Report (1997 data)		2001 Report (1999 data)	
	Life Expect.	**HDI (Rank)**	**Life Expect.**	**HDI (Rank)**	**Life Expect.**	**HDI (Rank)**	**Life Expect.**	**HDI (Rank)**
Botswana	65.	0.741 (71)	52.3	0.673 (97)	47.4	0.678 (97)	41.9	0.577 (114)
Nigeria	50.6	0.400 (137)	51.0	0.393 (141)	50.1	0.391 (142)	51.5	0.455 (136)
South Africa	63.2	0.649 (100)	63.7	0.716 (90)	54.7	0.717 (89)	53.9	0.701 (94)
Swaziland	57.8	0.586 (110)	58.3	0.582 (114)	60.2	0.597 (115)	47	0.583 (113)
Zimbabwe	53.4	0.534 (124)	49.0	0.513 (129)	44.1	0.507 (130)	42.9	0.554 (117)

Also badly affected are mortality rates for infants and children under five years of age. In the absence of interventions, an infected mother has about a 30 percent chance of transmitting HIV to her infant. Most infected children will not reach their fifth birthdays. In addition, some mothers of uninfected children will die of AIDS and evidence is that orphans have higher mortality rates. The economic and social stress associated with having AIDS in a household further reduces life chances of infants and young children. This indicator will take time to show the effect of AIDS, but it is starting to become apparent in the UNDP data.

Table 6: Infant and child mortality (UN HDP, 1996, 97, 99, 2001)

	UNDP 1996		**UNDP 1997**		**UNDP 1999**		**UNDP 2001**	
	Infant Mortality	**Child Mortality**	**Infant Mortality**	**Child Mortality**	**Infant Mortality**	**Child Mortality**	**Infant Mortality**	**Child Mortality**
Botswana	42	54	55	52	39	49	46	59
Nigeria	84	91	82	191	112	187	112	187
South Africa	52	68	51	67	49	65	54	69
Swaziland	74	107	72	107	66	94	62	90
Zimbabwe	67	81	70	74	53	80	60	90

These indicators are imperfect in many ways: they are based on information provided by national governments with all the biases this entails, they reflect events rather than processes, but most importantly, they are outdated. They show what happened a few years ago, not what is going to happen. Given the nature of the HIV/AIDS epidemic, it is inevitable that the number of adult illnesses and deaths will rise dramatically. Also likely but less inevitable is that there will be an increase in infant and child mortality. In order to look into the future, we need models and fortunately these are available from the US Bureau of the Census. Figure 5 shows modelled life expectancies for 2000 and 2010 whilst Figure 6 and Figure 7 illustrate modelled infant and child mortalities respectively, for the same years for our selected countries. This picture is devastating.

Figure 5: Life expectancy 2000 and 2010

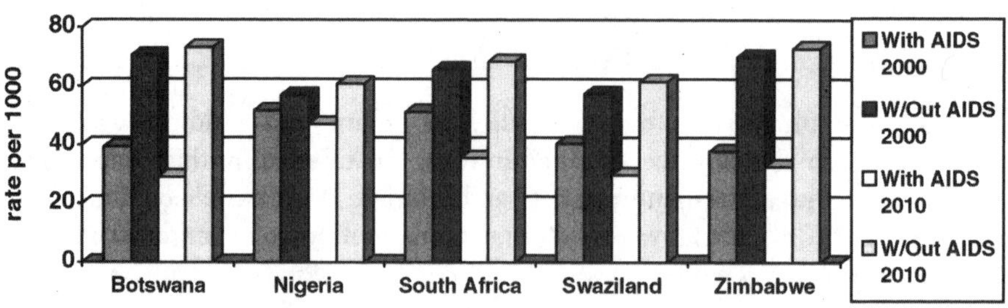

Figure 6: Infant Mortality for 2000 and 2010

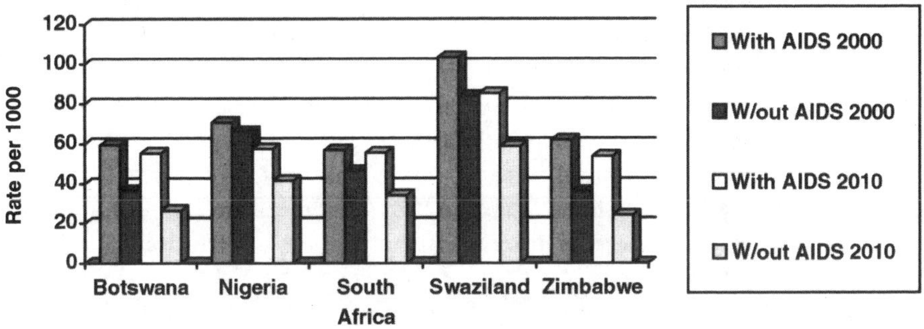

Figure 7: Child Mortality for 2000 and 2010

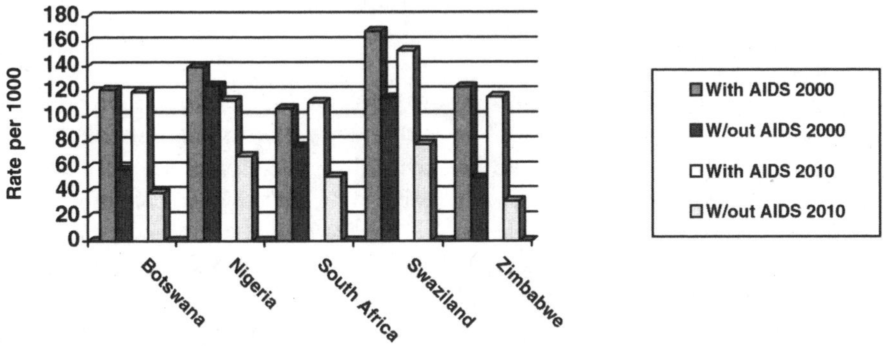

Conclusions

This article makes two main arguments. The first is that we are somewhat cavalier with our data about the scale and scope of the epidemic. We do not make it clear that we are working from limited data sources and what the implications of such limitations are. We suggest that people working in this field have allowed the urgency around the epidemic, and need to respond to lead us to accept data of lower quality and certainty than we would otherwise have done so. In addition, our presentation of the data has not been as critical as it might have been.

However, set against that is the need to convey the impact this disease will have. Here we have UN figures but these reflect the situation in the past, not the present or the future. In addition, in South Africa, there has been an analysis that provides a harbinger of what is to come, and our work in Swaziland shows that non-standard data sources can be mined for useful information. If we want to look ahead, then the modelling done by the US Bureau of the Census provides a sobering window into the future. In the absence of cheap, effective and deliverable treatments, adult deaths are inevitable but child deaths are not. We know that there are cheap and effective treatments that can greatly reduce mother-to-child transmission rates and it would be criminal if these were not made available as rapidly as possible.

People working in policy and planning in this field face a reality that is unique. There is a lot we don't know about the epidemiology of HIV/AIDS, but we know enough to predict potentially devastating developmental, social, economic and possibly political impacts. Our problem is to convince leaders at all levels that this is what we are facing; to show that there are things that can be done; and to persuade them to put responses in place. All this has to be done with imperfect data and where there are no precedents!

There is, therefore, an urgent need for more research that will hopefully yield more reliable data. Insufficient data has two consequences that are of moral import in the current crisis surrounding HIV/AIDS in the developing world. The first is that the scientific assessment of the scope and impact of the pandemic is thwarted. Given the extent to which scientific advances have benefited mankind over the past century, particularly in the area of medicine, this is a consequence that is lamentable.

Science is no infallible royal route to happiness and riches for all; some of the morally most problematic events of the past century (Hiroshima, Auschwitz and Chernobyl) occurred because of an irresponsible application of scientific knowledge. Yet, these hardly measure up to what we know science can produce if applied responsibly. There is little excuse for haphazard knowledge when we are dealing with a problem as calamitous as AIDS. The real extent and scope of what we are dealing with must be known. This is important in order to enable policy makers, planners and health care managers to make well-informed, rational decisions about the use of resources and preferential areas of action.

There is also a second consequence of insufficient data, which, in turn, suggests a further reason why more research is a dire moral requirement. As has often been referred to in this article, in Africa (specifically) we are dealing with policy makers on the level of national governments (particularly in South Africa) that seem to be in perpetual denial about the scope and seriousness of the pandemic. These people could easily abuse the findings of this article, interpreting it as oil to the fire of their state of denial. If data are scientifically judged insufficient, why take seriously what accredited scientists tell us about the pandemic? If such denial is part of the social and political context in which the pandemic has to be managed, there is an additional moral responsibility on scientists to attain as much reliable data as possible. Of course, the moral responsibility is not only on the scientists, but also on those who question their findings. An argument in support of denial has no moral standing if it does not suggest and enable imaginative and credible efforts to yield data that will settle the current disputes beyond reasonable doubt.

Enough research that will yield sufficient data is furthermore of the utmost importance, not only to counter the denials by African leaders, but also, and probably more importantly, to enable policy makers, once they face up to the real problem, to make informed policy decisions. There are so many things that, as yet, we still do not know about the pandemic. Some have already been suggested in this article. To these can be added the question about whether the health care infrastructures in Africa are able to administer antiretroviral drugs effectively and safely countrywide with adequate monitoring. It is, in addition, not really known whether preventing a maternal transmission of HIV does indeed save a life in the long term. It should (and can) be firmly established that lives saved from HIV will not in any case be taken by other ailments such as measles or diarrhoea in early childhood. And if this were the case, what are the policy implications? It is also a question whether more children's lives will be saved by improving maternal education and literacy than by antiretroviral treatment.[7]

The fact is: informed policy decisions have to be made which imply choices that must be motivated by sound scientific data. Of course, as has been forcefully argued by Karl Popper[8] and others, certainty is not and cannot always be an achievement of science. Most of our theories are never certain, and only corroborated, pending further evidence. But that does not mean that all efforts to establish the things that can be established must not be pursued. The need for more research and more reliable data is therefore beyond question.

It is commonplace nowadays to argue that science is not value-free, and that scientists must accept the moral responsibility for and the moral consequences of their work. The HIV/AIDS pandemic has created an almost unprecedented opportunity for this. Almost all scientific work done on this epidemic creates the opportunity for applications that will hopefully benefit mankind – if only in the sense of influencing policies that are required by the most rational and optimal use of resources. In that sense, the pandemic also creates a unique opportunity for scientists and policy makers to co-operate in a concerted effort to fight the plague of HIV/AIDS. Wherever this opportunity is not utilised to the fullest extent, moral blame is in order.

Endnotes

1 1 Corinthians Chapter 13, The Bible.

2 For the way this denial has been phrased, cf. Thabo Mbeki: Reciting comfortable catechisms on AIDS is not good enough. *The Sunday Times*, 23rd April 2000: 25. In this article, Mbeki asks a number of questions about the apparent differences between the way AIDS presents in Africa, and in other Western countries, and claims that 'we will not, ourselves, condemn our own people to death by giving up the search for specific and targeted responses to the specifically African incidence of AIDS'. He claims that this search for 'targeted responses' has been viewed as a 'criminal abandonment of the fight against HIV/AIDS'. He continues: 'Some elements of this orchestrated campaign of condemnation worry me very deeply. It is suggested, for instance, that there are some scientists who are 'dangerous and discredited' with whom nobody, including ourselves, should communicate or interact. In an earlier period in human history, these would be heretics that would be burnt at the stake!' He then continues to sing the praises of these discredited scientists. The people he is referring to are dissident scientists like Duesberg and Rasnick who, for many years, have denied the causal relationship between HIV and AIDS, claiming that HIV is, in fact, harmless (cf. Duesberg, P. & Rasnick, D. 1997. The drug-AIDS Hypothesis. *Continuum*, 4(5)). What exactly the reason for Mbeki's sympathy

with these dissidents is, is not entirely clear. However, he did give a rather sinister hint as to his motive in this regard in a widely reported address to the University of Fort Hare in 2001 (cf. Forrest, D. & Streek, B. Mbeki in bizarre Aids outburst. *Mail & Guardian* 26 October to 1st November 2001: 4–5). We quote Mbeki's words from this latter report: 'Thus does it happen that others who consider themselves to be our leaders take to the streets carrying their placards, to demand that because we are germ carriers, and human beings of a lower order that cannot subject its [sic] passions to reason, we must perforce adopt strange opinions, to save a depraved and diseased people from perishing from self-inflicted disease . . . Convinced that we are but natural-born promiscuous carriers of germs, unique in the world, they proclaim that our continent is doomed to an inevitable mortal end because of our unconquerable devotion to the sin of lust'. From these words it seems that his and other members of the governing party's denial springs, not only from scepticism about accepted scientific facts, but also from concerns about what these facts imply about continued racism as well as the sexual mores of African people.

[3] There are two reasonably easily useable models – the first a locally developed one from the Actuarial Association of South Africa www.assa.co.za. The second one was developed in the USA by The Futures Group International and is available from www.tfgi.com.

[4] For some countries, a third source of data is available: the Demographic and Health Surveys conducted by Macro International Inc. of Calverton, Maryland, USA. These surveys have been carried out and repeated in a number of countries.

[5] The limitations of demographic information are clear from the 2000 World Development Indicators (World Bank 2000). These include a mass of figures in numerous tables and graphs. It provides a table showing what primary data are available and when they were produced – no comment is made on their accuracy or reliability. Thus we learn that the latest population census data from Botswana was 1991, and the most recent Demographic and Health Survey available to the Bank was 1988. Cameroon had a census in 1987 and a DHS in 1998; Nepal a census in 1991 and DHS in 1996; and in India the last census was in 1991 but a national family health survey was carried out in 1992–93.

[6] The 1998 UNDP report has the following statement. 'The 1996 revision incorporates the demographic impact of HIV/AIDS in the population estimates and projections for developing countries where HIV seroprevalence had reached two percent in 1994 or where the absolute number of infected adults was large: Benin, Botswana, Brazil, Burkina Faso, Burundi, Cameroon, the Central African Republic, Chad, the Congo, Côte d'Ivoire, Democratic Republic of the Congo, Eritrea, Guinea-Bissau, Haiti, India, Kenya, Lesotho, Malawi, Mozambique, Namibia, Rwanda, Sierra Leone, the United Republic of Tanzania, Thailand, Togo, Uganda, Zambia and Zimbabwe' (p. 127). The 1999 report added Cambodia, Ethiopia, Gabon, Liberia, Nigeria and South Africa. The note has been dropped from the 2000 report so we must assume no new countries have been added. This means that in Swaziland with HIV prevalence at over 30 percent the life expectancy is recorded at over 60 years! UN data may be imperfect but so are those provided by the World Bank. Up to 1998, the World Development Report contained a mass of statistics in its World Development Indicators. In 1998, the report changed and many statistics were left out, as indeed are a number of countries. The result: comparisons can no longer be made between countries. Instead, the user of this data is required to purchase the new document, 'World Development Indicators' (in 2000, this cost $60). However, even the new, 'comprehensive' publication's user guide states, 'Selected indicators for 58 other economies – small economies with populations of between 30,000 and 1 million, smaller economies if they are members of the World Bank, and larger economies for which data are not regularly reported – are shown in Table 1.6'. ***In other words, detailed data on 58 countries are omitted.*** It is perhaps not surprising that countries like Afghanistan, Liberia and Somalia do not have data. It is a source of concern, however, that the only data available for places like Bahrain, Swaziland and Fiji, are gross national product, life expectancy, adult illiteracy and carbon dioxide emissions (all 'where available').

[7] Cf. S. Benatar, A.A. van Niekerk, W.A. Landman & T. Fleischer: Laying down AIDS gauntlet: there are some things that must be accepted so that HIV/AIDS can be defeated. *The Sunday Independent*, 7th April 2002, page 7.

[8] Cf. his *The Logic of Scientific Discovery*. London: Hutchison of London, 1959.

References

Adetunji, J.A. (1997). Assessing the mortality impact of HIV/AIDS relative to other causes of adult deaths in sub-Saharan Africa. *The Socio-Demographic Impact of AIDS in Africa Conference*. International Union for the Scientific Study of Population, and University of Natal Durban. February.

Barnett, T. & Whiteside, A. (2000). *Guidelines for Studies of the Social and Economic Impact of AIDS*. UNAIDS, Geneva.

Benatar, S., Van Niekerk, A.A., Landman W.A. & Fleischer, T. (7th April 2002). Laying down AIDS gauntlet: there are some things that must be accepted so that HIV/AIDS can be defeated. *The Sunday Independent*.

Boerma, J.T., Ngalula, J., Isingo, R., Urassa, M., Senkoro, K., Gabone, R., Mkumbo, E.N. (1997). Levels and Causes of Adult Mortality in Rural Tanzania with Special Reference to HIV/AIDS. *The Socio-Demographic Impact of AIDS in Africa Conference*. International Union for the Scientific Study of Population, and University of Natal Durban. February 1997.

Brieve. (2000). HIV Surveillance – What Grounds for Optimism? *South African Medical Journal, 90*(11). November.

Carel, M. & Schwartlander, B. (Eds.). Demographic impact of AIDS. *AIDS, 12*. Supplement 1.

Chong S. F. (1999). *A Critical Review of Household Survey Methodology: assessing the cost effectiveness of household responses to the economic impact of HIV/AIDS*. Masters dissertation. School of Development Studies, UEA Norwich.

Dorrington, R., Bradshaw, D., Bourne, D., Karim, S. A. (2000). HIV surveillance results – little grounds for optimism yet. *South African Medical Journal, 90*(5), May.

Dorrington, R., Bourne, D., Bradshaw, D., Laubscher, R., Timaeus, I. (2001). The impacts of HIV/AIDS on adult mortality in South Africa. *MRC Technical Report*. September.

Dorrington, R. et al. (2002). Some implications of HIV/AIDS on adult mortality in South Africa. *AIDS Analysis Africa, 12*(5).

Duesberg, P. & Rasnick, D. (1997). The drug-AIDS Hypothesis. *Continuum, 4*(5).

Forrest, D. & Streek, B. (2001, 26th October–1st November). Mbeki in bizarre Aids outburst. *Mail & Guardian*.

Greenhalgh, S. (1996). The Social Construction of Population Science: An Intellectual, Institutional, and Political History of Twentieth-Century Demography. *Comparative Studies in Society and History, 38*.

Kwaramba, P. (1998). *The Socio-economic Impact of HIV/AIDS on Communal Agricultural Production Systems in Zimbabwe*. Working paper No 19. Economic Advisory Project. Friedrich Ebert Stiftung. Harare.

Loewenson, R. & Whiteside, A. (1997). Social and Economic Issues of HIV/AIDS in Southern Africa: A review of Current Research. *SAfAIDS Occasional Paper Series, 2*. March. Harare.

Mbeki, T. (2000, 23rd April). Reciting comfortable catechisms on AIDS is not good enough. *The Sunday Times*.

Petersen, W. & Petersen, R. (1985). *Dictionary of demography: multilingual glossary*. Westport: Greenwood Press.

Popper, K. (1959). *The Logic of Scientific Discovery*. London: Hutchinson of London.

Sewankambo, N. K., Gray, R. H., Ahmad, S. et al. (2000). Mortality associated with HIV infection in rural Rakai District, Uganda. *AIDS, 14*.

South African Medical Journal, Brieve, HIV Surveillance – What Grounds for Optimism? November 2000, vol. 90, No. 11, pages 1062–1064.

Stover, J. & Way, P. (1998). Projecting the impact of AIDS on Mortality. *AIDS, 12*. Supplement 1.

Swaziland National AIDS/STDs Programme. *Sixth HIV Sentinel Surveillance Report* (1998). Ministry of Health and Social Welfare Mbabane, Swaziland. September 1998.

Swaziland National AIDS/STDs Programme. *Seventh HIV Sentinel Serosurveillance Report (2000).*

Ministry of Health & Social Welfare Mbabane. Swaziland. October 2000.

Timæus, I. M. (1998). Impact of the HIV epidemic on mortality in sub-Saharan Africa: evidence from national surveys and censuses. *AIDS, 12*. Supplement 1.

UNAIDS. (2000). *Report on the Global HIV/AIDS epidemic.* June. Geneva.

UNAIDS. (2001). *AIDS Epidemic Update.* December.

UNAIDS. (2002). *Report on the global HIV/AIDS epidemic.* Geneva.

UNDP Human Development Report. (2001). Oxford: Oxford University Press.

United Nations. Human Development Reports. New York. Oxford University Press. 1996, 1997, 1999 and 2001.

Whiteside, A. & Wood, G. (1994). *Socio-Economic Impact of HIV/AIDS in Swaziland.* National Development Strategy. Ministry of Economic Planning and Development. Government of Swaziland. April.

Whiteside, A., Desmond, C., King, J. & Tomlinson, J. (2001). Evidence of AIDS mortality from an alternative source. Swaziland case study. *AIDS Analysis Africa, 11*(5).

Chapter 3

Rolling out antiretroviral treatment in South Africa: economic and ethical challenges

Nicoli Nattrass *argues that the South African government can afford to implement a large-scale AIDS treatment intervention because the costs of the programme are balanced by the savings to the health sector (in terms of fewer opportunistic infections). However, she points out that this needs to be accompanied by changes to the welfare system and that there is a strong argument in favour of a Basic Income Grant (BIG).*

In August 2003, the South African government finally bowed to public pressure and agreed to provide highly active antiretroviral therapy (HAART) through the public health sector. However, implementation has been slow and remains hamstrung by resource constraints and insufficient political commitment (especially from the Minister of Health). Given the discourse of 'unaffordability' which has dogged South African AIDS policy-making over the past five years (Nattrass 2004a), it is likely that South Africa will opt for a limited rollout on the grounds that resources are best spent elsewhere.

Studies showing that in Africa AIDS prevention is more cost-effective than providing HAART (see e.g. Creese et al. 2002; Marseilles et al. 2002) offer some support for the South African government's apparent reluctance to implement a large-scale rollout. The problem with this literature, however, is that it does not take into account the link between treatment and prevention, and does not, for the most part, consider the savings for the public health sector (i.e. fewer hospital admissions) arising from the introduction of a HAART intervention. The South African costing exercise summarised here avoids both these limitations. It draws on earlier work (e.g. Geffen et al. 2003, Nattrass and Geffen 2004, Nattrass 2004a) and provides updated estimates where appropriate.

This chapter comprises three sections. The first highlights the reasons why a HAART rollout is likely to contribute to fewer new HIV infections. It also considers (and rejects) the counter-argument that a HAART rollout could result in increased 'HIV optimism', riskier sex and thus more new HIV infections. The second section turns to the issue of cost-effectiveness, showing that once HIV-related hospital costs are included in the calculation, the cost per HIV infection averted is lower in a treatment plus prevention intervention scenario than in a prevention-only scenario. It concludes by arguing that it is economically feasible to fund a large-scale comprehensive intervention and that the constraints on doing so are political. The third and final section draws attention to a specific dilemma posed by a HAART rollout, namely the potential trade-off between a disability grant income and antiretroviral treatment. The disability grant is an important source of income for many people living with AIDS. HAART restores health, thereby rendering AIDS patients ineligible for a disability grant. This trade-off between income and health threatens to undermine the success of the rollout and comprises an additional reason why a Basic Income Grant (BIG) should be considered in South Africa.

The link between AIDS prevention and treatment

The ASSA2000 Interventions Model was developed to take account of the demographic impact of a large-scale AIDS prevention and treatment rollout .[1] Drawing on data from developing and developed countries (e.g. VTCESG 2000, De Vincenzi 1994), the model assumes that people who have experienced voluntary counselling and testing (VCT) subsequently modify their sexual behaviour, but that this effect wears off over time for those who test HIV negative (Johnson and Dorrington 2002). Following medical studies (Vernazza et al. 2000, Hart et al. 1999), the model assumes that people on HAART have lower viral loads and thus are less infectious. This, together with the behavioural assumptions, results in the model predicting that a large-scale rollout of HAART will prevent many more HIV infections than any other single AIDS intervention. More specifically, the model predicts that over 80 000 new HIV infections would be averted per year between 2002 and 2015 if a large-scale HAART rollout was added to South Africa's existing suite of prevention interventions (see Table 1).

It is now widely accepted that more people are likely to participate in voluntary counselling and testing (VCT) if there is hope of treatment.

Marseille et al. (2002), however, caution against concluding that HAART helps prevent new HIV infections. They warn that the preventative benefits of reduced viral load have to be balanced against longer life expectancy for people on HAART. The ASSA2000 Interventions Model addresses this concern by assuming that HAART patients remain sexually active throughout their extended lives.

It is now widely accepted that more people are likely to participate in VCT if there is hope of treatment (see e.g. Harvard Consensus Statement 2001, De Cock et al. 2003). Farmer et al. (2001) found that the provision of HAART in rural Haiti resulted in a greater demand for VCT. A pilot HAART programme in Khayelitsha (a township in Cape Town) has similarly resulted in an uptake in VCT, AIDS activism and lower stigma (Coetzee and Boulle 2003). In other words, implementing a HAART programme is likely to create a social environment less conducive to the spread of HIV than would be the case in the absence of treatment possibilities. Some analysts [including Marseille et al. (2002)] however, worry that the presence of a HAART treatment programme will result in people becoming *less* fearful of HIV infection because of treatment possibilities, i.e. that they will start manifesting 'HIV optimism', and thus practice riskier sex. If so, HAART could contribute to the spread of HIV.

Studies in developed countries showing that HAART may have contributed to the increase in risky sexual behaviour amongst a minority of men who have sex with men (MSM) (Page-Shafer et al. 1999, Stolte et al. 2002, Perez et al. 2002, CIDPC 2002, Dubois-Arber et al. 2002) are the source of this concern. However, these results have to be treated with caution as they are typically cross-sectional and subject to selection bias. The best available study of the relationship between the availability of HAART and possible HIV optimism amongst MSM is that by the International Collaboration on HIV Optimism (2003). This study found that mean optimism scores were low in all places and that most gay men were realistic about the benefits of HAART (Ibid: 548).

In short, the view that HAART could easily result in a significant increase in risky sexual behaviour amongst MSM appears to be little more than a 'moral panic'. There is no scientific basis for assuming that the advent of HAART has resulted in a significant increase in risky sexual behaviour amongst MSM in high-income countries. There is even less basis for assuming that a possible behavioural response of a small minority of MSM is likely to be replicated on a significant scale in most developing countries where the dynamics of the HIV pandemic are very different. The fact that MSM on HAART are far more likely to engage in high-risk sex than heterosexuals on HAART (Laporte 2002: 15), together with evidence showing that MSM of non-Western nationality are less likely to engage in high-risk sex than their Western counterparts (Stolte 2002: 20), suggests that the problem (to the extent that it exists at all) may be located within a particular sexual sub-culture - and that this sub-culture has little obvious relevance for the African epidemic. It is too great a leap of logic to argue that because of a hypothetical link between HAART and risky sexual behaviour (for which there is little, if any, evidence) we should not consider the widespread use of HAART in developing countries. Nevertheless, it is important that the impact of HAART on sexual behaviour is monitored carefully, and educational programmes implemented where necessary.

The cost-effectiveness of providing HAART

One of the key differences between the South African study reported here and most other cost-effectiveness studies in Africa (see summary in Creese et al. 2002), is that all the hospital costs associated with AIDS are included in our calculation. According to the ASSA2000 Interventions Model, an AIDS intervention (over 13 years) comprising VCT, the improved management of sexually transmitted diseases (STDs) and mother-to-child transmission prevention (MTCTP) saves fewer new HIV infections (1.8 million as opposed to 2.9 million in total between 2002 and 2015) than an intervention that also includes a large-scale national HAART rollout. But the direct cost differential between the two programmes is substantial.

Figure 1: The drop in prices paid for antiretroviral treatment by the Western Cape Provincial Government between November 2003 and June 2004

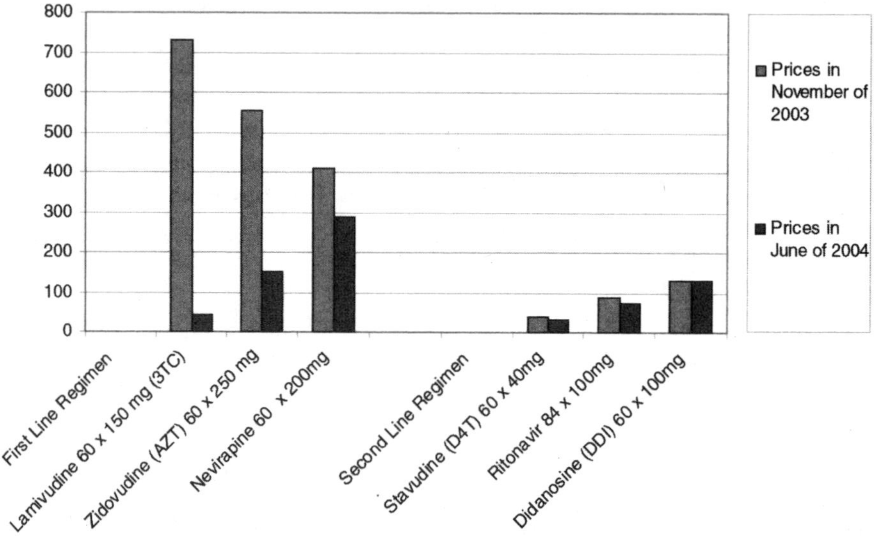

Source: Data provided by the Western Cape Provincial Government.

The first column of Table 1 on page 43 provides estimates for a prevention-only intervention (i.e. for VCT, MTCTP and improved management of STDs). The second column provides an estimate for a prevention plus treatment intervention. This is drawn from earlier work (see Nattrass and Geffen 2003 and Nattrass 2004a). All prices reflected in these two columns are 2001 prices. The third column takes into account the fact that antiretroviral drug prices have declined massively since 2001 (see Figure 1) and deflates the 2001 drug price estimate accordingly by 70 percent. The table shows that even taking into account the recent drop in drug prices, the direct costs of rolling out treatment in addition to an AIDS prevention intervention are substantially higher than a scenario in which only prevention interventions were implemented. Even though fewer HIV infections take place if HAART was rolled out, the cost per HIV infection averted is still four times higher in the prevention plus treatment scenario than in the prevention-only scenario.

Such findings are in line with the standard cost-effectiveness literature. If, however, we include the hospital costs associated with AIDS-related illness in all calculations, then the picture changes significantly – especially where a relatively high level of care is provided for those suffering from AIDS-related opportunistic infections. It is, unfortunately, very difficult to obtain an accurate measure of the costs of treating AIDS-related illnesses as this depends on the level of care provided in different hospitals and clinics and on the number of times people actually seek treatment for their illnesses. For this reason, Table 1 includes an upper- and lower-bound estimate for AIDS-related hospitalisation costs. The upper-bound estimate was based on information (updated to 2001 prices) from an urban hospital of the costs of treating people at different stages of AIDS illness (see Geffen et al. 2003). It assumes no rationing of treatment for AIDS patients and is thus a reasonable approximation of the 'worst-case' scenario from a cost perspective. The lower-bound estimate is based on a World Bank estimate of the cost of treating opportunistic infections (in Stage 4 of the disease) in higher-income developing countries (Haacker 2001). The actual cost experienced by South Africa will probably lie somewhere between these two estimates. A mid-point estimate is provided in parentheses.

The total cost figure in Table 1 includes the direct costs of the various programmes *and* the hospitalisation costs experienced by the public sector as a result of the AIDS pandemic. This is a very important addition to the costing exercise. With regard to MTCTP, it has been demonstrated that once total health costs (i.e. the costs of the intervention plus the costs of treating HIV-positive children for opportunistic infections) are compared to a no-intervention scenario (i.e. just the cost of treating HIV-positive children for opportunistic infections), then it becomes clear that government would actually *save* resources by introducing MTCTP (Skordis and Nattrass 2002, Nattrass 2004a). This is simply because the costs of treating HIV-positive children are high in relation to the cost of preventing them from becoming HIV positive in the first place.

Does the same logic hold for a HAART intervention? Table 1 shows that the average annual mid-point hospitalisation cost estimate is *lower* for the intervention that includes HAART (R18.8 billion) than it is for the one that does not (R22.5 billion). This is because of lower morbidity for people on HAART and fewer new HIV infections (and associated hospitalisation costs). Is this cost saving sufficient to compensate for the cost of providing HAART? The answer to this depends on the level of hospital care provided for people living with AIDS. Table 1 shows that if the upper-bound hospital cost is included in the total cost calculation, then total cost is lower for the prevention plus treatment scenario (R31.8 billion) than it is for the prevention-only scenario (R34.4 billion). This implies that the government would actually save money (through averting AIDS-related hospital costs) if a large-scale antiretroviral treatment rollout were implemented.

However, if hospital costs are closer to the lower-bound estimate, then total costs would be higher for the prevention plus treatment scenario (R12.9 billion) than is the case for the prevention-only scenario (R11.8 billion). In other words, the greater the level of hospital care provided to people living with AIDS, the greater the likelihood of government actually saving money by implementing a large-scale rapid national HAART rollout.

Table 1 also shows that the total cost (direct cost plus mid-point estimate for hospitalisation costs) per HIV infection averted is lower for the prevention plus treatment scenario than it is for the prevention-only scenario. If the objective was to save lives as cheaply as possible, then adding a HAART rollout to an existing suite of AIDS prevention interventions makes sense. This was the case before the antiretroviral drug prices fell, and is even more the case today.

Table 1: Average annual cost of AIDS intervention scenarios between 2002 and 2015 in 2001 prices

Prevention-only	Prevention-only intervention (VCT + STD + MTCTP)	Prevention plus treatment intervention (VCT + STD + MTCTP + HAART) - assuming 2001 drug prices	Prevention plus treatment intervention (adjusted to take into account recent decreases in drug prices)
MTCTP + VCT + Improved treatment of STDs + Additional infrastructure, public education and condom distribution	R0.6 billion	R0.6 billion	R0.6 billion
HAART	R0	R9.9 billion	R3.0 billion
Total Direct Costs	R0.6 billion	R10.5 billion	R3.6 billion
Public Hospitalisation Costs (upper and lower bound)#	R33.8 – R11.2 billion *(R22.5 billion)	R28.2 – R9.3 billion *(R18.8 billion)	R28.2 – R9.3 billion *(R18.8 billion)
Total costs (direct cost plus upper and lower-bound hospitalisation costs)	R34.4 – R11.8 billion *(R23.1 billion)	R38.7 – R19.8 billion *(R29.2 billion)	R31.8 – R12.9 billion *(R22.3 billion)
Average HIV infections averted each year	139 539	220 231	220 231
Average direct cost per HIV infection averted each year	R4 221	R47 550	R16 138
Average total cost per HIV infection averted each year (using the mid-point estimate)	R165 495	R132 693	R101 280

Source: Costing exercise done in conjunction with the ASSA2000 Interventions Model. See Nattrass, 2004a, 2004b; Geffen et al. (2003). # Lower-bound hospitalisation costs reduce the upper-bound costs by two-thirds [in line with World Bank data provided in Haacker (2001: 9)].
** Mid-point estimate.*

Note that the argument only considers the benefits of HAART for the public health sector. It does not consider human rights issues or try and put a value on the fewer orphans, the extra years of life gained by those on HAART or on the lives saved through HIV infections averted. If these benefits had been valued, the economic case in favour of adding HAART to an existing set of AIDS interventions would be even stronger. The strength of the finding is that *even* within this narrow fiscal frame of reference, there is a strong economic case to be made in favour of providing HAART for those who need it.

Cost-effectiveness calculations in health economics are typically designed to help answer the question: how should the marginal dollar be allocated in order to save the greatest number of lives? However, if the *only* objective was to design an AIDS-intervention strategy that saved the most years of life for the least amount of money, then a purely technocratic (albeit untenable from human rights, public health and legal perspectives) approach might be not to treat the opportunistic infections of HIV-positive people (on the grounds that the few extra years of life saved by treating their opportunistic infections are not worth the extra cost). The huge bill for hospitalisation costs (see Table 1) would then be reduced significantly. Once this decision was made, the next step (in terms of this kind of logic) would be to consider which intervention saves the most lives for the least amount of money (measured in direct costs).

The problem with this marginalist logic of cost-effectiveness is that it fails to question the very framework which made it necessary in the first place – i.e. the budget constraint. As such, it deflects attention away from a larger, prior question: 'How much would it cost South Africa to combat AIDS *inter alia* by providing HAART to all those who need it?' Given the scale of the AIDS epidemic in South Africa, and the government's recent acceptance of the need to provide HAART in the public sector, there is an urgent need for social deliberation over what sacrifices are required (in terms of additional taxation) to treat everyone living with AIDS (Nattrass 2004a).

There is an urgent need for social deliberation over what sacrifices are required (in terms of additional taxation) to treat everyone living with AIDS.

Earlier costing exercises using 2001 prices suggested that a full-scale rollout would require an extra 1.4 percent–3.2 percent of GDP per year (Nattrass and Geffen 2003, Nattrass 2004a). The estimate deliberately assumed no rationing in the public sector and (following the ASSA2000 Interventions Model) a rollout to 90 percent of those who need treatment. It was thus a high social benefit, high cost scenario and as such was the most expensive of the available South African costing studies (see review in Boulle et al. 2003). If such a programme were funded through an increase in taxation, total taxation as a percentage of GDP would rise from 24.6 percent to a maximum of 27.8 percent (which is not out of line with world averages). It has been argued previously that this is economically feasible and that ultimately the decision as to whether this is 'affordable' is a political issue (Nattrass 2004a).

The recent decline in drug prices has made this argument all the more compelling. As can be seen from Table 1, antiretroviral drug prices comprise over 90 percent of total direct costs, and between 25 percent and 50 percent of total costs (i.e. including hospital costs) depending on what level of care is provided for treating the opportunistic infections of HIV-positive people. Taking into account the recent drop in antiretroviral prices, the amount of extra spending required drops to between 0.9 percent and 2.6 percent of GDP (depending on the level of hospital care for HIV-positive people), thus lowering the required additional tax burden significantly.

Figure 2: A slow and limited versus a fast and comprehensive HAART rollout

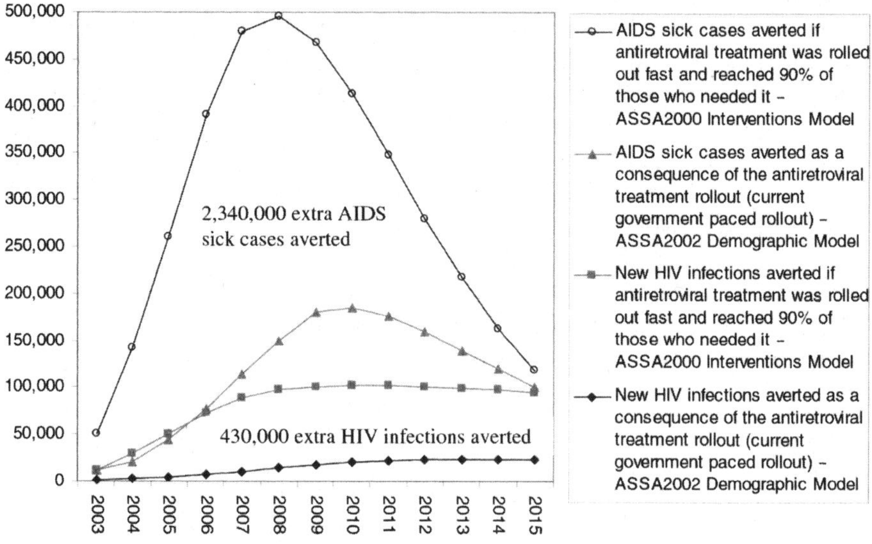

Source: ASSA2000 Interventions Model; ASSA2002 Model.

One of the limitations of this costing exercise is that it assumes, following the ASSA2000 Interventions Model, a rapid rollout reaching 90 percent of those who need it. Such a rapid rollout is unlikely to take place. The recently released ASSA2002 model incorporates many of the features of the ASSA2000 Interventions Model, but assumes a much slower rollout reaching only 50 percent of those who need treatment. It is, in other words, a much closer approximation of what is actually likely to materialise given the government's reluctance to prioritise the rollout.

Figure 2 plots output from both the ASSA2000 Interventions Model and the ASSA2002 model. It shows that almost half a million new HIV infections and almost two and a half million new AIDS cases could be averted if the faster rollout modelled by the ASSA2000 Interventions Model was adopted rather than the current sluggish programme. It would appear, however, that the South African government is reluctant to mobilise the necessary resources to save these additional lives. I have suggested elsewhere (Nattrass 2004a) that the government is effectively practising triage and sacrificing a large part of the current generation to HIV. Two out of three macroeconomic models of the impact of AIDS on the South African economy predict that per capita income will rise as a result of the AIDS pandemic. A cold-hearted economic calculus on the part of the elite may thus conclude that it is more efficient to let people die than to raise taxes to try and save them. Whether this was ever discussed explicitly in government circles is impossible to know. However, the existing policy stance is consistent with such logic.

The potential trade-off between disability grants and antiretroviral treatment

The discussion so far assumes that antiretroviral treatment is an unambiguous benefit for people living with AIDS. However, this may not be the case for those who as a result of their illness obtained access to disability grants and who subsequently stand to lose them as a result of restored health (Nattrass 2004b). Disability grants need to be renewed by medical officers, either every six months or five years depending on the grant (Simchowitz 2004). Someone on antiretroviral treatment who becomes well enough to work should thus expect to lose their disability grant.

Disability grants can be an important source of household income as it is the only welfare grant available in South Africa for adults of working age. According to survey evidence from Khayelitsha, Cape Town, disability grants comprise between 40 percent and 50 percent of household income for those households in receipt of a disability grant (Nattrass 2004b). Unsurprisingly, then, the disability grant is a major source of relief for poor AIDS-affected households. A respondent interviewed as part of a broader study went as far as to say 'I love this HIV' because of it (loc. cit).

The notion that someone might 'love this HIV' seems shocking. But it is understandable (albeit in a terrible way) when one considers the desperate circumstances that households can find themselves in when they lack access to an income-earner. The advent of a disability grant can be a significant lifeline for the entire family. The threat of its removal as a result of antiretroviral treatment is thus serious indeed. If the data from Khayelitsha is anything to go by, it suggests that average household income could fall by at least a third if a disability grant is lost through restored health.

It is, of course, possible that some of those individuals who lose their disability grant through restored health will in fact find a job, thereby contributing to an increase in household income. However, with over a third of the labour force in South Africa without work, the vast majority are likely to remain unemployed. As there is no significant welfare support for unemployed adults of working age besides the disability grant, the loss of such a grant has serious implications for household income.

Given such a scenario, it is possible that a small, but significant, proportion may opt to discontinue antiretroviral treatment so as to become AIDS-sick again in order to qualify once more for the disability grant – and then once it is reinstated, go back onto treatment (and when the grant expires once more, perhaps try to repeat the cycle). Besides the negative impact on the health of the individual, such behaviour will dramatically increase the growth of drug-resistant strains of the HIV virus, thereby rendering the entire antiretroviral rollout less effective. Put differently, the more that people switch from being on and off treatment, the greater the numbers of AIDS sick, and the greater the number of new HIV infections. In other words, the beneficial outcome in terms of HIV infections averted as a result of the rollout would be unlikely to be as dramatic. The final impact will depend on how many people choose to yo-yo between the disability grant and antiretroviral treatment, the rate at which resistant strains of HIV develop, and the extent to which such resistant strains spread through the population.

One response to the potential trade-off between disability grant and HAART is to remove the grant altogether for HIV-positive people. This would at least eliminate the perverse incentives described above. The cost, however, is that it is discriminatory (because people disabled by AIDS should not be any less entitled to government support than any other disabled person) and cuts away an important income lifeline for poor AIDS-affected households. And, to the extent that lower household income translates into lower food expenditure, it may also adversely affect the nutritional status of people on antiretrovirals – thereby reducing the effectiveness of the treatment rollout via a different route. Furthermore, to the extent that AIDS is driven by poverty (Stillwaggon 2002), this could also exacerbate the AIDS epidemic.

Allowing access to the disability grant for people whose health has been restored may result in some people desiring to become HIV positive.

An alternative response is to allow HIV-positive people to maintain their disability grants – even after their health has been restored. There are two problems with this strategy. The first is that the problem of perverse incentives remains. Allowing access to the disability grant for people whose health has been restored may result in some people desiring to become HIV positive. Although this may sound far-fetched, there is anecdotal evidence from the Western Cape, the Eastern Cape and KwaZulu-Natal indicating that some people become angry when they test negative – saying that they were hoping to get the grant.[2] In the Eastern Cape, there is a saying that you have 'won the Lotto' if you test HIV positive because it is seen as a ticket to the disability grant.[3] If antiretroviral treatment is regarded (incorrectly) as a 'cure' for HIV, then it is possible that some people may desire to become HIV positive under the mistaken notion that they will be able to get access to the disability grant and obtain antiretroviral treatment.

The second problem with allowing HIV-positive people to keep their disability grants even when their health has been restored through antiretroviral treatment is a moral one: why should they be privileged over other people who may be equally needy, but HIV negative? Put this way, the immediate question that poses itself is: why not get rid of the disability grant altogether and introduce a Basic Income Grant (BIG) for all? Although such a grant would need to be at a much lower level (probably in the region of R100 to R200) than the R780 maximum grant for the disabled, households relying on the disability grant as an important source of income will at least be partly compensated for its loss by the fact that everyone in the household would receive a BIG (and pensioners would continue to receive R780 a month).

Towards a Basic Income Grant in South Africa

There is a range of arguments, both moral and economic, in favour of a BIG in general (see e.g. Van Parys 2001) and for South Africa in particular (see e.g. Standing and Samson 2003). This is not the place to review these arguments, or the arguments against the introduction of a BIG. The point is simply that given the context of AIDS and the perverse incentives associated with the removal of the disability grant, this amounts to one more argument in favour of the introduction of a BIG.

Previous research and financial simulations have shown that even a modest BIG of R100 per month for all South Africans could contribute substantially to reducing poverty and inequality in South Africa (e.g. Bhorat 2002). This is why the Taylor Committee report on comprehensive welfare reform argued in favour of BIG (Taylor Committee 2002). According to Le Roux (2002), a BIG could be financed by a 7.3 percentage point increase in value added tax (VAT) and a 50 percent increase in excise and fuel taxes. This proposal is broad-based and redistributive: those who spend more than R1 000 a month end up paying more in consumption taxes than they benefit from the R100 BIG.

In earlier work, I estimated that implementing a full-scale AIDS prevention and treatment intervention which provided HAART to all those who needed it (i.e. with a rapid rollout and no rationing of antiretroviral treatment), would require an increase in resources equivalent to raising VAT by between three and seven percentage points depending on what level of care is provided to those suffering from AIDS-related illness (Nattrass 2004a).[4] Given the subsequent dramatic decrease in the price of antiretrovirals, the revenue which would need to be raised would now probably require an increase of between two and six percentage points on VAT. If we take the mid-point estimate (an increase of four percentage points in VAT), then it would appear that a 12-percentage point increase in VAT would be sufficient to finance a BIG *and* a large-scale national AIDS prevention and treatment intervention.

This, of course, is a significant increase in taxation. Is it feasible? There is no exact technical answer to this question as different societies tolerate different levels of taxation, and at different times. Welfare expenditure as a proportion of GDP has risen with economic development, and in times of crisis (such as war) citizens have accepted large increases in taxation as legitimate (Seekings 2003). The notion of what is and is not 'affordable' thus varies according to the social and economic context. Given the scale of the unemployment problem and the AIDS epidemic, it is possible that reasonable South Africans might agree to an increase in taxation so as to deal with it. Whether one appeals to Rawlsian logic to protect the lives and livelihoods of the poor – or to more radical left libertarian ideas of providing each citizen with a social dividend as a basic right – the issue ultimately boils down to whether reasonable people can tolerate living in a society that forces people living with AIDS to choose between income and health.

Endnotes

[1] The ASSA2000 Interventions Model was designed by Leigh Johnson and Rob Dorrington at the University of Cape Town. It includes various parameters of heterosexual behaviour (such as the probability that a partner comes from a particular risk group, the number of sexual partners per annum, the age of the partner and the probability that a condom is used during intercourse). Relevant South African data was obtained from the Demographic and Health Survey, the antenatal clinic survey and the best available estimates regarding mortality.

[2] Reported by social workers and peer counsellors.

[3] Correspondence with a journalist in the area.

[4] The money could, of course, be raised through income tax rather than VAT. The discussion about taxation is presented here in terms of VAT simply to keep the argument simple.

References

Bhorat, H. (2002). *A universal income grant scheme for South Africa: An empirical assessment*. Paper presented at the 9th International Congress of the Basic Income European Network, Geneva.

Boulle, A., Kenyon, C. and F. Abdullah. (2003). A Review of Antiretroviral Costing Models in South Africa, in Moatti, J., Coriat, B., Souteyrand, Y., Barnett, T., Dumoulin, J. and Flori, Y. (Eds.), *Economics of AIDS and Access to HIV/AIDS Care in Developing Countries: Issues and Challenges*, Paris: ANRS.

CIDPC (Centre for Infectious Disease Prevention and Control, Canada). (2002). HIV Infections Among MSM in Canada. *HIV/AIDS Epi Update*, April. Available on http://www.hc-sc.gc.ca.

Coetzee, D. and Boulle, A. (2003). *Adherence: Balancing Ethics and Equity, Selection Criteria and the role of DOT*, presentation at the Seminar on Scaling Up the Use of Antiretrovirals in the Public Health Sector: What are the Challenges? Hosted by the University of the Witwatersrand, School of Public Health and Perinatal HIV Research Unit, 1st August, 2003.

Creese, A., Floyd, K., Alban, A. and Guinness, L. (2002). Cost-effectiveness of HIV/AIDS Interventions in Africa: A Systematic Review of the Evidence. *The Lancet, 359*, 1635–1642.

De Cock, K., Mbori-Ngacha, D., and Marum, E. (2002). Shadow on the Continent: Public health and HIV/AIDS in Africa in the 21st Century. *The Lancet, 360*, 67–72.

De Vincenzi (for the European Study Group on Heterosexual Transmission of HIV). (1994). A longitudinal study of human immunodeficiency virus transmission by heterosexual partners. *New England Journal of Medicine, 331*, 341–6.

Dubois-Arber, F., Moreau-Gruet, and Jeannin, A. (2002). Men having sex with men and HIV/AIDS prevention in Switzerland. *Euro Surveillance: European Communicable Disease Bulletin, 7(2)*, February.

Farmer, P., Leandre, F., Mukherjee, J., Sidonise Claude, M., Nevil, P., Smith-Fawzi, M., Koenig, S., Castro, A., Becerra, M., Sachs, J., Attaran, M., Yong Kim, J. (2001). Community-based approaches to HIV treatment in resource-poor settings. *The Lancet, 358*, August.

Geffen, N., Nattrass, N. and Raubenheimer, C. (2003). *The Cost of HIV/AIDS Prevention and Treatment Interventions*, Centre for Social Science Research Working Paper no.29, Centre for Social Science Research, University of Cape Town. Available on www.uct.ac.za/depts/cssr.

Haacker, M. (2001). *Providing Health Care to HIV Patients in Southern Africa*. IMF Policy Discussion Paper, October, 2001. Available from mhaacker@imf.org.

Hart, C. et al. (1999). Correlation of Human Immunodeficiency Virus Type 1 RNA Levels in Blood and the Female Genital Tract, in *Journal of Infectious Diseases, 179*, 871–82.

Harvard Consensus Statement (2001). *Consensus Statement on Antiretroviral Treatment for AIDS in Poor Countries*. Individual Members of Harvard University, Harvard University.

International Collaboration on HIV Optimism (2003). HIV Treatments – Optimism among Gay Men: An International Perspective. *Journal of Acquired Immune Deficiency Syndromes, 32*, 545–550.

Johnson, L. and Dorrington, R. (2002). *The Demographic and Epidemiological Impact of HIV/AIDS Treatment and Prevention Programmes: An Evaluation Based on the ASSA2000 model*. Paper presented at the 2002 Demographic Association of Southern Africa Conference, Cape Town. Available on: www.commerce.uct.ac.za/care/Research/Papers/DEMSApaper.doc.

Karstaedt, A., Lee, T., Kinghorn, A. and Schneider, H. (1996). Care of HIV-infected Adults at Baragwanath Hospital, Soweto: Part 11: Management and Costs of Inpatients. *South African Medical Journal, 86*, 1490–3.

Kinghorn, A., Lee, T., Karstaedt, A. (1996). Care of HIV-infected Adults at Baragwanath Hospital, Soweto: Part 1. Clinical Management and Costs of Outpatient Care. *South African Medical Journal, 86*, 1484–9.

Laporte, A. (2002). A New Decline in Preventative Behaviours among Homosexual Men: The Role of Highly Active Antiretroviral Therapy. *Euro Surveillance: European Communicable Disease Bulletin, 7(2)*, February.

Le Roux, P. (2003). Financing a Universal Income Grant in South Africa. *Social Dynamics, 28(2)*.

Marseille, E., Hofman, P. and Kahn, K. (2002). *HIV Prevention before HAART in Sub-Saharan Africa*. In *Lancet*, 2002, 359, May 25, 1581–6.

Nattrass, N. (2004a). *The Moral Economy of AIDS in South Africa*. Cambridge: Cambridge University Press.

Nattrass, N. (2004b). AIDS and the Disability Grant: Further Reasons for Introducing a Basic Income Grant in South Africa, paper presented to the Basic Income European Network Conference, Barcelona Forum, 20th September 2004.

Page-Shafer, K., McFarland, W., Kohn, R., Klausner, J., Katz, M., Wohlfeiler, D., Gibson, S. and the Stop AIDS Project. (1999). Increases in Unsafe Sex and Rectal Gonorrhea among Men who have Sex with Men – San Francisco, California, 1994–97. *Morbidity and Mortality Weekly Report*, Centres for Disease Control and Prevention, 29th January. Available on: http://www.thebody.com/cdc/unsafe199/unsafe199.html.

Perez, K., Rodes, A. and Casabona, J. (2002). Monitoring HIV Prevalence and behaviour of men who have sex with men in Barcelona, Spain. *Euro Surveillance: European Communicable Disease Bulletin, 7(2) February*, 23–28.

Seekings, J. (2003a). *Providing for the Poor: Welfare and Redistribution in South Africa*, Inaugural Lecture, University of Cape Town, 23rd April.

Simchowitz, B. (2004). Social Security and HIV/AIDS: Assessing 'Disability' in the Context of ARV Treatment, draft paper presented at the Centre for Social Science Research, University of Cape Town, 29th July 2004.

Skordis, J. and Nattrass, N. (2002). Paying to Waste Lives: The Cost-Effectiveness of Reducing Mother-to-Child Transmission of HIV/AIDS in South Africa. *Journal of Health Economics, 21*, 405–421.

Standing, G. and Samson, M. (eds). (2003). *The Basic Income Grant in South Africa*, Cape Town: University of Cape Town Press.

Stillwaggon, E. (2002). HIV/AIDS in Africa: Fertile Terrain. *The Journal of Development Studies, 38(6)*, 1–22.

Stolte, G., Dukers, N., de Wit, J., Fennema, H. and Coutinho, R. (2002). A summary report from Amsterdam: Increase in sexually transmitted diseases and risky sexual behaviour among homosexual men in relation to the introduction of new anti-HIV drugs. *Euro Surveillance: European Communicable Disease Bulletin, 7(2), February,* 19–22.

Taylor Committee (2002). *Transforming the Present: Protecting the Future.* Report of the Committee of Inquiry into a Comprehensive System of Social Security for South Africa, RP/53/2002, Government Printer, Pretoria.

Van Parys, P. (2001). *What is Wrong with a Free Lunch?* Boston: Beacon Press.

VCTESG (Voluntary HIV-1 Counselling and Testing Efficacy Study Group). (2000). Efficacy of Voluntary HIV-1 Counselling and Testing in Individuals and Couples in Kenya, Tanzania and Trinidad: A Randomised Trial. *The Lancet, 356,* 103–112.

Vernazza, P. et al. (2000). Potent Antiretroviral Treatment of HIV Infection Results in Suppression of the Seminal Shedding of HIV: The Swiss Cohort Study. *Journal of Infectious Diseases, 28,* 117–121.

Chapter 4

Moral and social complexities of AIDS in Africa

When seen together, the many complexities surrounding AIDS in Africa represent a daunting challenge. In this chapter **Anton A. van Niekerk** *outlines some of these moral and socio-political complexities but warns against waiting for long-term solutions, arguing that there are opportunities for immediate action and response.*

AIDS has become the major reality of the African continent, despite the fact that this is still, incredibly, being denied by some of the continent's most prominent and influential leaders. According to the most reliable current opinion, AIDS is probably a fairly recent phenomenon, but might well have lingered relatively unobtrusively in small, undeveloped, yet stable rural communities in Africa for many decades because of their lack of contact with the wider world and their comparatively limited sexual behaviour patterns (Van der Vliet 1994). Developments such as increased trade, 'uhuru' (liberation from colonialism), urbanisation and more sexual freedom facilitated the recent epidemic spread of the disease. In Africa, women have turned out to be much more vulnerable to the epidemic than men.

Not since the Black Death of the mid-14th century[1] has a disaster of such magnitude confronted humanity. There are, however, significant differences between the AIDS pandemic and the Black Death. These are, amongst others:

- At the start of the 21st century, we know what we are dealing with, what its cause is, and how to prevent it.
- The speed at which the disease occurs and operates. Whereas the Black Death hit and killed within weeks or even days, AIDS is a slow-working ailment that can linger for years before it starts to destroy.
- Whereas the plague killed indiscriminately, AIDS targets certain groups (the sexually active and drug addicts) who happen to be among the young and economically active sectors of society.

In spite of massive global investments and efforts, neither a vaccine nor a cure for AIDS is currently available. In addition, even if a vaccine should eventually, after prolonged clinical trials involving almost unprecedented large groups of research subjects, be found, it is still unclear how accessible and effective it would be on a continent that faces such problems as Africa does.

Sub-Saharan Africa is the area that is by far the worst struck by this disaster.

The figures of the pandemic, which are more comprehensively dealt with in Chapter 1, are staggering, as illustrated by the following statistics:

> Of the 36 million adults and children in the world living with HIV/AIDS in 2000, more than 70 percent reside in sub-Saharan Africa . . . 17 million Africans have died since the AIDS epidemic began in the late 1970s, more than 3.7 million of them children. An additional 12 million children have been orphaned by AIDS. An estimated 8.8 percent of adults in Africa are infected with HIV/AIDS, and in the following seven countries, at least one adult in five is living with HIV: Botswana [with] the highest estimated adult infection rate – 36 percent – Swaziland, Zimbabwe, Lesotho, Zambia, South Africa and Namibia (McGeary 2001: 48–49).

It is, further, reliably estimated that 3.8 million Africans became HIV positive in the course of 2000 (McGeary 2001: 48). HIV/AIDS has superseded military conflict as the single biggest cause of death in Africa. In 1999, 1.4 million people died of AIDS in East and Southern Africa – twice as many as in the Rwandan massacre. Up to 70 percent of hospital beds in Africa are currently occupied by AIDS patients. Of the 25 million Africans due to die of HIV/AIDS, the majority will die within the next five to eight years (Swanepoel 2001).

The statistics in my own country, South Africa – the most developed economy in Africa – are particularly alarming[2]. South Africa has the largest number of people living with HIV/AIDS in the world, namely 5.1 million. That is one in nine of the total population, or about 20 percent of South Africa's adult population (http://www.unaids.org). It is reliably estimated that 420 000 children have been orphaned (cf. Cullinan 2001), and 250 000 people die each year from the disease (McGeary 2001: 49). By the year 2000, 500 000 South Africans had already died of AIDS. As far back as 1997, 50 000 new infections have occurred every month.

Projections are that the epidemic will reach its peak in 2010 with six million people infected by then. In such a situation, 52 percent of all deaths in South Africa will be AIDS related. More remarkable is the projection that 80 percent of all deaths in the 20- to 50-year-old range will be AIDS related. (Van der Vliet 1998). According to a UN report on AIDS (November 1999), less than half of South Africans will reach the age of 60, against a figure of 70 percent in other developing countries and 90 percent in developed countries. Life expectancy in South Africa has climbed from 44 in the early fifties to 59 in the early nineties. Because of AIDS, it will plummet to 45 in the next five years (Pretorius 1999). In fact, as predicted in a recent lecture by Alan Whiteside, there is a very real possibility that in the absence of meaningful interventions, life expectancy in South Africa could drop to 35 within the next decade. It is estimated that, at the current rate, South African population growth – once almost out of control at a whopping 3.2 percent – will drop to zero in 2025.

The purpose of this chapter is to identify and critically discuss some of the enormous complexities involved in trying to deal with a disaster of this kind in the context of under-development, as is manifested by most countries in sub-Saharan Africa. We shall be dealing with these complexities, the impediments they pose for constructive action in the face of the pandemic, and suggested solutions, if any.

A *complexity* refers to a kind of problem that not only has no clear-cut or self-evident answer, but is also often thus constituted that an analytical approach wherein we distinguish parts and whole, often with the expectation that addressing the parts will fix the whole, is not always successful either. In complexities or complex systems, the whole is more than the constituent parts; the approach to the solution of complex problems often requires a problem consciousness and a sense of interactive influences that defy our natural intuitions or analytical prowess (Cilliers 1998).

I shall, however, not be arguing that everything about AIDS in Africa is helplessly and uncontrollably complex. Much can be done about the problem in Africa – much more than is currently being done, particularly in South Africa, which, as was shown above, has become the epicentre of the pandemic in Africa.

The first and foremost of these complexities is the phenomenon of poverty.

Poverty as social context for HIV/AIDS in Africa

To talk of poverty in connection with AIDS in Africa is both necessary and confusing. According to the president of South Africa, Thabo Mbeki, poverty is the main cause of AIDS. This blunt statement fails to take into account a very basic distinction often lacking in the public discourse on AIDS in Africa. This is the distinction between the *cause* of the epidemic, and the *social context* within which the epidemic thrives[3]. There can be no doubt that AIDS is caused by a retro-virus which shows an unprecedented ability to undermine the human body's immune system, and for which neither a cure nor a vaccine has as yet been found. Viral diseases, as we know, do not all become epidemics. To become an epidemic, a niche or social context is required. In Africa, besides factors such as relatively recent urbanisation, migrant labour, natural and man-made disasters (such as war, floods and famine) and trade (sex tourism and the movement, above all, of truckers across the continent) (cf. Van der Vliet 1999: 1–4), poverty is the main aspect of this niche or social context.

> *Poverty has accompanying side-effects that are major contributing factors to the current spread of HIV/AIDS.*

Poverty has accompanying side-effects, such as prostitution (i.e. the need to sell sex for survival), poor living conditions, education, health and health care, that are major contributing factors to the current spread of HIV/AIDS. It is, for example, estimated that six million South Africans live in informal settlements or shanty towns. With the advent of South Africa's new democracy in 1994, the country still had one of the worst records in terms of social indicators and income inequality. About half (44 percent) of South Africans were regarded as poor, and still are[4]. Unemployment in South Africa is rife; fewer than 30 percent of poor working age adults are working in the formal sector of the economy. Almost 80 percent of the poor in 1994 had no piped water to their homes, no modern toilets (90 percent) or electricity (85 percent). More than a third (35 percent) of children under the age of five are nutritionally stunted, compared to six percent in richer households (*South African Health Review* 1999: 3).

As far as the provision of health services is concerned, it must be borne in mind that South Africa does not have a history of a very effective health system. In 1992/3, the country was spending 8.2 percent of its GDP on health care – comparatively much in global terms. In spite of that, South Africa ranked below 60th in terms of 'health status indicators'. This could be attributed to the fact that the private sector spent over 60 percent of the total spending on health care on less than 20 percent of the country's total population. The remaining 80 percent of the population are dependent on the public health services, which were spending the remaining 40 percent of the resources (Ibid. 70). The annual per capita expenditure on health care in the public sector currently is R1 000, as against R5 100 in the public sector (Benatar 2005). In 1998, 62 percent of South Africa's general practitioners, 77 percent of its specialists, 88 percent of pharmacists and 89 percent of dentists worked in the private sector (*South African Health Review* 1999: 72).

Benatar writes as follows about the serious deterioration in the quality of South African health services:

> Fifteen years ago South Africa had the potential to develop a strong public health system offering balanced primary, secondary and tertiary services. Such a system would have been aided and strengthened by a small and strong private sector with many private medical practitioners also doing part-time work in public hospitals. But the pace and extent to which privatisation has been allowed [in South African health care services] has largely destroyed this potential (Benatar 2005).

What is the solution? I would like to make two points in this connection:

First, we should be careful to resist the temptation of becoming so overwhelmed by the reality of poverty in Africa that the analysis becomes disempowering, i.e. that we start to believe that AIDS will be brought under control only if Africa is miraculously transformed into a set of economically prosperous, Western-like countries. That, to use an understatement, is not going to happen soon, and if that is the definitive condition for relief, Africa is irreversibly doomed. The 'all or nothing approach' should be abandoned and realistic aims must be set and pursued.

To stress only the poverty aspect of the problem is, expediently, to avoid facing up to matters that can make a difference, such as:

- addressing and criticising conventional sexual and religious mores;
- making condoms available on a massive scale;
- co-operating with multinational pharmaceuticals and Western governments to make antiretroviral drugs available and more affordable;

- exploring the import of generic equivalents without burning all bridges carrying patent rights;
- imaginatively introducing sex education to school curricula; and
- drawing on the influence of important societal role models.

The second point is that the AIDS catastrophe compels us to reflect critically on the massive imbalance between the wealth of Africa and the West, and thereby to rethink the requirements for human well-being on a global scale. The fact of the matter is that sub-Saharan Africa generates no more than one percent of the total wealth produced in the world. The buying power of all the countries south of the Sahara, excepting South Africa, in total just about matches that of a country such as Norway.[5] The developed world can no longer ignore the fact that Africa is the home of ten percent of the world's population, lives on one percent of the global economy, and carries 70 percent of the world's HIV/AIDS burden. Furthermore, 'annual per capita expenditure on health care is less than US$10 in many African countries, as compared with between US$ 2000–$4200 in industrialised nations' (Benatar 2001: 5).

African countries also carry extremely heavy debt burdens – often, as in the case of South Africa, incurred by an illegitimate previous regime. It is indeed a serious ethical question whether this catastrophe does not compel us to rethink the requirements for human well-being on a global scale. As Benatar argues:

> Perpetual economic growth for some cannot continue at the expense of others without sacrificing our humanity. The root causes of poverty should be openly acknowledged and studied more seriously, and powerful nations should be required to address these. Crucial to a new approach will be the recognition that it is not merely altruism that is called for, but rather a long-term perspective on rational self-interest in an increasingly interdependent world (Benatar 2001: 6).

Denial, lack of leadership and the politicisation of HIV/AIDS

The management and possible curbing of the AIDS pandemic on the African continent is immensely exacerbated by the denial of its seriousness and the lack of political will on the part of the leadership to tackle the problem. There are a few exceptions. In Senegal and Uganda, comprehensive national programmes were launched to address the problem, and they yielded considerable success (for discussion, cf. World Bank 2000: 18–22). But they remain exceptions. The lack of political will on the part of the leadership in South Africa, in its turn exacerbated by President Mbeki's flirtations with the views of discredited 'dissident' scientists such as Duesburg, Rasnick and Mhlongo (cf. Duesberg & Rasnick 1997), who challenge the theory that AIDS is caused by a virus, remains a serious impediment to the creation of an imaginative yet workable national strategy for approaching a problem which clearly is evolving into a national, if not global, disaster.

One can only speculate about the reasons for this state of denial. One theory is that the financial implications of a comprehensive AIDS strategy are so enormous that African leaders shrink from facing the challenge. Another theory is that the denial is born from a deep-seated, post-colonial scepticism about the structure of the global economy and the role of large, multinational conglomerates, in this case represented by the pharmaceutical corporations. Difficult as it might seem to believe in the light of the statistics mentioned at the beginning of this chapter, the perception is rife within the ruling party in South Africa that information about the AIDS pandemic is either unreliable[6] or is created to serve the interests of the pharmaceutical companies, who have a monopoly on effective antiretroviral drugs. South Africa, unlike countries such as India, does honour the international patent regulations protecting the pharmaceutical companies' interests. Consequently, the production and distribution of generic equivalents for these drugs are illegal in South Africa, although efforts have recently been made to change this, particularly by an organisation called the Treatment Action Campaign (TAC), a militant NGO campaigning for affordable treatment of HIV/AIDS.[7]

In 2000, a cohort of major drug companies challenged South Africa's alleged right to import or produce generic equivalents of their patented medicines in court, but dropped the action soon afterwards. Reasons were not given, but one can imagine that such an action turned out to be a serious public relations risk for these companies, given the extent of their business in the developing world and the criticisms such action might evoke amongst their (often quite vocal) critics back home.

The hesitation and denial of the leadership is, to a certain extent, understandable, though hardly pardonable.

Reacting to criticism and to the prospect of increased generic competition, Merck became one of the pharmaceutical corporations to declare that it would dramatically reduce the price of HIV drugs to the developing countries (*Time*, March 19 2001: 17). Following suit, Bristol-Meyers Squibb announced that it cut the cost of the two drugs that it manufactures, Videx and Zerit, to a combined price of US$1 per day. In 2001, an American AIDS patient paid US$16 per day. But even with these huge price decreases, African countries are still not able to afford these drugs without significant aid from abroad.[8]

As suggested earlier, the hesitation and denial of the leadership is, to a certain extent, understandable, though hardly pardonable. Just at the time when an intellectually gifted leader such as Thabo Mbeki was ready to launch his idea of an 'African Renaissance' (cf. Mbeki 1998 and Makgoba 1999) and to promote Africa as the continent of the 21st century, there arose the challenge of one of the severest health nightmares a politician could imagine. In the process, as is persuasively argued by Van der Vliet, all the existing prejudices against Africa were reinforced, if not exacerbated. One of the cruel effects of AIDS, as was realised from the outset, is that it often afflicts people who are already victims of prejudice and discrimination: homosexuals (initially), drug addicts, and eventually the poor and the wretched. 'The coincidence of a new disease, in marginalised communities, in troubled and insecure times, was a recipe for a new wave of prejudice' (Van der Vliet 1996: 53).

This reinforcement of old prejudices has now shifted from individuals and communities to a whole continent. AIDS is increasingly called 'the African epidemic'. This inevitably fosters a politicisation of the discourse about the pandemic which, in turn, complicates its effective management considerably. In a somewhat inflammatory article, Simon Watney articulates the kind of resentment that the identification of AIDS and 'Africanness' have fostered in many intellectual and leadership circles on the continent:

> . . . Africa has been effectively demonised in a post-colonial discourse of perpetual catastrophe and unnatural disasters. This undifferentiated apocalyptic Africa has proved an ideal site in which to find and 'see' disease. 'African AIDS' thus condenses ancient fears concerning contagious disease, together with vengeful fantasies concerning 'excessive' sexuality, understood in essentially pre-modern terms as both the source and the cause of AIDS . . . The racism and homophobia which Western culture has visited on racial and sexual minorities for millennia now threaten to turn back on heterosexuals themselves, in their seeming refusal and inability to acknowledge the realities of HIV infection and disease. It would appear that we are witnessing a fundamental reorganisation of Western racism, as the constitutive colonial analogy between race and class is dissolved, and African blackness is reconceptualised as an analogue of the sexually perverse (Watney 1989: 59).

Although some of these emotional allegations may not be devoid of truth, they are not very helpful when we are confronted with the question of how, in practical terms, to go about assisting in the relief of the suffering of real people living with HIV/AIDS. One of the main complexities facing the management of the disease in Africa, is, therefore, this kind of consistent politicisation of the discourse about AIDS – a politicisation that raises the level of inflammatory rhetoric and moral outrage about the injustices of the universe and the global economy but is irrelevant to the devising of practical programmes to assist ordinary and not always politically conscious sufferers: those who are the real victims of the denial and hesitant leadership of those who have it in their power to do something about the crisis in Africa.

The solution, as I see it, is twofold:

1. Acknowledge, for once, the crisis and stop obfuscating its understanding or management by undue politicised rhetoric about an alleged social outrage which, essentially, is a health problem and can significantly be curbed if primarily addressed as such.
2. Seek optimal partnerships and co-operation with the pharmaceutical multinationals as well as other supportive governments who have it in their power to facilitate the provision of essential antiretroviral drugs at more affordable prices.[9]

Behaviour changes under conditions of deprivation and illiteracy

I have written above about the need for a comprehensive AIDS prevention campaign in (South) Africa and the tragedy of its persistent delay by the national authorities. However, one of the most serious problems facing the issue of prevention in the African context, is how to effectively communicate with the people most vulnerable, viz. the masses of relatively uneducated, often illiterate people living in the rural areas.

Africa in general, and South Africa in particular, is an under-urbanised environment. One of the destructive consequences of apartheid is that that system's declared intention of discouraging urbanisation (in order to keep people in their 'homelands', even if it meant forcibly moving people to these arid, uninhabitable and over-populated regions). Verwoerdian social engineering (cf. Johnson 1983: 523–526) succeeded in keeping, until fairly recently, the majority of people in the rural areas. Currently, the figure is still in excess of 40 percent of the total population. In addition, 75 percent of the poor live in the rural areas (*South African Health Review* 1999: 3).

A rural existence in South Africa is by and large an existence devoid of opportunity or resources. Life is, for the large majority, a continuous struggle to get hold of one's next meal. Education and health care facilities are either non-existent or in a state of perpetual collapse. Something as basic as clean, disease-free drinking water is regarded as a luxury. In 2001, KwaZulu-Natal was hit by a cholera epidemic, simply because of the inaccessibility of clean water for tens of thousands of people living in areas that are very difficult to furnish with water storage tanks, where the only access to water is from the contaminated rivers flowing through the region.

Effective communication with people is, to a significant extent, a function of their ability to read, and, on the basis of that reading, to grasp concepts that are not self-evident. Literacy, however, is a huge problem in South Africa. If literacy is defined as the ability to read, write and numerate (normally conditional on seven years of schooling), then 41 percent of the adult population of South Africa is illiterate (Bot, Wilson & Dove 2000: 73). Macfarlane, reporting on a recent conference on this topic, claims that the figure is 45 percent (Macfarlane 2000). A map in the *Education Atlas of South Africa* shows that in one third of the country's 354 magisterial districts – all located in the rural areas – the illiteracy rate is between 60 percent and 80 percent. In the majority of the magisterial districts, over a third of the adults are illiterate. Urban and developed residential areas have the lowest illiteracy rates of between 11 percent and 20 percent. KwaZulu-Natal, where the AIDS pandemic is at its worst (according to the latest Dept. of Health figures the infection rate rose from 32.5% in 1999 to 36.2% in 2000), is also the province with the highest number of illiterate adults (1 982 845), while the Northern Province is proportionally the worst off (where 52% of all adults are illiterate).

Virginia van der Vliet rightfully asks in her book: 'How do you reach a poor, isolated, illiterate rural or urban woman, who is not at school, at work, or at church or a clinic attender?' (1996: 97). One has to go further and ask: If you reach her, how do you start communicating the complexities of HIV to this woman? How, first of all, do you explain that she might become devastatingly ill simply from having sex with her husband, who is a migrant labourer, and that it is best to have them both tested? She might be ill already, but she'll not yet know it, since the disease might take long to present with symptoms. There are drugs that can help her, but they are unaffordable for a person in her position. She, if HIV positive, can infect her husband or lover(s), but they will not be ill immediately, etc. The point is: understanding and explaining the phenomenon of HIV/AIDS is a complex matter. This woman will, in all probability, either not understand what is being communicated to her, not believe it, or shrug it off as just one of the many hazards that she has to face in order to continue her struggle for survival.

Most rural Africans lack the material, social and educational resources, even to understand, let alone to foster, their interests.

To get ordinary people to change their behaviour is, as we know, difficult enough. When AIDS originally struck in the gay communities of San Francisco and New York in the early eighties, a change of behaviour was effected, albeit only after a spirited campaign, utilising media of all sorts. The gay men who were at particular risk were mostly well-educated people who read newspapers, watched television and, most importantly, were sufficiently empowered to mobilise themselves and lobby for support and accelerated research about this life-threatening disease.

The complexity of dealing with the epidemic in Africa is that these kinds of resources are simply absent. Most rural Africans lack the material, social and educational resources, even to understand, let alone to foster, their interests in a way even remotely comparable to what happened in the US in the eighties. In addition, even if they are able to do this, the society in which they live does not have the resources to rise to this kind of challenge as US and Europe have done.

The solution to this complexity is not self-evident. Clearly more and better education is needed. But that will mainly benefit the younger generation, not the adult population referred to above. Adult education is, therefore, also clearly required, but the resources for that, and the motivation of the people who stand to benefit from it, are limited. It may be that the sheer brutality and extent of suffering and death that people from these communities experience in the near future will cause an outrage that provides the opportunity for education that focuses the mind. However, by then most of the damage will have been done for the foreseeable future. On what exactly to do about this problem, the jury is unfortunately still out.

Women's vulnerability

In the example above of the difficulty of informing and empowering people in Africa about their predicament, it was for good reason that the case of a poor rural woman was used. The position of women in Africa adds another burden to the spectrum of complexities that confront us when trying to deal with HIV/AIDS.

The situation in Africa has shown definitively that AIDS flourishes most demonstrably in a society where women are particularly vulnerable. In Africa, there are currently two million more women than men infected by AIDS (Pretorius 1999). Not only are these women physically more prone to become infected than men during normal sexual encounters, but their status and role put them at considerably greater risk. Women, because of their devalued status in the traditional African homestead, have significantly less control over the nature and frequency of their sexual contacts than their normal Western counterparts. They are, typically, in underdeveloped societies, much more likely to be illiterate. Before and after marriage, they are perceived to be, and often also perceive themselves to be, totally dependent on men. Consequently, if and when they opt out of marriage or concubinage, they have very few marketable skills. In this case, commercial sex is often their only option.

Van der Vliet also points out how vulnerable monogamously married women are:

> . . . raised in [a] strongly patriarchal society, with a tradition of polygamy, macho ideas of masculinity, and an emphasis on her duty to bear children to ratify bridewealth contracts, [the married woman's] rights to demand fidelity or the use of condoms, or to refuse sex, are, for most women, not negotiable. Economic dependency on her partner weakens her position further (1999: 3).

Add to this the grim evidence of a rapid increase in so-called 'sugar daddy' relationships, in which older men seek out younger sexual partners (often mere children) – partly because of their (the men's) perception that young girls might not be infected, while they themselves, of course, often are – and a scary picture of the moral depravity of sectors of South African society emerges. This is an environment very conducive to the flourishing of the AIDS epidemic.

The position of women in the current HIV/AIDS epidemic in (South) Africa is made all the more precarious by the severe forms of stigmatisation that people who acknowledge their HIV status currently have to face in that region.[10] In an issue of *Time*, Johanna McGeary tells the story of Laetitia Hambahlane (not her real name), a 51-year-old woman with AIDS (McGeary 2001: 48–50). The narrative starts with the observation that, in Africa, 'to ackowledge AIDS in yourself is to be branded as monstrous' (p. 48). Once Laetitia was diagnosed after falling sick in 1996, her employers:

> . . . fired her without asking her right diagnosis. For weeks she could not muster the courage to tell anyone. Then she told her children, and they were ashamed and

> frightened. Then, harder still, she told her mother. Her mother raged about the loss of money if Laetitia could not work again. She was so angry she ordered Laetitia out of the house ... When Laetitia ventures outside of the house, neighbours snub her, tough boys snatch her purse, children taunt her ... One day local youths barged into her room, cursed her as a witch and a whore and beat her (she contracted the disease from her husband). When she told the police, the youths returned, threatening to burn down the house (McGeary 2001: 50).

Women's disempowerment in Africa is, to a significant extent, the result of insufficient education.

In 1998 Gugu Dlamini, a young woman in KwaZulu-Natal, decided to 'come out of the closet' about her HIV-positive status and started to campaign on her own and other sufferers' behalf. She was stoned to death in her neigbourhood (SA Health Review 1999: 309).

Women's disempowerment in Africa is, to a significant extent, the result of insufficient education. UNICEF has recently made available figures that show that many African women are dangerously ignorant about HIV and its perils. More than 70 percent of adolescent girls in Somalia between the ages of 15 and 19 – an age, as has often been proved, when women are almost at their most vulnerable – and more than 40 percent in Guinea Bissau and Sierra Leone have apparently never heard of AIDS. The overwhelming majority of Africans who are HIV positive, do not know that they are carrying the virus, and are blissfully continuing to infect other people.

One study has shown that 50 percent of Tanzanian women know where they can be tested for HIV, but that only six percent of these women have in fact been tested. In Zimbabwe, only 11 percent of women have been tested for the disease. Many of those that have been tested prefer not to be informed of the results, mainly because of fear of stigmatisation. In the Côte d'Ivoire, it has been found that of all women who discover that they are HIV positive, less than 50 percent return for treatment to prevent mother-to-child-transmission (*UNAIDS AIDS Epidemic Update* December 2001: 17).

As regards women's power over their sexuality, the identity of their sexual partners, the frequency of sexual intercourse and the use of condoms, the most that can be said is that this is an area where there is dire and urgent need for more research. Too little is known about the culture of African sexual practices and the curbs on sexual behaviour that would be conducive to the prevention of AIDS. This is a highly sensitive area where concerns about political correctness often obfuscate reliable and relevant knowledge. One often hears about the natural resistance to condoms in many African communities, but I am not aware of solid research that has been done about this. It is claimed that improved education had a significant impact on the situation in Uganda, also as regards condom use. For example, UNAIDS report that 'in the Masindi and Palissa districts ... condom use with casual partners in 1997–2000 rose from 42 percent and 31 percent, respectively, to 51 percent and 53 percent. In the capital, Kampala, almost 98 percent of sex workers surveyed in 2000 said they had used a condom the last time they had sex' (*UNAIDS AIDS Epidemic Update* December 2001: 17).

It remains a question how reliable these findings are or could be. The problem, however, is not only the frequency of condom use. The more problematic issue is the status of women, their knowledge of HIV and its dangers, particularly to themselves, and their power to determine and structure their own sexual contacts. This issue cannot be divorced from their general status and empowerment in society. Everything possible, therefore, has to be done to enhance that status and power.

What can we do about these problems? They are complex, because both social roles and perceptions are deeply ingrained in the psyche of members of underdeveloped communities. South Africa has made impressive efforts to legislate in favour of more gender equality; e.g. one third of all members of parliament in the country must be women. But this has little effect on the situation in the rural areas. Gender equality is an ideal that has been attained almost nowhere in the world. We have to speed it up – everywhere.

The situation surrounding AIDS in Africa is one of many examples of the way in which women's health is threatened by inadequate social status. How to address the problem of stigmatisation[11] remains unclear. Education remains a paramount need. In addition, I would stress the importance of role models going public about their HIV status – a move that has been suggested for politicians in SA, but has met with very little success. It has to be attempted on a wider scale; the crisis warrants even this possible intrusion of privacy, although such action must remain voluntary.

Lastly, one cannot but ask whether the almost inordinate emphasis that has been placed on the right to privacy in the management of AIDS, has not, even if inadvertently, contributed to the increased stigmatisation of the disease in society. The more HIV/AIDS patients see and hear AIDS activists and advocates insisting on the patient's paramount right to privacy and to his/her sole decision-making power about disclosure of status, the more the idea grows that, because AIDS is seemingly such a 'big deal', it must be a terrible shame to have the condition. Hence stigmatisation is reinforced in a vicious circle of rights-talk, privacy hang-ups, increased shame and persistent stigmatisation.

What should instead be encouraged is the perception that AIDS, although a very serious and potentially fatal disease, is nevertheless a disease like all others, something that is manageable and with which a person can live responsibly for an indefinite period of time, akin to the experience of so many patients who have cancer and live with it for many years. Only when this perception becomes general in society, will stigma disappear, management of the disease improve and surveillance and statistics about the disease become truly reliable.

HIV/AIDS and the disenchantment of intimacy

The last problem I wish to address has to do with the fact that AIDS is intimately linked with sex, and that this link constitutes a perplexing complexity when trying to manage the epidemic in conditions of social and economic deprivation.

In South Africa, the majority of the population leads a brutalised existence because of continuous and unrelieved poverty. In such circumstances, authority and order are often restored by appeals to the law of the jungle. This scheme, where everyone vies for him- or herself and the physically strongest often prevails, reinforces the vulnerability of women. Crime flourishes, and crime breeds increased dependence on kinship and patronage relations. Violence prevails, and a sense of civil responsibility disappears. Planning and perspective become extremely short term, and a disposition is fostered in which little more is of importance than the pleasure and profit of the present moment. A sense of hope and futurity, as the outcome of rational and responsible planning in the present, tends to evaporate.[12]

In such circumstances, sex remains one of the few avenues of intimacy and an accompanying sense of self-worth or dignity. In the sexual bond, a residue of personal warmth, care and privacy is kindled. Sex, as is persuasively argued by both Robert Nozick (1989: 61–67) and Igor Primoratz (1999: 34–40), can be a mode of communication. 'Sex also is . . . a way of saying or of showing something more tellingly than our words can say' writes Nozick (1989: 63). Moreover, sex is not only about pleasure, as the hedonist would argue. It's also about engaging other people in the sphere of intimacy, thus communicating in a special way. If pleasure were the only purpose of sex, argues Robert Solomon, ' . . . it would seem that our sexual paradigm ought to be masturbation, and sexual release with other people [then only becomes] an unnecessary complication' (Solomon 1994: 276). Writes Primoratz:

> These crucial traits of sex among human beings – its great importance in human life, and the fact that it is something humans do or experience with others – are best explained when sex is seen as a type of body language: a language in which we communicate to others our feelings and attitudes about them, and about ourselves too (Primoratz 1999: 36).

If all of this is true, the trauma of the AIDS epidemic within the culture of the poor is better understood. Sex remains an outlet, a dimension of privacy and intimacy, an opportunity of special communication (particularly for those whose powers of communication with others have been incurably depressed by sustained lack of opportunity) for the poor and the destitute – a recourse that the deprivation and brutalisation of their everyday lives might seem not be able to take away from them.

Once AIDS appeared, disaster not only lurked in the sphere of the public, where one in this condition is almost predisposed to expect it, but in the only remaining sphere where one might have hoped to retain some measure of control and dignity: the private and the intimate. Lee Grove shows how sex and death now, in fact, become identified:

> 'To die', 'to have sex' – that coupling has always been figurative, metaphorical, sophisticated wordplay, a literary conceit, out of those outrageous paradoxes dear to the heart of a racy divine like John Donne. Outrageous no longer. The coupling isn't figurative anymore. It's literal.

(Grove, quoted in Edelman 1989: 301).

HIV/AIDS carries forward the brutalisation of the everyday lives of the destitute in Africa into the sphere of the private. The result is the eventual brutalisation of intimacy itself. Now sex becomes the topic of a depersonalised, mechanised, instrumentalist discourse. Condoms – a kind of technology hardly reconcilable with African sexual practices – become the avenue to security. Control over the management of privacy is increasingly lost; it is sometimes even experienced by the victims as the loss of the right to privacy.

We ought to rethink, very carefully, the purpose and wisdom of all the taboos of public discourse.

Again, as in the case of most true complexities, it is almost fundamentally unclear what could be done about this problem. I'll stick to one remark. Many of us believe, and mostly for good reasons, that human sexuality represents the truly profound, some will even say sacred, dimension of human existence, and that the discourse on human sexuality therefore deserves some protection from the banalities of the public sphere. The AIDS epidemic in Africa, however, where sex often is even more of a taboo in public discourse than elsewhere in the world (Mabanga 2000), shows the limitations of such a view in a situation where a sexually transmitted disease attains pandemic proportions. Too much of a taboo mentality towards sex for the sake of, for example, protecting children from premature exposure to the risks and perils of adulthood, which results in an accompanying taboo on the public dispensing of fixtures such as condoms, can and does backfire when a sexually transmitted epidemic strikes. We ought to rethink, very carefully, the purpose and wisdom of all the taboos of public discourse. However useful in some contexts, they can become an obstacle that attains life-threatening proportions.

Conclusions

This chapter set out to identify and critically discuss significant complexities facing any effort to manage and curb the rampant AIDS pandemic in Africa. To stimulate a sense of the complexities involved is not to create a sense of hopelessness. As is argued above, many things can be done, and have indeed been done, to successfully curb or even halt the epidemic's current apparently unbridled spread.

A recent publication by the World Bank lists, to my mind prudently, initiatives that experience has proved work, and those that do not work. According to the publication, the following programmes have proven significant positive effects:

- Changing behaviour to reduce risks through communication, including mass media, peer education, theatre and counselling, especially among youth.
- Making STI diagnosis and treatment readily available and affordable.
- Treating opportunistic infections, including tuberculosis.
- Making condoms affordable and widely accessible.
- Ensuring a safe blood supply.
- Making voluntary counselling and testing (VCT) available and affordable.
- Preventing transmission from mother to child.
  (*Intensifying Action against HIV/AIDS in Africa* 2000: 20–21)

What does not work? According to the same publication, many years of experience have shown that the following strategies do not work and that some can actually be damaging to programme efforts:

- Expecting health-oriented national AIDS committees to lead an intensified response to the epidemic in the absence of adequate, sustained and high-level government support.
- Inadequately targeting interventions to small sections of populations at increased risk of both HIV infection and transmission.
- Withholding knowledge from young people that would protect them from infection, under the guise of 'cultural and social norms'.
- Targeting the vulnerable, especially women and young girls, without addressing the root causes of their vulnerability.
- Stigmatising and marginalising those infected and affected by this epidemic.
- Investing in expensive pilot studies that have no chance of being sustained, replicated, or expanded.
- Building plans and programmes that are externally driven, based on available funding or donor interest rather than well-coordinated programmes based on need and proven strategies.
- Designing programmes without community involvement.
  (*Intensifying Action against HIV/AIDS in Africa* 2000: 21)

Whatever might be said or found to be the best available strategies, the complexities discussed in this chapter must be considered. Otherwise the effort of reaching the heart of Africa in its current predicament is bound to fail.

The phenomenon of HIV/AIDS has, probably more than anything else, proved our vulnerability to disaster, in spite of the unprecedented advances in medical science at the beginning of the 21st century. Joseph Wayne Smith even writes of a 'crisis of civilisation' in this regard - an expression that, to my mind, is too alarmist. But we might well bear in mind Smith's reminder of:

> ... a fundamental truth that has been lost to the mind of modern Western techno-industrial society, but was well known and accepted by ancient civilisations - human beings, despite intelligence and culture are still biological organisms in an environment which by no means requires human beings to exist, and does not guarantee the eternal existence of the human race (Smith 1991: 5).

We as humans, despite our ability to transplant hearts and kidneys, to cure many forms of cancer, and even to map the human genome, are currently confronted by a disease that can only be controlled at massive cost, and that has turned out to be a mass-killer for those without the resources required to keep its effects at bay. One question, amongst others, is: if AIDS can appear and destroy at the rate at which it is currently occurring in sub-Saharan Africa, what other dangers are lurking in the future? The achievements of medicine and medical technologies over the past century are unprecedented and rightly infuse a sense of security and optimism for the future. However, we are well advised not to over-estimate ourselves and our achievements in this regard.

HIV/AIDS is a disconcerting fact of our time, place and situation in the world. It is hoped that this chapter has conveyed something of the way in which disease is a function of our total human condition – biomedical, yet also social, political and behavioural. Above all, HIV/AIDS has demonstrated not only our vulnerability, but also the limits to our powers. Even though the disease may one day be conquered entirely, its message, in an age of unprecedented medical power and technological prowess, remains for all times singularly appropriate: we are human, and our humanity is a function of the dialectic between limited insight and as yet inconceivable opportunity and creativity. Let us seek to overcome, bolstered by the confidence of the numerous successes of the past. And yet, let us not forget or forsake humility, for we are not gods and our power to master and to heal can easily become a self-destructive force. Only in this ambiguity between our might and our limits can we pursue the adventure of human living.[13]

Endnotes

[1] Tuchman (1979, pp. 92–125) remains one of the most interesting and comprehensive narratives of this event. See also Jay 2000.

[2] Figures on HIV/AIDS in South Africa are largely based on surveys made at antenatal clinics. These findings are annually reported in the Dept. of Health's *National HIV and Syphilis Sero-Prevalence Survey of Women Attending Public Antenatal Clinics in South Africa* (references in this article indicated as *SA Dept. of Health*). The latest of these reports was released on 20th March 2001. According to this report 80 percent of pregnant women, of whom 85.2 percent are African, attended antenatal clinics provided by the Public Health Sector in South Africa. About sixteen and a half thousand women who visited these clinics in the previous year were tested for the first time at the 400 clinics that operate in all nine provinces of South Africa. The report further shows that about 24.5 percent of the women were found to be HIV positive by the end of 2000. These figures were 22.4 percent at the end of 1999, and 22.8 percent at the end of 1998. The rate of increase of these infections has therefore been curbed in comparison with the situation over eight years preceding 1998. For example, in 1992, the percentage of infected women at these clinics was 2.2 percent. In 1996 it was 14.2 percent, in 1997 17 percent and in 1998, as indicated, 22.8 percent. (This last jump represented a 33.8 percent rate of increase in the prevalence of HIV infection since the previous year.) Of particular concern was also the increase in the rate amongst 15–19-year-old girls from 12.7 percent in 1997 to 21.0 percent in 1998. According to a report in *The Cape Times* of 21st March 2001, South Africa's Minister of Health, Dr. Manto Tshabalala Msimang, was quite pleased with the lower escalation rate of infection over the past three years, in comparison to what happened before. She is even quoted as saying: 'We're on top of issues. We're getting there'! When one takes account of the magnitude of the problem in South Africa and the

rest of Southern Africa, as is argued in the rest of this chapter and in all other reliable literature, such a statement gives ample proof of the extent to which the current South African government has lost track of reality.

[3] In this connection, Virginia van der Vliet writes of the 'ecology' of a disease (Van der Vliet 1996: 77–116 and Van der Vliet, undated). She quotes Guenter Risse's definition of this concept: 'the dynamic relationship between the biosocial environment and humans' (1996: 78). Epidemics need to find the correct niche in which to flourish. The ecology of AIDS refers to the 'interaction between social, biomedical, environmental and behavioral conditions which allow for the rapid transmission of HIV' (Van der Vliet, 1999, p. 1).

[4] 'Poor' in this context refers to an *annual* income of below ZAR10 000 (US$ 1538) per household of 4.5 people.

[5] This was disclosed to me by a colleague in the Dept. of Economics at Stellenbsoch University, South Africa.

[6] About the problem of the alleged unreliability of data on the AIDS pandemic, see Chapter 2 of this volume.

[7] For a comprehensive discussion of the way the TAC has handled their protest against the South African government's hesitance to address the AIDS problem, see Friedman & Mottiar 2005.

[8] For a comprehensive discussion of the recent cuts in the prices of antiretroviral drugs in South Africa, see Nattrass's discussion and figures in Chapter 3 of this volume.

[9] For a persuasive argument in this regard, cf. Resnik 2001.

[10] For an extended discussion of this issue, cf. Van der Vliet, 1996, pp. 52–76.

[11] In a recent Masters dissertation for the M.Phil (Bioethics) degree at the University of Cape Town, Paul Roux argues persuasively for the thesis 'that the process of informed consent, although appropriate in Africa as an exercise in the recognition of autonomy, when applied in the case of African women may have the unexpected and deleterious effect of isolating her from a traditional support base and enhance the likelihood of non-disclosure of HIV status, and should therefore be adapted to meet the needs of this special situation' (Roux, 2001, p. 10). This 'adaptation', according to the author, mainly entails involving the family much more in the process of obtaining consent. Roux argues that his research has shown that this approach greatly contributes to a lesser risk of stigmatisation.

[12] For a compelling, though disconcerting account of the excesses that violent crime have attained in South Africa, see Venter 2001: 31–116.

[13] I wish to thank Loretta M Kopelman for her valuable comments on earlier drafts of this article.

References

Benatar, S.R. (2001). *Global Issues in HIV Research* (Unpublished Paper), 1–9.

Benatar, S.R. (2005). The lost potential of our health system. *The Cape Times*, 14th January 2005, 9.

Bot, M., Wilson, D. & Dove, S. (2000). *The Education Atlas of South Africa*. Johannesburg: Education Foundation.

Cilliers, F.P. (1998). *Complexity and Postmodernism. Understanding complex systems.* London: Routledge.

Codrington, G. (1999). *12 Sentences that define Generation X.* Edenglen: The Edge Consulting.

Coetzee, E. (2001). Impak van VIGS blyk uit inkomste per kop. *Die Burger*, 23rd March 2001, S2.

Cullinan, K. (2001). The AIDS Orphans that Slip through the Red Tape. *The Sunday Times*, 18th March 2001.

Duesberg, P. & Rasnick, D. (1997). The drug-AIDS Hypothesis. *Continuum*, 4(5).

Edelman, L. (1989). The Plague of Discourse: Politics, Literary Theory and AIDS. *The South Atlantic Quarterly*, 88 (1), 301–317.

Friedman, S. & Mottiar, S. (2005). *A Moral to the Tale: the Treatment Action Campaign and the Politics of HIV/AIDS.* Durban: Centre for Civil Society Research Report no. 27.

Intensifying Action against HIV/AIDS in Africa: Responding to a Development Crisis. (2000). Washington D.C.: The World Bank, Africa Region.

Jay, P. (2000). A distant mirror: Europe's Black Death is a history lesson in human tragedy - and economic renewal. *Time*, 17th July 2000: 38.

Johnson, P. (1983). *A History of the Modern World.* London: Weidenfeld and Nicholson.

Mabanga, T. (2000). The fear that keeps the families silent. *Mail & Guardian*. 1st–7th December 2000: 9.

Macfarlane, D. (2000). Almost half of SA is illiterate. *Mail & Guardian*, 1st–7th December 2000: 18.

Makgoba, M.W. (Ed.) (1999). *African Renaissance: The New Struggle.* Cape Town: Mafube & Tafelberg.

Mbeki, T. (1998). *Africa: The Time has Come: Selected Speeches.* Cape Town: Tafelberg & Mafube.

McGeary, J. (2001). Death Stalks a Continent. *Time*, 12th February 2001.

National HIV and Syphilis Survey of Women attending Public Antenatal Clinics in South Africa (Abbreviated to *SA Dept. of Health*). 2001. Pretoria: SA Department of Health.

Norton, R., Schwartzbaum, J., & Wheat, J. (1990). Language Discrimination of General Physicians: AIDS Metaphors used in the AIDS Crisis. *Communication Research*, 17 (6), 809–826.

Nozick, R. (1989). *The Examined Life: Philosophical Meditations.* New York: Simon & Schuster.

Primoratz, I. (1999). *Ethics and Sex.* London & New York: Routledge.

Pretorius, W. 'SA lewensverwagting val tot 45 j. weens Vigs', *Die Burger*, 24th November 1999.

Resnik, D. (2001). Developing drugs for the developing world: an economic, legal, moral and political dilemma. *Developing World Bioethics*, 1, 11–32.

Roux, P. (2001). *Informed Consent for Voluntary Counselling and Testing for HIV Infection in South African Mothers and Children: An Assessment of Burdens and Consequences and an Argument for a Modification in the Process of Informed Consent.* Unpublished M.Phil. (Bioethics) Dissertation, University of Cape Town.

Schindler, J. & Bot, M. (1999). Literacy in South Africa - An Update. *EduSource Data News*, 24th March 1999, 1–3.

Smith, J.W. *AIDS, Philosophy and Beyond.* Aldershot: Avebury.

South African Health Review (1999). Durban: Health Systems Trust.

Steyn, P. (2001). VSA-Firma sal nie patente afdwing in Suid-Afrika. *Die Burger*, 16th March 2001.

Swanepoel, T. (2001). Regop graf toe? *Die Burger*, 15th March 2001.

Tuchman, B.W. (1978). *A Distant Mirror.* Harmondsworth: Penguin Books.

Van der Vliet, V. (1996). *The Politics of AIDS.* London: Bowerdean Publishing Company.

Van der Vliet, V. (1998). *Aids: the economic and social implications for South Africa.* (Unpublished Paper), 13–14.

Van der Vliet, V. (1999). The ecology of South Africa's AIDS epidemic. *Pulse Track*, 15th July 1999, pp. 1–5.

Venter, L. (2001). *In the Shadow of the Rainbow.* Johannsburg: Heinemann Publishers.

Watney, S. (1989). Missionary Positions: AIDS, 'Africa' and Race. *Critical Quarterly*, 31 (3), 46–62.

Chapter 5

The HIV/AIDS pandemic: a sign of instability in a complex global system

The first world has a great deal to answer for. In this chapter **Solomon Benatar**[1] *argues that for the sake of world stability and common decency, more affluent countries should realign their development aid priorities and help Africans create a better quality of life by responding to poverty, hunger and disease on the continent.*

In the previous chapter, Anton A van Niekerk justifiably focuses on those issues that can and should be addressed in resource-poor countries faced with the devastation of the HIV/AIDS pandemic. He argues that diverting attention away from what can be done in the short-term by addressing longer-term solutions to complex system effects is potentially disempowering. His approach, appropriately, encourages severely afflicted communities to do whatever they can to ameliorate the effects of this plague, and overcome the paralysis that may follow a sense of hopelessness associated with a victim image.

I wish to offer a perspective that complements and extends this approach by acknowledging the need to begin to reverse the disempowering effects of the exploitation, discrimination and imperialism that characterise the current world system (Gilbert 1992, Hosle 1992, Lee & Zwi 1996, Alexander 1996, Katz 2003). Drawing the attention of scholars to the complex deeper issues that must be faced when considering the implications of HIV/AIDS in an unstable world could also be coupled to discrediting, through shaming, those nations that believe that their military and economic strength imbues them with incontestable power. While their confidence may be justified in terms of destructive and coercive military and economic power, they cannot justifiably claim to be morally superior when their interests in continuous economic growth and wasteful lifestyles take precedence over the basic living needs of billions of 'others' (Dower 1991, O'Neill 1992, Aitken & La Follette 1996, Unger 1996, Pogge 2002).

In an era in which the emergence of severe infectious diseases, the development of biological weapons and the potential for subversive use of genetic and information technology may render military might less influential, new concepts of power and security are required to ensure secure lives for all (Falk 1999, 2000, Benatar 2003). The suggestion that HIV/AIDS is one of several signs of instability in a complex world system at a crucial time in history should not be dismissed lightly (Garrett 1995, Benatar 2001). Working for greater global solidarity holds the key to the future health and security of the majority of the world's people.

Globalisation and the legacy of the 20th century

Globalisation is a popular term used to refer to a complex and ambiguous concept with social and ecological manifestations that reflect a long, interwoven economic and political history in which peoples, economies, cultures and political processes have been subject to international influences. The pace of globalisation has escalated during the past 40 years under the influence of advances in information and transport technology, decreasing barriers and homogenisation of activities, and through the imposition of a set of neo-liberal ideas seemingly closely associated with the propagation of democracy and human rights. However, in reality over-emphasis on the market has somewhat eclipsed considerations of democracy and social justice (Barnet & Cavanagh 1994, Amin 1997, Teeple 2000, Gray 1998, Gill 1990, Falk 1999 & 2000, Ralph 2001, Ellwood 2003).

Negative effects of globalisation include widening economic disparities between rich and poor . . . and increases in both absolute and relative poverty.

Exploitation, a long-standing feature of human life, is thus covert because globalisation is only superficially linked to democracy and human rights. Much has been achieved to promote human rights since the promulgation of the Universal Declaration of Human Rights in 1948, and many agree that there is no plausible alternative to democracy (Dunne 1992). However, it is becoming clear that neither the flourishing of modern democracy – even in developed nations (Ralph 2001) – nor sincere propagation of a coherent human rights agenda are features of a world in which economic globalisation is pervasively imposing a set of ideas and beliefs that favour market transactions above all other values (Falk 2000, Royal Danish Foreign Ministry 2000, Heywood and Altman 2001).

Positive and widely appreciated manifestations of progress associated with globalisation include advances in science and technology; increased life expectancy; enhanced economic growth; greater freedom and prosperity for many; improvements in the speed and cost of communications and transport; and popularisation of the concept of human rights. About 20 percent of the world's population has benefited maximally from such progress. The positive impact of globalising forces in South Africa has been to promote the demise of apartheid.

Negative effects of globalisation include widening economic disparities between rich and poor (within and between nations) and increases in both absolute and relative poverty. At the beginning of the 20th century, the wealthiest 20 percent of the world's population were nine times richer than the poorest 20 percent. This ratio grew slowly to 30 times by 1960, and more rapidly to

60 times by 1990 and to over 74 times by 1997. World debt grew from $0.5 trillion in 1980 to $1.9 trillion in 1994 and $2.2 trillion in 1997.

The 'debt trade' (and the way in which this has been created and its relationship to the arms trade), a major factor in perpetuating and intensifying poverty and ill health (Sivard 1996), has been described as the modern equivalent of slavery (Pettifor 1996). Most countries that were required by the World Bank to pursue structural adjustment programmes are in greater debt than ever before. Third world debt, although accounting for a small proportion of total world debt, has reached obscene levels in relation to income levels in the third world, and is indeed unpayable (Pettifor 1996, Pettifor 2003). These adverse effects are felt most severely by 80 percent of the world's population.

The development of a complex web of material, institutional and ideological forces and powerful massive multinational corporations in a globalising world has profound implications for the accumulation of capital and for the way in which resources are controlled. In 1970, 70 percent of all money that exchanged hands on a daily basis was payment for work, while speculative financial transactions accounted for 30 percent. By 1998, massive growth in speculative exchanges to $1,500 billion daily (Ellwood 2003) had changed these proportions to five percent and 95 percent respectively. Such striking shifts in the distribution of money arguably reflects devaluation of the lives and labour of most people in the world, and have particularly serious implications in Africa where unemployment rates are extraordinarily high.

The influence of a shift in the locus of economic power from the nation state to global corporations alters the balance of power in the world. Boundaries between states, and between foreign and domestic policies become blurred, in the process undermining small states' control over their own economies, and threatening their ability to provide for their citizens. Economic disparities have become so marked and their adverse effects so apparent that a very significant degree of incompatibility has arisen between neo-liberal economic policies and the goals of democracy (Gill 1990, Brecher 2000, Ralph 2001).[2]

In addition to progressive widening of the economic divide between nations, and growing external control over the economies of small countries through the 'debt trade' and markets that are increasingly global, other powerful forces are generating new patterns of inclusion and exclusion. Evidence is accumulating that, associated with globalisation, there has developed a large (but little discussed) illicit global economy comprising an uncontrolled arms trade, money laundering, an illicit drugs trade (now an industry worth over $500 billion annually), massive migration and smuggling of people, trafficking in endangered species, toxic waste dumping, prostitution, sexual exploitation and child labour (Friman & Andreas 1999, Bales 1999).

The latter half of the 20th century has been characterised by more striking changes than ever before (Hobsbawm 1994). The world's population has doubled from three billion to six billion. Economic disparities have widened dramatically with billions of people now living under dehumanising conditions of poverty and squalor. New patterns of war and ethnic conflict have resulted in displacement and migration of millions of people. Changing spatial dimensions of human relations resulting from war, migration, travel and new forms of communication have radically disrupted the social lives of many. Widespread ecological damage is resulting from escalating consumption of the earth's resources far out of proportion to population growth (McMichael 1993).

It is against this background of rapid and profound change, contributing to the creation of new ecological niches and to the adaptive evolution of microbes with resistance to many antimicrobial drugs, that dozens of new infectious diseases have emerged since 1973 to afflict humankind. These include Legionnaires' disease, Lyme disease, various forms of encephalitis, bovine spongiform encephalopathy, Hantaan virus disease, Ebola fever and other haemorrhagic diseases, new forms of E. coli and Vibrio cholerae, HIV/AIDS and most recently SARS. In addition, many other infectious diseases that had become localised, limited or controlled have broken out again with serious adverse implications for all. Examples are tuberculosis, malaria and measles (Garrett 1995, World Health Organisation 1996).

Contemplating the third world

Rather than taking the 'third world' for granted and ignoring its plight, Vitorio Hosle, a German philosopher, has examined the concept of the 'third world' through its historical origins, and its presumed hierarchical relation to, and aim towards, approximating the 'first world'. He criticises the failure to examine the increasing gaps between it and the first world, and argues that unless we address elementary ideas of justice in relation to the third world, the ecological crisis and the accumulation of weapons of mass destruction, all other questions regarding our moral behaviour will become obsolete. In writing eloquently about 'the third world as a philosophical problem', he has explicated how appalling conditions of life in many countries are intimately linked to powerful historical forces and to ongoing discriminatory attitudes, and he has made a cogent case for efforts to ameliorate third world problems (Hosle 1992).

Hosle's ideas are enhanced by Anthony Richmond's description of the pervasive effects of racism (Richmond 1994); Titus Alexander's analysis of how similar forces to those that have marginalised and oppressed blacks under apartheid South Africa are operative at a global level, revealing the pervasive discrimination against vast numbers of people, most especially those of colour (Alexander 1996); and Thomas Pogge's moral analysis of world poverty and human rights (Pogge 2002).

Sub-Saharan Africa (home to about ten percent of the world's population) has been most severely affected by the temporal relationship of the abovementioned powerful social forces to its economic and political development (Davidson 1992, Ungar 1992, Michaels 1992/3, Logie & Benatar 1997, Sandbrook

2000, Lancaster 1999, Schwab 2001). It is also the poorest area (consuming less than one percent of the world's economy), and the most severely affected by the HIV/AIDS pandemic (bearing over 70 percent of the global burden of HIV/AIDS). The desperate condition of Africa, a continent desired, exploited and eventually discarded, has been reviewed (in the medical literature) from differing but complementary perspectives (Elmore-Meegan & O'Riordan 1993, Benatar 1994). HIV/AIDS has refocused attention on Africa but action has been limited (Stillwagon 2001).

The tragedy of Africa has been aggravated in recent decades by its elimination from the foreign policy agendas of powerful countries.

Africa has long been central to the aspirations of industrialised nations. Initially presenting a challenge to circumnavigation, it became a sub-continent inviting exploration and adventure resulting in a clash of civilisations, colonisation, brutal enslavement of its people and relentless extraction of its rich resources. After initiation of the process of independence in Africa in the 1960s, powerful nations pursuing their ongoing interests colluded with selfish African leaders who were co-opted into neo-liberal economic policies and corrupt practices. Economic slavery propagated through covert and sophisticated guises replaced physical slavery and colonial oppression, and will in due course be recognised as such (Pettifor 1996).

The tragedy of Africa has been aggravated in recent decades by its elimination from the foreign policy agendas of powerful countries, passivity towards genocide, and tardy and inadequate responses to HIV and AIDS. The withdrawal of industrialised nations from even attempting to deal with the dire condition of the African continent is reflected in the writings of political scientists. 'The crisis is so diffuse and of such magnitude that the United States and the world at large shrink from engaging with it ... In fact, history mocks the very idea of an international coalition to save Africa' (Michaels 1992/3). Economic analysts noted that after the Cold War ended, Africa lost whatever political lustre it might once have had. The Association of Concerned Africa Scholars continues to work towards restoring Africa to an appropriate status within US foreign affairs (ACAS 2000).

The recently announced World Health Organisation's programme to provide antiretroviral treatment for three million people by 2005 (WHO 2004), together with President Bush's emergency plan for AIDS relief (PEPFAR) and other philanthropic endeavours, offer a glimmer of hope that required action will be taken.

Africans must clearly take some responsibility for the state of their continent since post-colonial independence. Poor governance, corruption, internal exploitation, nepotism, tribalism, authoritarianism, military rule and overpopulation through patriarchal attitudes and disempowerment of women have all contributed to its sad state. However, to be fair, these shortcomings must be seen in the context of powerful external disruptive forces acting over several centuries to impede progress in Africa (Davidson 1992, Unger 1992, Lancaster 1999,

Sandbrook 2000, Schwab 2001). The call for more responsible government and other activities embraced within the New Economic Plan for African Development (NEPAD 2001) offers additional hope that the depredations of African government to date could be reversed.

The role of the World Bank, the IMF and the G8 countries in global health

Over the last 20 years, the World Bank and the IMF have held the balance of power in formulating global health policy (Pauly 1997). They have encouraged liberalisation of economies, cut subsidies from basic foods and shifted agricultural policy to promote exporting crops to the detriment of home-grown food production, all of which has resulted in devastating malnutrition and starvation that have caused billions to suffer, especially in Africa (Lurie, Hintzen and Lowe 1995, Amin 1997, UNDP 1999, Lancaster 1999, Wade 2001).

It is an indictment of the IMF and World Bank's structural adjustment programmes that they required governments to reduce expenditure on health care, education and other social services and encouraged privatisation, even within health care (Ellwood 2003). Availability of condoms, STD treatments, anti-tuberculosis therapy and treatments for co-infections of HIV are subject to user-charges introduced and still encouraged by the World Bank in many African countries. The whole Public Health Agenda (information surveillance, epidemiology, research and behavioural surveillance) has thus been radically curtailed. Structural adjustment programmes, debt repayments, cuts in foreign aid budgets (especially by the US), discrimination against African trade, increasing malnutrition and the cold-war activities of the great powers have all played a significant part in fanning the AIDS pandemic. Illness and death from AIDS in families result in loss of breadwinners, substantial funeral and mourning costs and the removal of children from school to increase household income (Abbasi 1999, Nandy, Scott, Logie & Benatar 2000). In recent years, hope has diminished that an enlightened approach by the G8 countries (that dominate decision-making at the IMF and World Bank) would facilitate recovery from debt and poverty (Labonte et al. 2004).

Regrettably even the World Health Organisation, which promotes public health, has not adequately acknowledged or discussed these adverse forces (Navarro 2004). The somewhat naïve surprise that, despite considerable global attention to HIV/AIDS, so little has been achieved in slowing the pace of the pandemic in sub-Saharan Africa, reflects denial and neglect of the effects of profound social forces and human behaviour on the environment and how these have contributed to the emergence and spread of new plagues. Failure to recognise the pervasive social, economic, behavioural and political aspects of HIV/AIDS, both in terms of its origins and its control, is self-defeating. The complexity of the scientific endeavour required to understand the pathobiology of the disease, and to develop appropriate treatment and vaccines, is more than matched by the complexity of understanding and dealing with the social underpinnings of HIV/AIDS and other plagues locally and globally (Garrett 1995, Lee & Zwi 1996, McNeill 1998, Benatar 2001).

HIV/AIDS cannot be dealt with adequately unless efforts are made to ameliorate these underlying conditions progressively. Recognition of the adverse effects of overt racial apartheid in South Africa, while failing to recognise the adverse effects of covert economic apartheid at a global level, regrettably reflects a form of 'selective moral blindness'. Moreover, it is not necessary to go beyond considerations of the rational long-term interest of the world's privileged people to appreciate this (Hosle 1992).

It is also predictable that unless the conditions that promote the emergence of new infectious diseases are addressed, other new diseases will in all probability emerge in the future with potentially devastating effects worldwide (Garrett 1995, Benatar 2001). Appreciation of this prospect has led former US President Bill Clinton to declare HIV/AIDS a security threat to the industrialised world. In 1999, the Commonwealth Heads of Government Meeting declared HIV/AIDS a global emergency. The importance of this insight lies in understanding that more is needed than the mere development of 'drugs as weapons' to combat the pandemic. Acknowledgement of and attention to both the immediate and ultimate causes of plagues are essential (Garrett 1995, McNeil 1998, Katz 2002).

An expanded concept of bioethics and its relevance to HIV/AIDS

Most of the debate about medical ethics generally, and about HIV/AIDS specifically, has focused on ethical issues at the *micro level* of the doctor/patient relationship – most especially confidentiality, informed decision-making, individual human rights and the harm/benefit balances for individuals involved in clinical research. At this level, basic human needs can be identified as respect for human dignity, and self-determination of individuals conceived of as rational and autonomous. In this context, the physician is viewed as committed to the care of each individual patient within various models of the doctor/patient relationship embracing the concepts of contract, respect for autonomy, covenant and trust in beneficence.

At the *meso level* of ethical considerations, human needs extend towards such considerations as order and justice within the communities in which individuals are socially embedded and 'constructed' (Doyal & Gough 1991, Taylor 1992). The responsibility of physicians here is viewed more broadly and includes concern for equitable access to health care, public health and the common good. Considerations of justice, the 'social contract' and utilitarian considerations necessarily impact on the physician/patient relationship. Morality here requires an institutional component embracing attention to public health and the management of resources. Interpersonal relationships are broadened to encompass the concept of civic citizenship with primary responsibilities complementing the primary rights of individuals and the correlative duties of others in order to achieve rights in practice.

The justified focus on ethical issues at the micro level that have profound implications for individuals, and especially those at risk of stigmatisation, has somewhat eclipsed ethical issues that need to be addressed in dealing with threats to public health. However, the era of genetic medicine and lessons learnt from the HIV pandemic are prompting recognition that some information about individuals cannot belong exclusively to individuals. The web of relationships and responsibility extends to family members for whom knowledge of familial genetics or transmissible disease may be crucial to their future well-being. It is also becoming apparent that research on HIV/AIDS requires consideration of the ethics of relationships between communities, trial sponsors, industry, ministries of health and between the private and public sectors in the process of protecting and promoting public and population health.

Lack of attention to civic responsibilities allows individuals and powerful groups to place their own needs above those of all others.

Such considerations raise the perennial problem of how to strike a balance between the rights and needs of individuals and the common good of societies. While the focus on individual rights is vital and necessary for the well-being of individual persons and has a high social utility value, such focus is not sufficient for the achievement of improved public health. Scholarly debates on public health ethics are inadequately developed and require greater attention (Beauchamp 1999, Buchanan 2001). Eloquent arguments have been offered in favour of a language of public health that 'speaks to the reciprocity and interdependence which characterise community' (Robertson 1998).

There is also a need to go beyond advocacy for rights to include consideration of the duties necessary for rights to be widely satisfied. Lack of attention to civic responsibilities allows individuals and powerful groups to place their own needs above those of all others – and thwarts the achievement of such goals as universal access to health care (Benatar 1996), and curbing the spread of infectious diseases.

Achieving an improved balance between the needs and rights of individuals and the requirements for advancing public health will require a shift in mindset away from exclusive and often selfish individualism towards respect for individuality that is combined with a strong sense of community and civic citizenship. Essential steps will include:

- acknowledging the need for a new balance (Jennings 1987, Margalit 1998);
- involvement of the community to be researched in the design and acceptance of such public health endeavours as vaccine trials (reducing stigmatisation and promoting admiration of those who are willing to participate);

- dealing with conflicts of interest between communities and trial sponsors; and
- seeking longer-term economic and social justice when balancing the harms and benefits of vaccine research.

Clearly public debate and education needs to proceed simultaneously with processes that ensure accountability and protection of individuals (Benatar 2000). Recent articles on public health ethics (Thompson 2003), new approaches to public health (Beaglehole et al. 2004) and responses to the crisis of global human resources for health (Narasimhan 2004), illustrate imaginative ways of thinking required to deal with public and population health issues.

In the same way that embarking on vaccine research in developing countries will require going beyond micro-ethical considerations to include the meso level of ethics mentioned above, so dealing with global pandemics requires ethical considerations at the *macro level* – that is, at the level of the global economy and of the relationships between nations that have profound effects on human health and well-being (O'Neill 1992, Benatar 2003).

The importance of physical and moral interdependence is so great that self-interest alone should be sufficient to drive policies toward sustainable development.

At the macro level, human need extends to encompass security and a safe environment. The desired conception of the individual becomes that of an autonomous person sharing equal rights with all other citizens in the world, in a relationship of interdependence in which the rights of some should not be acquired at the expense of the rights of even distant others. The level of complexity here is much greater because of the ways in which the foreign policies of some countries may covertly enhance the lives of their own citizens through exploitation of unseen persons elsewhere. The role of physicians, scientists and all health care professionals needs to be broadened further to include commitment to global professional ideals, to the continuing advancement of knowledge and to concern for the health of populations globally, as well as the health of future generations (Rotblat 1997, Alberts 2000). The moral perspective is thus extended from 'interpersonal morality to civic morality and to an ethics of international relations that has dimensions intimately linked to political, military, cultural and economic issues (O'Neill 1992, Elfstrom 1997, 1998, Benatar 1998, Paul & Hall 1999, Dunne and Wheeler 1999, Pogge 2002).

Why should we bother to go beyond the micro level of ethics? Modern communication, transport, methods of money exchange, the creation of nuclear and other weapons of mass destruction and the emergence of new infectious diseases have shrunk distances and differences in many senses, and created common global risks. In this context, and with a deeper understanding of the impact of historical forces on shaping the wealth and health of nations, we need to appreciate how we are all implicated in the lives of others, and that it is increasingly impossible to hide with credibility behind the barrier of physical distance while billions of people live impoverished lives. Altruism and reparations aside, the importance of physical and moral interdependence is so great that self-interest alone should be sufficient to drive policies toward sustainable development (Hosle 1992). Unless such progress is made, the prospects for dealing adequately with the HIV/AIDS pandemic and indeed for our humanity seem bleak. Recent progress towards provision of antiretroviral treatment to millions of people offers much hope for improving global health (Institute of Medicine 2004).

Conclusions

New infectious diseases such as HIV/AIDS, the recurrence of tuberculosis and malaria in multi-resistant forms, ecological degradation, escalating ethnic conflict and persistent poverty and hunger in the midst of plenty are all signs of an increasingly unstable world at the end of a period of major progress (Hobsbawm 1994, Amin 1997, Falk 1999, 2000, Wallerstein 2000). At this time in history when the dark side of progress is becoming so obvious, old ways of linear thinking about progress, in particular when this is defined only in economic terms, are becoming obsolete. It is unlikely that relying solely on advances in scientific knowledge, free-market forces, simplistic notions of human rights and interpersonal ethics will provide sufficient solutions to problems within an unstable complex system (Homer-Dixon 2000).

Imaginative and creative new practical approaches, associated with the wise application of scientific and social knowledge using systems theory and supported by a broader ethics framework, are required to ameliorate the adverse effects of rampant market forces (Elfstrom 1997, Rist 1997, Paul & Hall 1999, Dunne and Wheeler 1999, Falk 2000). In a complex interdependent world, averting the potential for setting back the clock of progress by ensuring better quality of life for all is the 21st century's challenge to human society (Wallerstein 1999).

Endnotes

[1] Benatar S R. (2002). The HIV/AIDS pandemic: A sign of instability in a complex global system. *Journal of Medicine and Philosophy*. 27: 163–177.

[2] Several mechanisms are operative: the influence of transnational corporations on the power of governments of small/weak nations to pursue development, full employment or other national goals; lack of corporate accountability at the national level; trade agreements such as North America Free Trade Agreement and the World Trade Organisation; and the restrictive power of international financial institutions such as the World Bank and International Monetary Fund over national, state and local governments' control over their economies; and the complicity of these organisations in the denial of human rights.

References

Abbasi, K. (1999). The World Bank and health. *Brit Med J.* 318: 1132–35.

Aitken, W., La Follette, H. (eds). (1996). *World hunger and morality.* Prentice Hall, New York.

Alberts, B. (2000). Science and human needs. Presidential address. 137th Annual Meeting of the US National Academy of Sciences. Washington DC.

Alexander, T. (1996). *Unravelling global apartheid: an overview of world politics.* Polity Press. Cambridge

Amin, S. (1997). *Capitalism in the age of globalisation.* London: Zed Books.

Association of Concerned Africa Scholars. (2000). Special Issue: progressive Africa action for a new century. *ACAS Bulletin.* 57/58.

Bales, K. (1999). *Disposable people: new slavery in the global economy.* University of California Press, Berkeley.

Barnet, R.J. & Cavanagh, J. (1994). *Global dreams: imperial corporations and the new world order.* Simon and Schuster, New York.

Beaglehole, R., Bonita, R., Horton, R., Adams, O., McKee, M. (2004). *Public health in the new era: improving health through collective action. Lancet.* 363: 2084–86.

Beauchamp, D. E., Steinbock, B. (eds). (1999). *New ethics for the public's health.* Oxford University Press.

Benatar, S.R. (1994). Africa and the world. *S Afr Med J.* 84: 723–6.

Benatar, S.R. (1996). Just health care beyond individualism: challenges for North American Bioethics. *Cambridge Quarterly of Healthcare Ethics.* 6: 397–415.

Benatar, S.R. (1998). Millennial challenges for medicine and modernity. *J Roy Coll Phys London. 32: 160–65.*

Benatar, S.R. (2000). Global issues in HIV research. *Journal of HIV Therapy.* 5: 85–92.

Benatar, S.R. (2001). South Africa's transition in a globalising world: HIV/AIDS as a window and a mirror. *International Affairs.* 77: 347–75.

Benatar, S.R. (2001). The coming catastrophe in international health: an analogy with lung cancer. *International Journal.* LV1 (4) 611–31.

Benatar, S.R. (2003). Bioethics: power and injustice. *Bioethics.* 17: 387–398.

Benatar, S.R. (2003). Ethics and tropical disease: a global perspective. In: Manson's Tropical Diseases. 21st Ed. G Cook, A Zumla (Eds). Elsevier Science Edinburgh, Chapter 8 pp. 85–93.

Buchanan, D. (2001). *An ethic for health promotion.* New York: Oxford University Press.

Davidson, B. (1992). *The black man's burden: Africa and the curse of the nation state.* James Currey, London.

Dower, N. (1991). World poverty. In: *A companion to ethics.* Singer P (Ed). Blackwell, Cambridge.

Doyal, L., Gough, I. (1991). *A theory of human need.* Macmillan Press London.

Dunne, J. (1992). Democracy: the unfinished journey 508 BC to AD 1993. Oxford University Press, Oxford.

Dunne, T, Wheeler, N.J. (eds). (1999). *Human rights in global politics.* Cambridge University Press, Cambridge.

Elftsrom, G. (1997). *New Challenges for Political Philosophy.* Macmillan Press London.

Elfstrom, G. (1998). *International Ethics: a reference handbook.* ABC Clio-Press. Santa Barbara California.

Ellwood, W. (2003). *No-Nonsense Guide to Globalization.* Verso London.

Elmore-Meegan, M. & O'Riordan, T. (1993). Africa on a precipice: an ominous but not yet hopeless future. *JAMA.* 270: 629–31.

Falk, R. (1999). *Predatory globalisation: a critique.* Cambridge UK: Polity Press.

Falk, R. (2000). *Human rights horizons: the pursuit of justice in a globalising world.* Routledge, New York.

Friman, H.R. & Andreas, P. (eds). (1999). *Illicit global economy and state power.* New York: Rowan & Littlefield.

Garrett, L. (1995). *The coming plague: newly emerging diseases in a world out of balance.* Harper Collins, Canada.

Gill, S. (1990). Globalisation, democracy and the international financial institutions. Seminar on World Bank, structural adjustment and Nordic visions: welfare and development co-operation. Session 3. Helsinki 27th March.

Gill, S. (2000). The constitution of global capitalism. (Paper presented to International-Studies Association Annual Convention, Los Angeles, 15th March).

Gilbert, A. (1992). *An unequal world: the links between rich and poor nations.* 2nd Edition, London: Nelson.

Gray, J. (1993). *False Dawn: the delusions of global capitalism.* London: Granta Books.

Heywood, M., Altman, D. (2001). Confronting AIDS: human rights, law and social transformation. Health and Human Rights. 5: 149–179.

Hobsbawm, E. (1994). *The age of extremes.* Pantheon Press, New York.

Homer-Dixon, T. (2000). The ingenuity gap: how can we solve the problems of the future? Alfred A Knopf, New York.

Hosle, V. (1992). The third world as a philosophical problem. *Social Research.* 52: 227–262.

Institute of Medicine 2004, *Scaling Up Treatment for the Global AIDS Pandemic: Challenges and Opportunities*, James Curran, Haile Debas, Monisha Arya, Patrick Kelley, Stacey Knobler, and Leslie Pray, Editors, http://www.nap.edu/catalog/11043.html.

Jennings, B., Callahan, D. & Wolf, S. M. (1987). The professions: public interest and common good. *Hastings Center Report.* 17 (1) Special Supplement 3–11.

Katz, A. (2002). AIDS, individual behaviour and the unexplained remaining variation. *African Journal of AIDS Research.* 1:125–142.

Labonte, R., Schrecker, T., Sanders, D., Meeus, W. (2004). *Fatal Indifference: the G8 and global health.* UCT Press and International Development Research Centre. Ottawa.

Lancaster, C. (1999). *Aid to Africa: so much to do so little done.* University of Chicago Press, Chicago.

Lee, K. & Zwi, A.B. (1996). A global political economy approach to AIDS: ideology, interests and implications. *New Political Economy.* 1: 355–373.

Logie, D. & Benatar, S.R. (1997). Africa in the 21st century: between hope and despair. *Brit Med J.* 315: 1444–6.

Lurie, P., Hintzen, P. & Lowe, R.A. (1995). Socio-economic obstacles to HIV prevention and treatment in developing countries: the roles of the International Monetary Fund and the World Bank. *AIDS.* 9: 539–46.

Margalit, A. (1998). *The decent society.* Harvard University Press, Cambridge MA.

McMichael, A. (1993). Planetary overload: global environmental change and the health of the human species. Cambridge University Press.

McNeil, W.H. (1993). *Plagues and peoples.* New York: Anchor Books, Doubleday.

Michaels, M. (1992/3). Retreat from Africa. *Foreign Affairs.* 72: 93–98.

Nandy, S., Scott, R. & Logie, D. E. & Benatar, S. R. (2000). Realistic priorities for AIDS control *Lancet.* 356: 1525–6.

Narasimhan, V., Brown, H., Pablos-Mendez, A., Adams, O., Dussault, G., Nordstrom, A., et al. (2004). Responding to the global human resources crisis. *Lancet.* 363: 1469–72.

Navarro, V. (2004). The world situation and WHO. *Lancet.* 363: 1321–3.

New Partnership for African Development (NEPAD) Abuja 2001. http://www.nepad.org.

O'Neill, O. (1992). International justice: distribution. In: *Encyclopedia of Ethics.* L.C. Becker, C.B. Becker (Eds) Garland New York. pp 624–628.

Paul, T.V., Hall, J.A. (eds). (1999). *International order and the future of world politics.* Cambridge University Press. Cambridge UK.

Pauly, L. (1997). *Who elected the bankers? Surveillance and control in the world economy.* Cornell University Press. Ithaca and London.

PEPFAR. (2003). The White House, Office of the Press Secretary.. *The President's Emergency Plan for AIDS Relief Fact Sheet.* [Online]. Available: http://www.state.gov/g/oes/rls/fs/2003/22270.htm [accessed 2nd July, 2003].

Pettifor, A. (1996). *Debt, the most potent form of slavery.* London: Christian Aid Society.

Pettifor, A. (ed) (2003). *Real world economic outlook, the legacy of globalization: debt and Inflation.* Palgrave Macmillan.

Pogge, T. (2002). *World Poverty and Human Rights: Cosmopolitan Responsibilities and Reforms.* Polity Press, Cambridge UK.

Ralph, J. (2001). American democracy and democracy promotion. Review article. *International Affairs.* 77: 129–140.

Richmond, A. (1994). *Global Apartheid: refugees, racism and the new world order.* Oxford: Oxford University Press.

Rist, G. (1997). *The history of development: from Western origins to global faith.* Zed Books, London.

Robertson, A. (1998). Critical reflections on the politics of need: implications for public health. *Social Science and Medicine.* 47: 1419–1430.

Rotblat, J. (1997). *World citizenship: allegiance to humanity.* Palgrave Press.

Royal Danish Foreign Ministry of Foreign Affairs. (2000). Building a world community: globalisation and the common good. Copenhagen

Sandbrook, R. (2000). *Closing the circle: democratisation and development in Africa.* Zed Books, London.

Schwab, P. (2001). *Africa. A continent self-destructs.* Palgrave Macmillan, New York.

Sivard, R.L. (1996). *World military and social expenditures* 1996. 16th edition. Washington DC, World Priorities Press.

Stillwagon, E. (2001). Aids and poverty in Africa. Feature story. *The Nation,* 21st May.

Taylor, C. (1992). *Sources of the self: the making of modern identity.* Harvard University Press, Cambridge.

Teeple, G. (2000). *Globalisation and the decline of social reform: into the 21st century.* 2nd Edition (Aurora, Ontario: Garamond Press).

Thompson, A., Robertson, A., Upshur, R. (2003). Public health ethics: towards a research agenda. *Acta Bioethica.* 1X (2) 157–163.

Ungar, S.J. (1992). The once and future Africa. *Washington Post Guardian Weekly.* 12th August, pp. 20.

Unger, P. (1996). *Living high and letting die: our illusions of innocence.* Oxford University Press, New York.

Van Niekerk, A.A. Moral and social complexities of AIDS in Africa. (This issue).

Wade, R. (2001). Global inequality: winners and losers. *The Economist,* 28th April, 72–74.

Wallerstein, I. (1999). *The end of the world as we know it: social sciences for the 21st century.* University of Minnesota Press, Minneapolis.

World Health Organisation. (1996). *World Health Report 1996.* Fighting disease, fostering development. Geneva.

Chapter 6

Principles of global distributive justice and the HIV/AIDS pandemic: moving beyond Rawls and Buchanan

The appropriateness and contents of principles of global distributive justice (PGDJ) are a matter of debate, and highly relevant in view of the HIV/AIDS pandemic. In this chapter **Anton A van Niekerk** *explores the debate and goes on to offer two additional principles in reference to the current global response to HIV/AIDS.*

John Rawls's theory of justice (Rawls 1972) is indisputably the most renowned theory of justice associated with egalitarian sentiments developed in the course of the 20th century. Rawls is not a 'strict egalitarian' in the sense of someone who argues for the absolutely equal distribution of burdens and benefits in a society. Rawls's theory is more guarded in its claims. His celebrated version of egalitarian justice is: 'All social values . . . are to be distributed equally unless an unequal distribution of any, or all, of these values is to everyone's advantage'. Injustice, in turn, '. . . is simply inequalities that are not to the benefit of all' (Rawls 1972: 62).

People have a great variety of needs, as well as a great variety of means and backgrounds in terms of which those needs might be addressed and achieved. Rawls's theory focuses on those needs that are essential to people for the sake of successful functioning as a species. The desirability of the most equal possible distribution of the goods fulfilling these needs is a much more pressing requirement of justice. The needs that are absolutely essential in society are, for Rawls, 'primary goods'. He defines primary goods as 'things every rational man is presumed to want . . . the chief primary goods at the disposition of society are rights and liberties, powers and opportunities, income and wealth . . . These are the primary social goods' (Rawls 1972: 62). From 'primary social goods', he distinguishes 'natural goods'. He writes: 'Other primary goods such as health and vigour, intelligence and imagination are natural goods; although their possession is influenced by the basic structure, they are not so directly under its control' (Ibid.).

In egalitarian theories of justice, a case is made for as equal a distribution of certain primary and natural goods as is possible. At the same time, the most prominent egalitarian theories take care to avoid claiming that justice in fact requires that all possible societal benefits should be shared equally (Beauchamp

& Childress 1994: 339). Although such equal sharing or distribution may sound attractive, such a requirement would fly in the face of real life where the equal distribution of benefits such as intelligence, personal drive or ambition and entrepreneurial skills – all characteristics that significantly contribute to personal fortunes – is clearly not attainable. However, that does not necessarily apply to health care, which is a social benefit that resides considerably more in our power to distribute equitably through external and potentially enforced or enforceable means.

Justice in the provision of health care is broadly the subject of this chapter. But first, a short note: The principle of Justice has indeed been elevated to one of the four main principles of biomedical ethics espoused by Beauchamp and Childress in a book that has seen five editions[1] and that has attained an almost unprecedented status amongst the textbooks introducing students to the subject all over the world. In fact, the principle, together with Respect for Autonomy, dominates current debates in biomedical ethics. Moreno has pointed out how the principles of Respect for Autonomy and Justice have in fact overtaken the traditional Hippocratic emphasis on Beneficence and Non-Maleficence as the more conventional principles of biomedical ethics (Moreno 2001). In view of this development, it was to be expected that Rawls's theory of justice would have drawn considerable attention in attempts to give content to conceptions of justice in biomedical ethics.

By 'global bioethics' I mean the reflection that has in recent years gone into the question of the injustices pertaining to the massive inequalities of wealth and resources between countries of the developed and developing worlds.

This chapter will consider not so much the traditional applications of Rawls's contribution to issues of justice within single societies. I shall focus, rather, on the problem of the applicability of Rawls's ideas to the growing interest in developing what might now well be called 'global bioethics'. Within the context of this general need for the development of 'global bioethics', I shall, in the latter half of the chapter, concentrate specifically on the question as to whether Rawls's later work helps us to develop principles of distributive justice for such an alleged global bioethics. By 'global bioethics' I mean the reflection that has in recent years gone into the question of the injustices pertaining to the massive inequalities of wealth and resources between countries of the developed and developing worlds, and its implications for efforts to provide health care services more equitably to the developing world, particularly in view of the catastrophic dimensions that infectious diseases and other health problems have attained in the developing world over the past few decades.

My plan of action is therefore as follows:

- Firstly, I shall briefly review the main tenets of Rawls's theory, particularly as it concerns health care as a very important societal need, albeit not a primary, but a 'natural' good. In this respect, I shall draw on the work of Norman

Daniels that has applied, with certain important revisions, Rawls's theory to the issue of the provision of just health care.

- Secondly, I shall briefly argue for the necessity of a global approach to biomedical ethics in view of the need for a more equitable provision of health care between developed and developing worlds, drawing on the important work that Solomon R. Benatar and others have done in this regard.
- Thirdly, I shall discuss the main tenets of Rawls's *The Law of Peoples*, the book in which he extrapolated the implications of his theory of justice to the sphere of just international law. I shall also review Allen Buchanan's important criticisms of this Rawlsian enterprise.
- Finally, I shall evaluate this debate, arguing that, although I largely agree with Buchanan's identification of the shortcomings in Rawls's *The Law of Peoples*, I would like to add two additional principles of global distributive justice (PGDJ) to two of those formulated by Buchanan. (I have a problem with Buchanan's third principle, as will be shown.) The relevance and applicability of the first of these additional principles (the need for special measures in cases of catastrophic occurrences) will be fully illustrated by a discussion of aspects of the current HIV/AIDS pandemic in (Southern) Africa. The other emerges from a second problem that I have with Buchanan's otherwise excellent analysis: his tendency, when formulating PGDJ, to concentrate the burden of responsibility implied by these principles entirely on the wealthy 'peoples' (Rawls's term) or societies. I therefore argue that this principle involves the responsibility of poor societies to not only be on the receiving end of aid and to bask in continuous entitlements, but to also exert responsible policies that create sustainable conditions for the meaningful redistribution of global wealth and health. I also show how responses (and the lack thereof) to the HIV/AIDS pandemic on the level of public policy-making in the developing world illustrate the relevance and applicability of this principle.

Rawls and the theory of just intra-societal health care

The main tenets of Rawls's theory of justice are well known and hardly require extensive repetition.[2] Rawls's basic assumption is that a social arrangement is a communal effort to advance the good of all members of society. Inequalities of birth, natural endowment and historical circumstances are undeserved, and, in a society where the co-operative nature of action to promote justice is taken seriously, every effort should be made to make more equal the unequal situation of people who have been disadvantaged by the mentioned factors (Rawls 1972: 100–108). Advantages that people have over others that are the results of 'accidents of biology and history' seem, for Rawls, arbitrary from the moral point of view, and should therefore as far as possible be redressed.[3] 'The idea is to redress the bias of contingencies [i.e. the inequalities of birth and natural endowment] in the direction of equality' (Rawls 1972: 100–102).

Another central claim of Rawls (cf. the quote at the beginning of the chapter) is that all vital economic goods and services should be distributed equally, unless their unequal distribution works to everyone in the society's advantage. The distribution of these goods ought to be the result of a social contract to which all that are affected by its contents should contribute equally. How can this contract be set up in a way that will have an equitable outcome for everyone? It is in this respect that Rawls suggests the thought experiment of members of society freely negotiating the position of people accommodated by a future society behind a 'veil of ignorance' (Rawls 1972: 136–142). The argument in this respect is that the veil of ignorance will guarantee a process of mutual bargaining that will accomplish two things. First of all, it will maximise the fulfillment of the essential needs of everyone. Behind the veil of ignorance, everyone has a maximum interest to maximise the primary goods available in society in order to protect future society members' vital interests in potentially adverse contexts.

Behind the veil of ignorance there is no vital incentive to negotiate for luxuries that might well be forfeited when other essential needs crop up in real life.

Put differently, behind the veil of ignorance there is no vital incentive to negotiate for luxuries that might well be forfeited when other essential needs crop up in real life. Secondly, because no participant in the negotiations behind the veil of ignorance has any idea of what his/her position in society is likely to be (Rawls 1972: 137), there is every incentive to ensure that the position of persons that will be worse off in the actual society will be as tolerable as possible. As Rawls formulates it: 'The veil of ignorance makes possible a unanimous choice of a particular conception of justice. Without these limitations on knowledge the bargaining problem of the original position would be hopelessly complicated' (1972: 140).

Health and health care, in the sense of 'natural goods', can nevertheless be regarded as an essential need (i.e. a good that ought to be socially allocated and not gained by individual initiative).[4] Clearly not all health needs are equally basic or essential. Consensus must be reached in a society about which health needs are essential. Daniels, in his appropriation of Rawls's theory, shows that we have to work with a truncated scale of social goods. Arrangements are just when individuals are guaranteed a reasonable share of essential social goods. These goods constitute, for Daniels, 'the relevant, truncated scale for purposes of justice'. He argues that happiness is not the immediate object of justice. In the pursuit of justice, individuals maintain a responsibility for the choice of their ends. One could then argue that there is at least no injustice to refrain from providing people with means to reach 'extravagant ends' (Daniels 1985: 38).

Health care refers to that category of needs necessary to reach our goals as members of our species, i.e. it belongs to that which is necessary to achieve, restore or maintain adequate ('species-typical') levels of functioning (Beauchamp & Childress 1989: 270). Daniels's application of Rawls's theory therefore implies that each member of society, irrespective of wealth or position, must be, for the sake of justice as fairness, provided with equal access to *adequate* (though obviously, in the light of limits on resources, not *maximal* or the *best available*) levels of health care.

Daniels explores what role health care could play in giving content to the liberal principle of 'fair equality of opportunity' that Rawls also wants to accommodate in his theory (see Rawls 1972: 83–90). It is because meeting health care needs has an important effect on the distribution of opportunities of people in society that health care institutions ought to be regulated by a principle of fair equality of opportunity (Daniels 1985: 45). This principle is important because it guards against the futile goal of trying to eliminate or 'level' all natural differences between people. It is true that we do not deserve the advantages provided to us by the 'natural lottery', e.g. the social (rich parents) and genetic (IQ) advantages bestowed on us by birth. These advantages cannot wholly be allowed to determine opportunity; resources ought to be made available, e.g. through the educational system, to provide fair equality of opportunity (Daniels 1985: 46).

Daniels's argument then is that, if it is important to use resources to counter the advantages of opportunity that some have because of the natural lottery, it is equally important to administer resources to counter the natural disadvantages that people have because of their suffering from disease. This does not entail the futile goal of trying to extinguish all differences between people. Writes Daniels: 'Health care has normal functioning as its goal: it concentrates on a specific class of obvious disadvantages and tries to eliminate them. This is its limited contribution to guaranteeing fair equality of opportunity' (1985: 46).

Health simply is one of those current-day societal advantages that cannot, in any society, be available without limitations.

Another valuable point made by Daniels in his appropriation of Rawls's theory for defining justice in health care, is to note that Rawls's contractarian theory requires a 'thick veil' of ignorance in order to guarantee the impartiality of completely free and equal moral agents. However, in selecting principles to govern health-care resource-allocation decisions, Daniels makes the interesting and, to my mind, valid point that we need a 'thinner' veil of ignorance. This is the case because we cannot assume that the negotiations behind the veil of ignorance might be led by the assumption that health care resources in real life will be unlimited. We must know something more about the society in which the participants in the original position will eventually live – in particular its resource limitations (Daniels 1985: 47). It would make no sense for individuals to negotiate behind the veil of ignorance for benefits in terms of health care that turn out, in real life, to be totally unaffordable. Health simply is one of those current-day societal advantages that cannot, in any society, be available without limitations[5].

Daniels then goes on to identify four levels at which health care institutions ought to be provided in order to operationalise the original idealisation under which Rawls's theory was constructed – this idealisation consisting in the ideal to enable normal, fully functioning people to complete their normal lifespan. The four levels are:

1. Preventative health-care institutions that minimise the likelihood of departures from the 'normality assumption'.
2. Institutions that deliver personal medical and rehabilitative services that restore normal functioning.
3. Institutions that offer more extended medical and social support services for people who are (moderately) chronically ill or disabled, including the frail elderly.
4. Institutions that take care of people who are seriously ill in the sense that they cannot be brought closer to the idealisation mentioned earlier (terminally ill people and mentally and physically disabled people) (Daniels 1985: 47–48).

These distinctions make a lot of sense. They not only show the variety of institutions that come into play in order to enable people requiring health care to restore their normal functioning. They also provide a scale of preference in the (hopefully exceptional and mostly avoidable) cases where rationing has to be considered. If Rawls's idea that health care ought primarily to restore 'species-typical' functioning is to be taken seriously, this demarcation by Daniels at least shows at which level (point 4 above) rationing, if required, ought firstly to kick in. Whereas, as will soon be apparent, rationing is much less of an issue in the developed world, it is an almost daily occurrence in developing world settings, and has therefore to be taken into account as a possibility when levels of health care provision are considered.

The need for a global bioethics

What has been discussed up till now are the main tenets of Rawls's theory of justice and its applications to *intra-societal* health care provision. This discussion was necessary in order to be reminded of the broad outline of Rawls's theory of justice, as well as of how Daniels's work helps us to apply his broad theory to the issue of justice in the provision of health care. But the discussion up till now had mainly been concerned with health care provision *within a single society*. I have little to add to Daniels's excellent analyses in this regard. What intrigues me, however, is what the implications of the Rawlsian conception of justice might be for problems generated by globalisation, and, in particular, how these bear upon the issues pertaining to health care provision on a global scale. I therefore now turn to the global dimensions of bioethics and the questions of justice raised by *inter-societal* health care provision. Before proceeding to the question of the specific relevance of Rawls's work for this aspect, I shall make a few brief remarks about (the need for) global bioethics, and the concomitant questions of justice raised by that need.

In a recent article, Solomon R. Benatar (who has done seminal work in this area in recent years[6]), Daar and Singer (2003) point out how profoundly the world has changed since the birth of modern bioethics. These changes pertain to widening international economic disparities, the emergence of new infectious diseases, new consumption patterns, new wars, advances in science in technology, and many others. One of the important implications of these changes is that bioethics is increasingly challenged to not only interest itself in the 'micro level of interpersonal relationships', but to also concern itself with the 'the meso level of institutions and nations and [with] the macro level of international relations' (Benatar, Daar & Singer 2003: 108).

The economic and health-care inequalities between developed and developing countries are truly stupefying.

If this happens, a 'new mindset' could be promoted that is currently required to improve health and well-being all over the world. The authors emphasise the increasing complexity and interdependence of the world in which we currently live. This growing complexity indicates how narrowly health, human rights and economic opportunities are related. (I shall refer to supporting facts and statistics in the next few paragraphs.) It is a serious question whether the models in terms of which human flourishing has mainly been understood up till the present, particularly in the West, have adequately espoused the value of the dignity of all people and the need to promote that dignity through optimal development, particularly in less privileged environments and societies (Ibid.)

The economic and health-care inequalities between developed and developing countries are truly stupefying. The following facts and statistics are relevant in this regard and starkly illustrate these inequalities. Firstly, we may note the indefensible general income disparities between people in the developed and developing worlds. 'At the beginning of the 20th century, the income of the richest 20 percent of the world's population was nine times that of the poorest 30 percent. By 1960, it was 30 times as large, and since then the gap has widened ever more rapidly to the point where at the end of the [20th] century the richest fifth had an income 80 times that of the poorest fifth ... Today, two billion people live on less than US$2 per day, and more than a quarter of the world's population lives under conditions of 'absolute poverty' (Benatar, Daar & Singer 2003: 112). Sub-Saharan Africa generates no more than one percent of the total wealth produced in the world. In fact, in a recent issue of *Time* (3 May 2004: 14), it is reported that there has been a 15 percent drop in GDP per capita in sub-Saharan Africa between 1981 and 2001. There has also been a 91 percent increase in the number of people living on less than $1 a day in the same region over the same period.

Income disparities between richer and poorer countries are therefore, in spite of inflated political rhetoric at international level in favour of their reduction, as well as initiatives such as the New Partnership for African Development (NEPAD), increasing all the time. The buying power of all the countries south of the Sahara, except South Africa, in total just about matches that of a country such as Norway[7]. African countries also carry extremely heavy debt burdens – often, as in the case of South Africa, incurred by an illegitimate previous regime. The debt situation in Africa is often described as 'the modern (and much more sophisticated) form of slavery'. These issues have been discussed in greater detail by Benatar in Chapter 5.

Apart from the general disparities of wealth and income, we might next note the extraordinary – in fact stunning – inequalities between developed and developing worlds in terms of health care needs and provision. Life expectancy is, for example, generally regarded as a relatively trustworthy indicator of health status in a society. To illustrate the discrepancy between first and third worlds: in Canada life expectancy is 80 years, whereas in some African countries it is dropping below 40.[8]

Spending on health care is probably the most pronounced indicator of inequalities in this regard. The USA spends above 50 percent (US$1.2 trillion per year) of the total health care expenditure in the world (which is approximately US$2.2 trillion per year). This expenditure covers only five percent of the world's population. Compare that to the fact that government expenditure on health in sub-Saharan Africa fell from 5.8 percent to 1.6 percent of GDP over the period 1980 to 1997 (Benatar, Daar & Singer 2003: 115). Furthermore: 'Annual per capita expenditure on health care is less than US$10 in many African countries, as compared with between US$2000–$4200 in industrialised nations' (Benatar 2001: 90).

Not only is there no comparison between the available resources and actual spending on health care between the richer and poorer parts of the world. There is also inequality in terms of health care provision, succinctly illustrated by a comparison of health care research spending, as well as the priorities that are revealed in the patterns of research spending. Ninety percent of global expenditure on medical research is on diseases causing ten percent of the global burden of disease. Of the 1 223 new drugs developed between 1975 and 1997, only 13 percent were for the treatment of tropical diseases so prevalent in Africa (Benatar, Daar & Singer 2003: 110).

It is indeed a serious ethical question whether these immense inequalities do not compel us to rethink the requirements for human well-being on a global scale. As Benatar argues elsewhere: 'Perpetual economic growth for some cannot continue at the expense of others without sacrificing our humanity. The root causes of poverty should be openly acknowledged and studied more seriously, and powerful nations should be required to address these' (Benatar 2001: 91). Although the argument cannot be developed in full here, there is a distinct need to move away from a vision of society which is by and large constituted by individuals who live for the fulfilment of ends that are primarily individual.

We are, much more than we would normally like to admit, the keepers of our brothers and sisters.

Our humanity is not only defined by individualist needs.[9] It is also, and, for some definitively, defined by our sense of belonging to a community. (Wo)man is (also) a social animal, as was first pointed out by Aristotle. The point about the communal dimension of the human personality is not only the empirical fact that people cannot physically survive on their own. It is, more particularly, that people develop their characteristically human capacities only in society. As Charles Taylor formulates it: 'The claim is that living in society is a necessary condition of the development of rationality ... or of becoming a moral agent in the full sense of the term, or of becoming a fully responsible, autonomous being' (Taylor 1985: 191). Outside of society we cannot hope to develop those capacities that make us distinctly human.

It therefore is our dependence upon and our commitment to society that, in an important sense, constitute our moral sense. We are, much more than we would normally like to admit, the keepers of our brothers and sisters. What has happened in the contemporary world is that our sense of 'society' is almost daily transformed as a result of more effective mass communication, advanced means of transport, vanishing traditional (particularly economic) borders, enhanced international awareness and a growing international sense of moral duty and responsibility. We live, as has been argued, in an interdependent world where trade agreements, exchange rates, mobile money markets and international agreements increasingly determine our economic position.

Particularly in a context where there is one superpower, closely associating with the eight or ten largest economies in the world, and where their combined buying and selling power dwarfs the economic leverage of the smaller and developing nations, it is imperative that a growing sense of global responsibility for the vulnerable 'wretched of the earth' is cultivated. The need for such a responsibility is enhanced by the legacy of the historical colonialism and exploitation to which the developing world has been subjected in the past. As never before, the inequalities of the international situation call for a new international consensus on values that will facilitate the alleviation of the suffering of the destitute and the enhancement of developing nations' capacity to transform the plight of their suffering masses.

Bioethics therefore has to be reconceived on a global scale. Benatar et al. argue that the first requirement is the development of a 'global state of mind' (2003: 129–133). The greatest moral challenge brought forth by globalisation is the need to think of humanity in more communitarian terms. Ann Robertson has argued for a new moral language of public health which is informed by the realities of reciprocity and interdependence as we experience them in our time.[10] It is even a question whether too much must be made of reciprocity in this regard. The moral value of community relates back to what the French philosopher and ethicist Emmanuel Levinas calls the unconditional claim that other people make on me in space and time to be available to them and to have their interests (which include their health and general well-being) at heart, irrespective of the question whether they, in their conduct towards me, act reciprocally, i.e. whether they always act morally and take care of my interests.

Levinas formulates it in the following way: '[The] intersubjective relation is a non-symmetrical relation. In this sense, I am responsible for the Other without waiting for reciprocity, were I to die for it. Reciprocity is *his* affair. It is precisely insofar as the relationship between the Other and me is not reciprocal that I am in subjection to the Other . . . I am responsible for a total responsibility, which answers all the others and for all in the others, even for their responsibility. The I always has one responsibility *more* than all the others' (Levinas 1985: 98–99, his italics). Accountability towards and responsibility for the other, which also imply accountability and responsibility on a global scale, offer a powerful and defensible basis for morality, as well as a perspective that ought to be taken into account in the grounding of a global bioethics.

In addition, it must be argued that enlarging our sense of responsibility for fellow human beings in the direst of needs not only requires a heightened sense of altruism. It indeed also implies a more enlightened sense of self-interest. As Benatar argues: 'Crucial to a new approach will be the recognition that it is not merely altruism that is called for, but rather a long-term perspective on rational self-interest in an increasingly interdependent world' (Benatar 2001: 91). Improving the health status of developing countries makes both moral and strategic sense. What is required is the avoidance of unnecessarily pessimistic or optimistic caricatures about globalisation.[11]

Realism that avoids these caricatures is called for. It is a realism that:

- accepts the inevitability of globalisation;
- accepts that free markets are the basis of growth in the world economy, but that these markets are often, because of the growth of multinational conglomerates, not free;
- promotes international deliberation in which the nature of the inequalities are recognised and imaginative measures are constructed to alleviate the plight of the worst off, and
- promotes the strengthening of capacity in the developing world to better provide for its own needs.

We might conclude this section with a succinct claim by Benatar et al.: 'A social democratic pattern of globalisation is considered to require two types of enforceable international agreements: one set to regulate international competition among firms and states so as 'to yield socially and environmentally desirable outcomes'[12]; another set to redistribute some of the economic gains from globalisation towards those who are vulnerable and most in need . . . Striking a balance between optimism and pessimism will require a platform for dialogue among stakeholders, and a space where people can share different views about globalisation. Bioethics offers such a space' (Benatar, Daar & Singer 2003: 135–136).

Buchanan on principles of global distributive justice (PGDJ) in response to Rawls's *Law of Peoples*

In his book *The Law of Peoples* (1999) Rawls extends his theory of justice to the international situation. Now the issue is no longer what justice means within an individual society, but rather what it means in the situation of the international or global community of states or nations (although, as will become clear, Rawls prefers not to use the terms 'state' or 'nation'). He argues that, instead of the individuals who, in the 'original position', bargain for a state of just distribution of advantages behind the 'veil of ignorance', the parties responsible for this bargaining in the global situation are the representatives of 'peoples'. Rawls comes to the conclusion that the outcome of these negotiations will yield the following eight principles or 'laws':

1. Peoples are free and independent, and their freedom and independence are to be respected by other peoples.
2. Peoples are to observe treaties and undertakings.
3. Peoples are equal and are parties to the agreements that bind them.
4. Peoples are to observe a duty of non-intervention.
5. Peoples have the right of self-defence, but no right to instigate war for reasons other than self-defence.
6. Peoples are to honour human rights.
7. Peoples are to observe certain specified restrictions in the conduct of war.
8. Peoples have a duty to assist other peoples living under unfavourable conditions that prevent their having a just or decent political and social regime (Rawls 1999: 37).

Particularly in view of principles 1, 4 and 5, this theory of Rawls has been suspected of betraying liberalism because it clearly recognises and respects inegalitarian regimes that do not necessarily honour human rights and that defend their unjust actions in the name of self-determination and the duty of other peoples to not intervene in their internal affairs, very akin to the kind of strategies prevalent in pre-1994 South Africa or in current-day Zimbabwe. The criticism leveled at Rawls in this respect, and with which authors like Allen Buchanan and Darrel Moellendorf (1996) are sympathetic, is the claim that Rawls makes a mistake to fundamentally regard peoples, and not individuals, party to the law suggested by these principles. As Buchanan formulates it: 'What this means is that there is a need for principles that track individuals across borders – principles that specify the rights that individuals have irrespective of which society they happen to belong to, and which reflect the independence of individuals from any particular society' (Buchanan 2000: 698).

Personally, in view of principles 6, 7 and 8, I again am not entirely convinced of this criticism. The criticism seems to suggest that the duty to protect human rights, as called for in principle 6, is set to be at odds with 1 ['Peoples are free and independent, and their freedom and independence are to be respected by other peoples'], 4 ['Peoples are to observe a duty of non-intervention'] and 5 ['Peoples have the right of self-defence, but no right to instigate war for reasons other than self-defence'], and I do not see why that needs to be the case.

'Peoples', for Rawls, are groups that are united by 'common sympathies and a desire to be under the same democratic government'.

Why does Rawls use the term 'peoples' and not 'states'? 'Peoples', for Rawls, are groups that are united by 'common sympathies and a desire to be under the same democratic government' (1999: 24). Of peoples he writes that they, like citizens in a domestic society, are 'both reasonable and rational, and their rational conduct, as organised and expressed in their elections and votes . . . is similarly constrained by their sense of what is reasonable' (1999: 25). Buchanan points out that Rawls uses the term 'societies' interchangeably with 'peoples', and understands 'peoples' as groups with their own states.

There are, however, two differences between peoples and states. Firstly, peoples do not have all the powers of sovereignty traditionally associated with states, and, secondly, whereas states have the right of noninterference in their internal affairs, peoples must meet certain minimal standards in their internal affairs – standards that Rawls might call human rights (Buchanan 2000: 698–699). Rawls claims that states do not have a moral character, whereas peoples do. 'The term "peoples", then, is meant to emphasise these singular features of peoples as distinct from states, as traditionally conceived, and to highlight their moral character . . . ' (Rawls 1999: 27).

Buchanan argues that he not only agrees with Rawls's critics that he (Rawls) has overlooked the need for international principles that apply to individuals as individuals, but that, in addition, principles are needed for determining relations between Rawlsian societies or 'peoples', as he calls them (Buchanan 2000: 700). Buchanan argues strongly in favour of the fact that there is a 'global basic structure' which, like the domestic basic structure, is a subject of justice because it has significant effects on the prospects of individuals and groups. Buchanan also argues that the populations of states are not 'peoples' in Rawls's sense. They are rather sometimes conflicting collections of 'peoples' as well as other groups, and they often only become 'peoples', in Rawls's sense, after massive and unjustifiable coercion (Buchanan 2000: 700–701).

These last two mentioned facts explain, for Buchanan, two puzzling omissions in Rawls's *Law of Peoples*:

1. 'the lack of principles of international distributive justice'
2. 'the lack of principles addressing intrastate group conflicts' (Buchanan 2000: 701).

Buchanan goes on to suggest, in an involved argument that I shall not further pursue here, that 'Rawls's Law of Peoples, even if understood as supplying only that part of the moral theory of international law dealing with relations among states, is a set of rules for a vanished Westphalian world[13] and hence is of limited value for our world' (701).

Buchanan shows quite compellingly how Rawls negates the relevance of what Buchanan calls the 'global basic structure' in his *Law of Peoples*. By 'global basic structure' Buchanan means 'a set of economic and political institutions that has profound and enduring effects on the distribution of burdens and benefits among peoples and individuals around the world' (Buchanan 2000: 705). There is such a structure, as is increasingly argued in a growing international literature.[14] Elements of this structure include, amongst others: regional and international economic agreements, international financial regimes, and the increasingly global system of private property rights (Buchanan 2000: 706).

Rawls seems to ignore the existence of such a structure. He claims, for example, that 'many societies with unfavourable conditions don't lack resources. Well-ordered societies can get on with very little; their wealth lies elsewhere; in their political and cultural traditions' (Rawls 1993: 76). And elsewhere: 'I would further conjecture that there is no society anywhere in the world – except for the marginal cases – with resources so scarce that it could not, were it reasonably and rationally organised and governed, become well-ordered' (Rawls 1999: 108). He refers to Japan as an example of a resource-poor country that is 'well-ordered', and to Argentina as a 'resource-rich' country that 'has serious difficulties'. But this clearly shows that by 'resources' he means no more than minerals and land – entities that have been proven inadequate in themselves for attaining success in the contemporary global economy.

It is hard to believe that someone who takes careful cognisance of the conditions of success of modern economies and the concurrent inequalities in the current world, as partially indicated earlier in this article, could claim what Rawls is in fact claiming. Take, for example, a country such as South Africa, which is by far the most prosperous in Africa – a country rich in some natural resources (like minerals) although poor in others (such as water). Of South Africa it might be claimed that, although its policies on HIV/AIDS have in the past been disastrous (we turn to these later), it is, economically speaking, arguably the best run (Rawls would say 'ordered') country on the African continent today. That does not, however, mean that it is able to escape the paralysing manifestations of poverty that seem to be enforced by the global structure on all countries in the developing world.

> *As far as income disparities between rich and poor are concerned, South Africa still has one of the worst records in terms of social indicators.*

Poverty can be well demonstrated in the fields of income levels, employment, basic infrastructure, housing and education, expressed in terms of literacy. South Africa, in spite of its current sound economic policies, fares quite badly on all of these scores, although it admittedly does considerably better than many other countries in the developing world. A few statistics on each of these areas support my claim.

As far as income disparities between rich and poor are concerned, South Africa still has one of the worst records in terms of social indicators. For many years the country's 'Gini coefficient' – a figure between 0 and 1 indicating the rich-poor divide – was the highest in the world (in the vicinity of .65); it has, in recent years, been overtaken by one or two South American economies. About half (44 percent) of South Africans are regarded as poor. 'Poor' in this context refers to an *annual* income of below ZAR10 000 (US$1538) per household of 4.5 people.

Unemployment – a second important indicator of poverty – is rife in South Africa; fewer than 30 percent of poor working age adults are working in the formal sector of the economy. The same goes for the availability of basic infrastructure in South Africa, although it must be admitted that things in this regard have improved markedly over the past ten years since democratisation. On the housing front, it is estimated that between five and six million South Africans live in informal settlements or shantytowns. Lastly, economic development and wealth creation is to a significant extent dependent on literacy, particularly in view of the need to be able to do skilled, let alone high-skilled labour – so essential for creating economic growth and welfare. The reader is in this respect reminded of the disturbing information on literacy levels in South Africa that I provide in Chapter 4.

I therefore tend to agree with Buchanan's claim that the mere occurrence of 'being well-governed' is not, in itself, a guarantee for a decent and worthwhile life for all its members. 'A well-governed society might [yet] be seriously disadvantaged by the global structure . . . The chief point is that, like a domestic global structure, the global basic structure in part determines the prospects not only of individuals but of groups, including peoples in Rawls's sense. It is therefore unjustifiable to ignore the global basic structure in a moral theory of international law – to proceed either as if societies are economically self-sufficient and distributionally autonomous (so long as they are well-governed) or as if whatever distributional effects the global structure has are equitable and hence not in need of being addressed by a theory of international distributive justice' (Buchanan 2000: 705, 706).

It therefore makes perfect sense to consider a full range of alternative conceptions of justice for the global basic structure, particularly conceptions of justice that require greater equality. Buchanan argues persuasively that parties who represent peoples would choose principles of justice for the global basic structure (708). This will happen for two reasons. Firstly, such parties will have a serious interest to ensure that the distributional effects of the global basic structure will not impede the capacities of the societies that they represent to achieve their own conception of justice and the good. Secondly, 'because the parties in the domestic original position are represented as "free and equal", they will avoid principles that might turn out to assign them to an inferior status. Similarly, the parties to the choice of the Law of Peoples would be concerned to choose principles that would ensure fundamental equality for their societies *vis-á-vis* other societies' (Buchanan 2000: 708).

It is therefore clear that Rawls, although he takes care to propose a law of peoples that recognises and affirms the equality of peoples, and although he remains concerned about such societies' right to non-interference from others, overlooks one salient possibility. This is that the global basic structure – the nature of which has been described – has the undeniable possibility of undermining the equality of peoples unless it is regulated by principles of distributive justice (Buchanan 2000: 709). Rawls believes that parties who choose the Law of Peoples would not choose such principles because doing so would pose the distinct possibility of imposing liberal principles on non-liberal societies who are nevertheless well governed and ordered – the so-called 'decent' societies.[15]

Buchanan claims that, in spite of the fact that Rawls formulates principle 8 ('Peoples have a duty to assist other peoples living under unfavourable conditions that prevent their having a just or decent political and social regime') of his Law of Peoples, this duty seems to resemble the 'imperfect duty of charity rather than a duty of justice'. This is because 'there is no indication that this duty of aid is to be understood as the collective responsibility of the society of peoples and no mention of a right on the part of the "burdened" societies' to receive it' (Buchanan 2000: 710).

It is in setting up these kinds of reproaches against Rawls that it seems to me as if Buchanan is going too far and is reading way too much in what Rawls says. I cannot see why Rawls's formulation (as quoted) could not be interpreted as a straightforward duty of justice. Why must what Rawls formulates as principle 8 ('Peoples have a duty to assist other peoples living under unfavourable conditions that prevent their having a just or decent political and social regime') be seen only as a duty of charity and not a duty of justice? If I have a duty to provide for my child's education and I am financially and socially in a position to do so, surely my child – the receiver of this benefit – can claim as his right, in terms of the demands of justice, that he receives this education from me?

It is interesting to note that the public health movement in the world gained momentum the moment it became common knowledge that disease is spread through microbial organisms that ignored geographical borders.

However, even if Buchanan is right and the duty to which principle 8 refers is not a 'duty of justice', but 'merely' a 'duty of charity', he seems to be inclined to disparage the moral worth and force of charity. I argued earlier in this chapter ('The need for a global bioethics') that bioethics ought to exploit its global dimension and implications precisely on the basis of the rediscovery of a global *sensus communis* and the mutual care and responsibility that privileged societies ought to take for the less privileged nations. I see no self-evident reason why the acceptance and execution of a 'duty of charity' has less of a moral force than the acceptance and execution of a 'duty of justice'. For these reasons, I do not accept Buchanan's criticism of Rawls's principle 8

('Peoples have a duty to assist other peoples living under unfavourable conditions that prevent their having a just or decent political and social regime').

Apart from concerns of justice and charity, a powerful case can, of course, also be made for principle 8 on the basis of mere prudence. If large-scale infections occur in a developing country with the overt possibility that the infections might spread to a richer, developed environment or even country, it seems to be in the interest of the rich country to help the poor one, not primarily in order to achieve 'justice' or to dish out charity, but because it becomes in the interest – health wise, economically, and otherwise – of the richer country to improve the situation in the poorer country. Pure prudence seems to suggest as much. It is interesting to note that the public health movement in the world gained momentum the moment it became common knowledge that disease is spread through microbial organisms that ignored geographical borders. People now realised that those from poor neighbourhoods, for whom they felt little charity earlier (let alone concerns of justice), have become a threat to their own well-being if they are not assisted. Prudence prescribed aid.[16]

Buchanan goes on to suggest that, although he does not see it as his task in his article that I am discussing to provide a theory of global distributive justice, the parties formulating the Law of Peoples would come up with at least three types of principles of global distributive justice – principles that go beyond the duty to aid burdened societies. These three principles, according to Buchanan, would be:

1. A principle of global equality of opportunity.
2. A principle of democratic participation in global governance institutions (the United Nations is presumably intended).
3. A principle designed to limit inequalities of wealth among societies (Buchanan 2000: 711 ff.).

I think that a very strong case can be made for the first two of these three suggested principles. In the next section, I evaluate these principles and add, discuss and illustrate two of my own.

Two new principles of distributive justice for the Law of Nations

The global basic structure mentioned earlier is certainly something that has both the potential and actual effect of impeding equality of opportunity between peoples. The growth of the 'Asian Tigers' over the past few decades has shown that imaginative investment from the side of the developed world can precipitate significant economic growth and a turnaround in the standard of living of people in societies earlier subjected to abject poverty. Combined with the prevalence and nurturing of a positive work ethic and enhanced levels of productivity, these societies have shown that the promotion of equality of opportunity can have extremely positive results. Argued purely on the basis of the demands of justice, such equality of opportunity would undoubtedly have to be demanded by parties bargaining behind the imagined veil of ignorance when setting up a law of peoples, since the parties would not be aware of the position of relative prosperity that their society would have in the real world.

As far as the principle of democratic participation in global governance institutions is concerned, it is as easy to agree with Buchanan. There seems to be no justifiable grounds for excluding developing nations from such institutions, unless the cynical consideration of access to and possible utilisation of weapons of mass destruction is regarded, in isolation, as sufficient ground for exclusive access to these institutions. There is, for example, no justifiable reason why no country in Africa has a permanent seat on the Security Council of the United Nations; in fact, the rationale for 'permanent seats' in itself seems to be a consideration that is increasingly losing its validity on the grounds of justice.

Whether it would be wise to accept a principle that would limit a society's acquisition of wealth, is more dubious as far as I am concerned. It is true that that is not strictly what Buchanan's formulation of his third suggested principle requires; it requires only that limits be set on the extent of the inequalities between societies. But could that mean anything but putting a stop to a prosperous society's wealth accumulation as soon as it moves too far ahead from others at a certain historical juncture? What remains of incentives to produce wealth if a certain level of wealth acquisition inevitably will result in a programme of redistribution in favour of societies that fall behind for whatever reason? Would the prudent way to go not rather be to maintain all possible incentives that can be morally justified, and to maintain help to lagging societies, irrespective of the size of the lag?

This brings me finally to the question of whether Buchanan's three proposed principles exhaust what is required for the parties formulating the Law of Nations to formulate in terms of principles of distributive justice. I am of the opinion that two principles might well be added to the first two suggested by Buchanan (I am, as argued above, doubtful about the third).

The first principle that I would like to see added would be a principle necessitating aid by wealthy, relatively unaffected peoples to support peoples in cases of social catastrophes. This principle – let's call it PC (the principle regarding catastrophes) – can formally be stated as: 'Justice in international relations requires that the burden of catastrophic events be distributed equitably between affected and unaffected peoples'. Note that this principle does not require the *equal* sharing of such burdens, but only its *equitable*, i.e. just, fair or reasonable sharing. That implies that a considerable share of the burden of catastrophes *will* be carried by the nation, country or people (for the purpose of the current discussion, I shall use these terms interchangeably) primarily affected. The principle merely points out the injustice of such entities carrying the burden of catastrophic events *alone*, or being subjected to an unjustifiable exploitation of their plight by unaffected entities.

The term 'equitable' also has a bearing on the extent of help that might be expected from countries or peoples. It seems to me that the weight of the burden to be carried under normal circumstances cannot be the same for the rich and the poor countries. In other words, there rests a heavier duty on the richer countries to aid in the case of catastrophes hitting poorer, developing countries or nations than the other way round. This is simply the outcome of the expected ability to and resources available for help. Of course, when catastrophes hit the rich world, the principle still applies. The idea of 'equitability' in the sense of fairness or reasonableness nevertheless also applies in order to help ensure that aid from poor to rich in these circumstances does not precipitate a comparable catastrophe in the economically more vulnerable societies. It is too ambitious to try and give more content to the concept of *equitable sharing of burden* apart from considerations emanating from the actual cases to which the principle is set to apply.

The next crucial term requiring definition is 'catastrophe'. By 'catastrophe' I mean an adverse event:

- that occurs in the existence of (a) nation(s) or country(ies) in such a way that it is a demonstrable threat to the health (in the earlier sense of people's ability to function effectively as a species) of a significant number of people (i.e. significant relative to the size of the country's population);
- whose impact is enhanced by the nature of the social and economic vulnerability to which the nation(s) are subjected due to their historical circumstances;
- that threatens to consume a disproportionate amount of the affected country's available resources; and
- that has the potential to destabilise not only the country(ies) concerned, but also (at least) the region, if not the world as such.

Catastrophes, particularly in the form of pandemics of infectious diseases, can of course hit more than one country/peoples at the same time, hence the need for the plural. Note, furthermore, that this principle calls for the transfer of benefits in the form of money, goods, aid workers and the like only in situations of catastrophe. It does not call for a 'general transfer of wealth' from richer to poorer countries. The latter issue, to my mind, is sufficiently addressed by Rawls's principle 8 ('Peoples have a duty to assist other peoples living under unfavourable conditions that prevent their having a just or decent political and social regime'), as argued above.

I shall now discuss the HIV/AIDS pandemic as a good illustration of what I mean by the kind of catastrophe to which the principle discussed above applies. I stress that this principle goes beyond the 8th principle formulated by Rawls (see last paragraph). The issue is by far not only that privileged peoples have a duty to assist other peoples living in unfavourable conditions in order to restore, for them, 'a decent political and social regime'. The need is for a principle that addresses the occurrence of real catastrophes. In such circumstances, the normal patterns of provision, trade, business and development aid must be eligible to be overturned in order to restore a semblance of normality of the affected societies.

There exists a need for a principle that addresses the occurrence of real catastrophes.

The first requirement of a catastrophe is that it 'occurs in the existence of (a) nation(s) or country(ies) in such a way that it is a demonstrable threat to the health (in the earlier sense of people's ability to function effectively as a species) of a significant number of people (i.e. significant relative to the size of the country's population)'. It is self-evident that HIV/AIDS is a catastrophe in this sense. I shall not here repeat the horrific statistics about the nature and scope of the pandemic. Readers are advised to remind themselves of the facts and figures identified and discussed in Chapters 1, 2 and 4 of this book.

The second criterion of a catastrophe delimited above is that it is an event 'whose impact is enhanced by the nature of the social and economic vulnerability to which the nation(s) are subjected due to their historical circumstances'. There can be no doubt that this criterion applies to the situation in the whole of the developing world, including, and in particular, South Africa. I shall not repeat it here, but I remind the reader of what was stated earlier in this chapter (section 3) about the levels of poverty as well as about the position of women *vis-á-vis* the AIDS pandemic in a country such as South Africa (note, in particular, the section on 'Women's vulnerability' in Chapter 4).

The third criterion of a catastrophe that I formulated above is that it is an event that 'threatens to consume a disproportionate amount of the affected country's available resources'. Few issues illustrate this danger better than the debate about the honouring of patent rights for AIDS drugs in the developing world, particularly antiretroviral drugs that can prevent mother-to-child transmission. The overriding figure to be kept in mind in this debate is that Africa has ten percent of the world's population, earns one percent of the world's income, and carries 70 percent of the world's HIV/AIDS burden. The other highly relevant figures are that government expenditure on health in sub-Saharan Africa fell from 5.8 percent to 1.6 percent of GDP over the period 1980 to 1997 (Benatar, Daar & Singer 2003: 115), and that annual per capita expenditure on health care is less than US$10 in many African countries, as compared with between US$2000–$4200 in industrialised nations (Benatar 2001: 90).

To insist, under these circumstances, that patent rights for the manufacturing and distribution of antiretroviral drugs should be honoured at all costs is morally indefensible. In fact, the issuing of compulsory licenses that could facilitate making these drugs much more affordable to countries in the developing world could indeed be seen as one way in which the aid required by the formulated principle PC could be made available to countries challenged by the HIV/AIDS catastrophe. The following arguments can be forwarded in this regard:

Firstly, HIV/AIDS represents not only a national emergency for the countries in Africa and elsewhere in the developing world, but indeed an international emergency of enormous scope and with clearly devastating potential and actual effects. Not since the Black Death of the 14th century or the Spanish Influenza Epidemic of 1918 has the world encountered a comparable health crisis. This is exactly the kind of emergency that the existing Trade Related Aspects of Intellectual Properties (TRIPS) agreement provides for in order to justify compulsory licensing in the countries concerned. The necessity to save as many lives as possible, or to ameliorate the suffering of millions whose lives cannot still be saved, is a moral duty overriding all other duties in these catastrophic circumstances. Desperate circumstances warrant measures that would, under normal circumstances, be morally and legally more spurious. In addition, the AIDS pandemic ought to be seen as nothing less than an international disaster in response to which those who have been less harmed by it, have a moral duty to come to the aid of the real victims, without any concern about the financial costs incurred by such aid.

HIV/AIDS represents not only a national emergency for the developing world, but indeed an international emergency of enormous scope.

Secondly, pharmaceutical companies would not be unduly financially harmed or disadvantaged by the developing world's 'free riding' (Brock 2001: 37) on its intellectual property by manufacturing and/or parallel importing/exporting of generic equivalents of HIV drugs. Two arguments are relevant here. The first has to do with the extent of the profits that multinational pharmaceuticals make. The second has to do with where they make those profits. As regards the first, Resnik, in spite of his concerns about a unilateral forfeiture of upholding intellectual property rights by the developing countries, quotes staggering figures about the size and scope of the companies' profits. The pharmaceutical industry is without any doubt one of the most profitable businesses in the world. 'In 1999, the top ten pharmaceutical companies had an average profit margin of 30 percent, and the pharmaceutical industry averages an 18.6 percent return on revenues ... a ten percent profit margin is considered to be excellent in most industries. In the United States, prices of prescription drugs have risen at a rate far greater than the inflation rate: the average cost of filling a drug prescription rose from $34 in 1990 to $61.33 in 1999. Pharmaceutical sales in the US rose from $59 billion in 1990 to $91.8 billion in 1999' (Resnik 2001: 13). Chapter 7 in this volume explores this issue in more detail.

The second argument in this regard is that the profits that multinational pharmaceuticals make in the third world, are hardly significant in comparison with what they make in the first world. Schüklenk and Ashcroft, in this regard, argue:

> 'The pharmaceutical industry, by any standard amongst the most profitable industries, makes its profits not in developing countries where the vast majority of people is unable to purchase its products, but in developed countries. IMS health, a leading global provider of market research, business analysis, forecasting and sales management services to the global pharmaceutical industry, predicts that the global pharma-

> ceutical market is worth $406 billion in 2002. Of this sum only $5.3 billion is contributed from African countries' (Schüklenk & Ashcroft 2002: 190–191).

A third argument against honouring the patent rights of pharmaceutical companies states that third world countries cannot abide by the often occurring philanthropic practice of handouts by these companies. The argument runs that these deeds, laudable as they might seem *prima facie*, are not necessarily motivated by duty, but only by charity. Charity, it is then argued, 'involves the liberty to divert one's giving elsewhere if it suits one, and to arrogate to oneself the right to desist if the recipient is "ungrateful" or "undeserving"' (Schüklenk and Ashcroft 2002: 186). In addition, it is argued that charity on its own is a rather unstable basis for international aid programmes. On the one hand, as argued earlier, there is nothing wrong with charity as such. The global community that we ought to aspire to become requires that charity should be a strong motivational force for mutual benevolent interaction. On the other hand, we should take seriously the point made by Schüklenk and Ashcroft in the last quote. Charity has the potential not only to morally degrade the receiver of aid by fostering dependence and an attitude of humility towards the giver, but also to disempower the receiver to co-operate in setting the terms and to negotiate the terms of receipt. Charity can thus be supererogatory and can foster an attitude of paternalism, although, as I argued, this need not necessarily be the case.

The fourth argument is more radical and concerns the historical relationship between developed and developing world. A statement by Dan Brock is pertinent in this regard:

> 'The enormous income inequalities between developed and poorer developing countries, which make it impossible for the latter to afford the prices of patent protected pharmaceuticals, are in my view . . . one of the most serious injustices in the world today. If that is correct, then pharmaceuticals are unaffordable in the developing world largely because of unjust global inequalities in income and wealth. When developing countries choose not to respect product patents as their only effective means of making available pharmaceuticals necessary to save lives and protect the health of their citizens, doing so is arguably a step towards greater justice between the developed and the developing world; this may be a case where two wrongs do make a right, that is where existing global injustices make not respecting product patents, which in the absence of those injustices would be wrong, all things considered, morally justified' (Brock 2001: 37).

To sum up: the above arguments, individually and collectively, suggest that the AIDS crisis represents so serious a situation that commercial concerns, particularly pertaining to intellectual property rights, cannot be held on a morally equal footing with the urgency of, at almost any cost, saving lives or relieving the suffering caused by the pandemic. In the words of Peter Piot, UNAIDS' Executive Director, 'in the north, in return for innovation, intellectual property is protected and profits are made. This has benefited both northern shareholders and society. But it doesn't work for the south, where 95 percent of the world's population of 36.1 million [the figure is much higher in 2004, my comment] with HIV/AIDS lives' (quoted by Schüklenk & Ashcroft, 2002: 184).

The AIDS crisis represents so serious a situation that commercial concerns . . . cannot be held on a morally equal footing with the urgency of . . . saving lives.

The last criterion for a catastrophe that I distinguish is that the event in question has to have the potential to destabilise not only the country(ies) concerned, but also (at least) the region, if not the world as such. From all that has been shown and argued above, it is clear that HIV/AIDS must be seen as an occurrence that can play exactly this kind of destabilising role, particularly in Africa, but also in the larger world. What happens to a society where the average life expectancy drops to 35? What happens when, as current projections show, we are in this country prone to handle no less than two million orphans by the year 2010 if some major intervention does not occur in the meantime to curb the further spread of the infection? What happens to public health services when it becomes in its entirety consumed by AIDS management? What will the reaction be in the populace at large? These questions, rhetorical as they are, envisage real possibilities for a country such as South Africa, and clearly indicate the devastating destabilising potential that the pandemic has for us.

The above serves as the justification for my proposal of a principle of distributive justice for the global basic structure necessitating aid by wealthy, relatively unaffected peoples to aid peoples in cases of natural and social catastrophes.

The last principle that I would like to propose is one that recognises that all responsibility for attaining more equity between societies in the face of the global basic structure does not lie with the richer, developed societies. It is a principle that requires societies in need to formulate and adopt policies that will optimise both the effect of aid received from more wealthy societies, and of efforts internal to a society to improve its level of wealth and health.

Formalised into a principle of distributive justice, this principle – call it PP (the principle regarding appropriate policies) – should read as follows: 'Justice requires that efforts at an equitable distribution of burdens at the level of international relations be met with policies from the beneficiaries that, as far as possible, sustain the benefits attained from these efforts'. The principle elevates to the level of justice the expectation and practice that require that just acts not be met by dismissive, irresponsible reactions that nullify the good established by the act. In other words, it elevates reciprocity of beneficial acts to a requirement of justice. As such, it seemingly contradicts the denial of the importance of reciprocity that was, as shown earlier in the article (section 3), argued by Levinas. The contradiction, however, is only seeming and not serious, since Levinas's argument was one that tried to ground morality, not justice.

When we are dealing with justice, we deal with relationships in which there are at least two parties and where actions are interactive. Particularly at the level of international relations, which constitute the context of the current argument, justice cannot mean a responsibility that resides, in its entirety, with the benevolent party. Too often we see circumstances where, for the sake of justice, good is done by the rich for the poor, only to be met by selfish, irresponsible and thoughtless acts of negligence or squander which nullify the justice-enhancing effects that could have been achieved by the good that was done. The suggested principle is intended to provide for the avoidance of such situations in the pursuit of justice.

Justice for all victims requires that policies be set in place to optimise help from whatever available quarters.

How this principle comes into play can be illustrated with specific reference to what, for many years, occurred in the (mis-)management of the HIV/AIDS pandemic at the level of public policy-making in South Africa. The story of public policy on AIDS in South Africa has been a tale of neglect and denial[17], resulting in the disastrous statistics mentioned in earlier paragraphs. In this regard, one is saddened by the sustained signs of reluctance by the South African government to launch, with vigour and conviction, not only a programme for rolling out antiretroviral drugs in the public health sector, but also to embark on a full-fledged programme of prevention of the unprecedentedly fast spreading HIV/AIDS pandemic. Justice for all victims requires that policies be set in place to optimise help from whatever available quarters, and to facilitate circumstances and infrastructure that could optimally create conditions for curbing the seemingly uncontrolled spread of the infection.

Examples[18] of steps that could be taken by developing countries in respect of the HIV/AIDS pandemic and the need for affordable drugs that would prove their *bona fides* in creating the conditions to optimise the effects of aid programmes include:

- The creation of an international fund, supported by governments, international agencies and multinational corporations of all kinds, from which the provision of affordable drugs to the developing nations is subsidised.
- Alternatively, significant tax reductions for pharmaceutical companies who cut prices of drugs for developing countries below agreed margins. Either of these measures ought to be explored in order to facilitate the provision of essential AIDS drugs, either free of charge or at actually affordable prices to the developing world.
- If free or affordable drugs turn out to be unattainable, other venues for acts of co-operation that will help the companies to drastically cut prices ought to be explored. In this, the developing countries can indeed help, for example: by providing a guaranteed market that will facilitate the production of a drug at significantly reduced costs; or by assisting with the developing of research protocols with recruitment of subjects, obtaining valid informed consent, monitoring of data, etc.

- Developing nations can also significantly assist drug companies in developing give-away programmes by providing an efficient, reliable and fair system for distributing these medicines – a very severe obstacle to the success of these programmes when attempted in a hostile host environment.
- Developing countries could also buy drugs directly from pharmaceutical companies in order to take advantage of bulk buying and sell them at discounted prices or provide them free to the very needy.

In this way, content can be given to the last suggested principle of distributive justice in the international relations between unequal societies that seek more justice in their mutual relationships, particularly in the face of global catastrophes, the danger of which is seemingly growing. Rawls's *The Law of Nations* has stimulated much-needed reflection on this matter. I hope to have added one or more useful ideas to this reflection by drawing on and responding to Buchanan.

Conclusions

In summary, my main aim in this chapter was to focus on the problem of the applicability of Rawls's ideas to the growing interest in developing what might now well be called 'global bioethics'. Within the context of this general need for the development of 'global bioethics', I specifically concentrated on the question of whether Rawls's later work helps us to develop principles of distributive justice for such an alleged global bioethics, drawing on and critically evaluating Allen Buchanan's critical discussion of Rawls's *The Law of Peoples*.

I started out by briefly reviewing the main tenets of Rawls's theory of justice, particularly as it concerns health care as one of our 'primary needs'. In this respect, I drew on the work of Norman Daniels that has applied Rawls's theory to the issue of the provision of just health care. Secondly, I argued for the necessity of a global approach to biomedical ethics in view of the need for a more equitable provision of health care between developed and developing worlds. Thirdly, I discussed the main tenets of Rawls's *The Law of Peoples*, the book in which Rawls extrapolated the implications of his theory of justice to the sphere of just international law. Allen Buchanan's criticisms of this Rawlsian enterprise were critically reviewed. My main aim was to evaluate this debate, arguing that, although I largely (but not wholly) agree with Buchanan's identification of the shortcomings in Rawls's *The Law of Peoples*, two additional principles of global distributive justice ought to be added to the two formulated by Buchanan with which I agree. (With one, suggested by Buchanan, I do not agree.)

I then formulated and discussed my suggested two principles. The first (PC) is: 'Justice in international relations requires that the burden of catastrophic events be distributed equitably between affected and unaffected peoples'. I discussed the implications of this principle, and complemented it with an extended definition of the concept of 'catastrophe'. Drawing on each component of that definition, I illustrated how the HIV/AIDS pandemic is the best current example of an international catastrophe, and how that calls for the implementation of the formulated principle.

I then formulated the second principle for distributive justice for the law of peoples. This principle is: 'Justice requires that efforts at an equitable distribution of burdens at the level of international relations be met with policies from the beneficiaries that, as far as possible, sustain the benefits attained from these efforts'. I ended by showing how this principle is being neglected by the denialism of, for example, the South African policy makers' lack of a responsible response to the HIV/AIDS pandemic over the past decade, and by making suggestions how this denial and neglect might be rectified in the area of the provision of antiretroviral drugs to prevent mother-to-child transmission of HIV.

My main conclusion is that Rawls's work does indeed help us to formulate principles of distributive justice for the law of peoples, although neither he nor Buchanan came to the complete formulation of such principles. It has been my effort to engage in such an exercise.[19]

Endnotes

[1] My references will mainly be to the 1989 and 1994 editions.

[2] Apart from drawing on Rawls's own work, I draw on the very useful brief exposition of Rawls's position provided by Beauchamp & Childress, 1989: 268–270 and 1994: 339–341.

[3] Rawls formulates two principles of justice: 1. Each person is to have an equal right to the most extensive basic liberty compatible with similar liberty for others. 2. Social and economic inequalities are to be arranged so that they are both (a) reasonably expected to be to everyone's advantage and (b) attached to positions and offices open to all (Rawls 1972: 60).

[4] Reasons for what is so special about health and health care are eloquently supplied by Daniels, 1985: 1–35. His conclusion is that we should use impairment of the normal opportunity range as a fairly crude measure of the relative importance of health care needs at the macro level. In general, it will be more important to prevent, cure, or compensate for those disease conditions which involve a greater curtailment of an individual's share of the normal opportunity range (Daniels 1985: 35). Or, put in other words, health is important because it is the absence of disease, and diseases are deviations from the natural functional organisation of a typical member of a species (28).

[5] The limitation of health care resources is, in spite of the massive imbalances between the North and the South, nevertheless a world-wide phenomenon. It is, for example, estimated that, if managed care had not been established in the USA in the early nineties, medical costs would have gone completely out of control. In the late 1970s and early '80s, medical costs were rising at a rate that straight mathematical projection indicated would eventually consume the entire gross national product (Church 1997:36). The defenders of managed care point out that the system in the USA, with all its admitted shortcomings (e.g. the danger that it provides incentives to doctors to treat too few patients) has brought about a very significant decrease of medical costs. In the USA in 1996, medical costs rose by only 2.5 percent, compared to the 3.3 percent rise in consumer prices (Ibid.).

[6] Cf. also Benatar, 2001 and 2002.

[7] Personal communication by Colin McCarthy of the Economics Department, University of Stellenbosch.

[8] In a recent lecture, Alan Whiteside projected that if the AIDS epidemic is not drastically curbed within the next decade, South Africa's average life expectancy is expected to drop to 35.

[9] For a compelling argument against atomism and in favour of the idea that human personhood is

constituted by communality, see Taylor 1985, on whose views I gratefully draw for the rest of this paragraph.

[10] As discussed by Benatar, Daar & Singer 2003: 129–133.

[11] For formulations of these caricatures, see Benatar et al. 2003: 134–135.

[12] A quotation from Sandbrook 2000.

[13] Buchanan refers, in this respect, to the international legal system that grew out of the Peace of Westphalia in 1648 that ended the Thirty Year European War.

[14] Cf. footnote 11 of Buchanan (2000: 705–706) where a review of this literature is provided. Cf., for example, the works of Gilpin (1987), Hout (1996) and Wallerstein (1974 and 1991).

[15] See Rawls 1999: 64–67 for his two criteria for decent hierarchical societies.

[16] This point was suggested to me by Loretta M Kopelman.

[17] For a comprehensive discussion of the extent of this denialism, which space here does not allow, cf. Van Niekerk 2003: 161–168.

[18] I am indebted to Resnik (2001: 31–32) for many of these ideas.

[19] I would like to express my sincere gratitude to Hennie Lötter as well as two anonymous referees for their perceptive and helpful criticisms of and comments on the original draft of this article. I also very sincerely thank Loretta M Kopelman who made valuable comments on the version of the article that has become this chapter. My assistant, Liezl Dick, provided valuable support in proofreading the manuscript.

References

Beauchamp, T.L. & Childress, J.F. (1989). *Principles of Biomedical Ethics*. Oxford: Oxford University Press, third edition.

Beauchamp, T.L. & Childress, J.F. (1994). *Principles of Biomedical Ethics*. Oxford: Oxford University Press, fourth edition.

Benatar, S.R. (2001). Global issues in HIV research. *Journal of HIV Therapy*, *5*, 89–91.

Benatar, S.R. (2002). The HIV/AIDS epidemic: a sign of instability in a complex global system. *The Journal of Medicine and Philosophy*, *27*(2), April 2002, 163–178.

Benatar, S.R., Daar, A. & Singer, P.A. (2003). Global health ethics: the rationale for mutual caring. *International Affairs*, *79*(1), 107–138.

Bot, M., Wilson, D., & Dove, S. (2000). *The Education Atlas of South Africa*. Johannesburg: Education Foundation.

Brock, D.W. (2001). Some questions about the moral responsibilities of drug companies in developing countries. *Developing World Bioethics*, *1*(1), 33–37.

Buchanan, A. (2000). Rawls's *Law of Peoples*: rules for a vanished Westphalian world. *Ethics*, *110*(4), 697–721.

Church, G.J. (1997). Backlash against HMOs. *TIME Magazine*, 14th April 1997.

Daniels, N. (1985). *Just health care*. Cambridge: Cambridge University Press.

Gilpin, R. (1987). *The Political Economy of International Relations*. Princeton, N.J.: Princeton University Press.

Hout, W. (1996). Globalization, regionalization and regionalism: a survey of contemporary literature. *Acta Politica*, *31*(2), 164–179.

Levinas, E. (1985). *Ethics and infinity: conversations with Philippe Nemo* [Tr. R.A. Cohen]. Pittsburgh: Duquesne University Press.

Macfarlane, D. (2000). Almost half of SA is illiterate. *Mail & Guardian*, 1st–7th December 2000, 18.

Moellendorf, D. (1996). Constructing the Law of Peoples. *Pacific Philosophical Quarterly*, *77*, 132–154.

Moreno, J.D. (2001). Goodbye to all that: the end of moderate protectionism in human subjects research. *Hastings Center Report*, *31*(3), 9–17.

Pretorius, W. (1999). SA lewensverwagting val tot 45 j. weens Vigs. *Die Burger*, 24th November 1999.

Rawls, J. (1972). *A theory of justice*. Oxford: Oxford University Press.

Rawls, J. (1993). *The Law of Peoples*. In: S. Shute & S. Hurley: *On human rights: the Oxford Amnesty Lectures*. New York: Basic Books.

Rawls, J. (1999). *The Law of Peoples*. Cambridge, Massachusetts: Harvard University Press.

Resnik, D.B. (2001). Developing drugs for the developing world: an economic, legal, moral and political dilemma. *Developing World Bioethics 1*(1), 11–32.

Sandbrook, R. (2000). Globalisation and the limits of neoliberal development doctrine. *Third World Quarterly, 21*(6), 1071–1080.

Schüklenk, U. & Ashcroft, R.E. (2002). Affordable access to essential medication in developing countries: conflicts between ethical and economic imperatives. *The Journal of Medicine and Philosophy, 27*(2), 179–196.

South African Health Review. (1999). Durban: Health Systems Trust.

Taylor, C. (1985). Atomism, in his *Philosophy and the human sciences: Philosophical Papers vol 2*. CambridgeL CUP, 187–210.

United Nations AIDS (UNAIDS). (2003). *AIDS Epidemic Update. http://www.unaids.org.*

Van der Vliet, V. (1996). *The politics of AIDS*. London: Bowerdean Publishing Company.

Van der Vliet, V. (1999). The ecology of South Africa's AIDS epidemic. *Pulse Track*, 15th July, 1–5.

Van Niekerk, A.A. (2002). Moral and social complexities of AIDS in Africa. *The Journal of Medicine and Philosophy, 27*(2), 143–163.

Van Niekerk, A.A. (2003). Mother-to-child transmission of HIV/AIDS in Africa: ethical problems and perspectives. *Jahrbuch für Wissenschaft und Ethik, 8*, 149–171.

Wallerstein, I. (1974). *The modern world-system*. Garden City: Academic Press.

Wallerstein, I. (1991). *Geopolitics and geoculture: essays on the changing world system*. New York: Cambridge University Press.

Chapter 7

Access to affordable medication in the developing world: social responsibility vs. profit

Do global pharmaceutical companies have a moral obligation to develop affordable drugs and to make these drugs accessible to the developing world? In this chapter **David Resnik** *claims they do, and argues that although pharmaceutical companies and developing nations are often in conflict, they need to work together to achieve these goals.*

Access to affordable medications is one of the most challenging moral, political and economic issues facing the developing world today (Benatar 2000). Most people in the developing world cannot afford medications used to treat or prevent infectious diseases, such as HIV/AIDS, malaria, tuberculosis, cholera and dysentery, and half the people in the developing world do not have access to even basic medications (Reich 2000). Many people blame the pharmaceutical industry for this problem. According to critics of the industry, pharmaceutical companies charge exorbitantly high prices on medications and have no sense of social responsibility (Angell 2004). Drug prices, according to this view, are based solely on greed, not on fairness (Chetley 1990, Angell 2000, 2004). If pharmaceutical companies had a greater commitment to social responsibility, then they would help people in the developing world obtain access to affordable medications.

The facts tend to support this view, as statistics in Chapter 6 show. I repeat some figures here. The pharmaceutical industry is one of the most profitable businesses in the world – in 1999, the top ten companies in this industry had an average profit margin of 30 percent, and overall industry average return on revenues was 18.6 percent (Gerth & Stolberg 2000). Drug companies continue to raise their prices higher than the rate of inflation, and the high price of prescription drugs plays a large role in the rising costs of health care in the United States and other countries (Angell 2004, Gerth & Stolberg 2000).

Critics also claim that the high prices of drugs cannot be justified as a way of making a return on research and development (R&D) investments, since the industry spends too much money on marketing (Angell 2004). The amount of money that the industry spends on marketing vs. R&D is difficult to determine. According to industry estimates, most companies spend twice as much on R&D as they do on marketing, but, according to other sources, most companies spend more money on marketing than on R&D (PhRMA 2004, Angell 2004). Finally, critics also point out that the industry tends to fund R&D that addresses problems of the developed world, not the developing one. Ninety percent of the money spent on health R&D focuses on medical conditions responsible for only ten percent of the world's burden of disease (Benatar 2000).

Even though one can make a strong case for blaming the pharmaceutical industry for the access problem, the complete story is not so simple. First, pharmaceutical companies have sponsored R&D on many of the medications used to treat diseases with a high impact on the developing world. Most of the new HIV/AIDS drugs were developed by private companies. About 60 percent of all biomedical R&D is industry funded (Shamoo and Resnik 2003). Even R&D devoted to solving a developed world problem, such as sexual dysfunction, can have an impact on the developing world. Moreover, developing nations cannot afford to develop their own drugs, since it costs $500 million, on average, to develop a new drug that will be sold in the US (Goldhammer 2001).

Ninety percent of the money spent on health R&D focuses on medical conditions responsible for only ten percent of the world's burden of disease.

Second, owing to the inadequacies of the developing world's health care infrastructure, there would be problems with access to affordable medications even if pharmaceutical companies drastically lowered their prices or gave away their medications. An HIV patient cannot receive the necessary medication if he or she does not have access to doctors, nurses, pharmacies, hospitals or clinics. Third, many developing nations have a high degree of social, economic and political instability. It is difficult to provide access to any type of health care in the middle of civil wars, ethnic conflicts, and so on.

Although the pharmaceutical industry is not the only reason why developing nations are having difficulties with accessibility to health care, it has become a convenient target as many governments in developing nations have taken steps to combat the industry. Some governments, such as Bangladesh, Thailand, and Brazil, honour patents on pharmaceutical manufacturing processes but do not honour patents on pharmaceutical products. This strategy allows generic companies operating in these countries to manufacture patented drugs without paying any royalties to the patent holders, as long as they use a manufacturing process that has not been patented (McNeil 2000a). Not surprisingly, the prices of drugs are much cheaper in these countries. For example, the wholesale price of Fluconazole is $6.38 per pill in South Africa, but $0.41 per pill in Bangladesh, because Madawa Pharmaceuticals manufactures the drug in Bangladesh and pays no royalties to Pfizer (McNeil 2000b). Most drug companies have abandoned efforts to obtain or enforce patents in countries that do not recognise pharmaceutical product patents. Countries that honour patents on pharmaceutical products can take advantage of the lower prices on drugs manufactured in countries that do not honour these patents. Kenya's parliament debated a law that would allow the health minister to declare a public health crisis and would allow the minister to allow importation of cheaper, generic drugs, even when the patent on drugs in Kenya had not expired (McNeil 2000a).

Some countries have also considered compulsory licensing as a strategy for lowering drug costs. In compulsory licensing, a government forces the holder of a patent to license its invention to other businesses at a reasonable price. This strategy increases the supply of the drug, which lowers the cost. The Trade Related Aspects of Intellectual Properties (TRIPS), a global trade treaty signed in 1994, allows countries to use compulsory licensing to deal with a public health crisis. South Africa has considered compulsory licensing as a way of making drugs more affordable for its citizens (McNeil 2000a).

Drug development for the developing world is an economic and moral dilemma for both pharmaceutical companies and for the governments of developing nations.

Thus, drug development for the developing world is an economic and moral dilemma for both pharmaceutical companies and for the governments of developing nations. Pharmaceutical companies must decide 1) whether and how to invest money for medications designed to treat disease epidemics that plague the developing world, and 2) how to address the problems of affordability and accessibility of medications for the developing world. Developing nations, on the other hand, must decide how best to respond to pharmaceutical companies and whether to use any of the tactics described above.

In arguing for cooperation between pharmaceutical companies and developing nations, I would like to stress that one should not underestimate the importance of other parties, such as the governments of developed nations, the United Nations, and non-governmental organisations (NGOs), such as private charities, in helping to address these problems (Daniels 2001). Ideally, the solution to the accessibility problem will involve cooperative efforts on many fronts, since the problem is too large to be solved by industry, government or NGOs alone. Even though I recognise that governments and NGOs should play a large part in addressing the problem, I will focus on the pharmaceutical industry's responsibilities.

The pharmaceutical industry and social responsibility

A popular conception of private businesses is that they are either immoral or amoral, operating outside the bounds of morality and barely within the scope of the law (DeGeorge 1995). During the 20th century, many business professors and economists provided a theoretical basis for this idea by arguing that companies have one primary obligation: to make profit. By pursuing profit, companies manage their resources effectively and produce goods and services that benefit society. Laws can be useful in regulating corporate conduct, but corporations have no moral obligations over and above the requirement to comply with law (Friedman 1970). I suspect that many people regard pharmaceutical companies in the same light: pharmaceutical companies are moral pariahs.

Although many, if not most, companies frequently ignore moral standards, there are solid arguments for holding that businesses have moral responsibilities beyond merely obeying the law. All businesses are shaped by and depend upon social values, such as honesty, integrity, fidelity, diligence and fairness. These values provide a social infrastructure for contractual arrangements, employer-employee relations, marketing, investing, trading, and so on. Values play a key role in creating a climate within and amongst companies for conducting business. Without these values in place, corruption, theft, fraud, disloyalty and other ethical problems would make it impossible to do business. Thus, most businesses today recognise the importance of ethical conduct in business and many adopt and enforce codes of conduct (Murphy 1998).

Although corporations do not have a mind that makes conscious choices, they can be held legally and morally responsible for their decisions and actions.

Many people would accept the idea that moral values play an important role within business, but they might argue that they play no role in the interaction between businesses and society at large. A business could adopt and enforce a code of ethics that applies to its dealings with employees, customers, stockholders and associates, yet show absolutely no respect for other social values not directly related to business. Although it is also probably the case that many businesses ignore these other values, many writers argue that businesses have social responsibilities. Businesses have these responsibilities because they exist within societies where people care about the environment, public health and safety, and other values.

There are at least two reasons why businesses have social responsibilities. First, businesses that ignore their social responsibilities may face the public's wrath. A company that wantonly pollutes, for example, will one day have to deal with additional pollution regulations. Companies that make unsafe products may have to deal with expensive lawsuits. Thus, social responsibility makes good business sense (DeGeorge 1995). Second, corporations are like moral agents in that they make decisions that have important effects on human beings. In making these decisions, corporations can decide to either accept or ignore social values. Although corporations do not have a mind that makes conscious choices, they can be held legally and morally responsible for their decisions and actions. If corporations are like moral agents, then they have some of the same duties that apply to other moral agents. In particular, corporations have obligations to avoid causing harm and to promote social welfare and justice (DeGeorge 1995).

Since pharmaceutical companies are corporations, they also have social responsibilities. At least two types of responsibilities apply to pharmaceutical companies:

1. *Beneficence:* Pharmaceutical companies should promote the greatest balance of benefits/harms for society. They should avoid doing harm and try to do good.

2. *Justice:* Pharmaceutical companies should distribute benefits and burdens equitably.

The rationale for a duty of beneficence is fairly straightforward and uncontroversial. Indeed, most countries have a variety of laws designed to regulate drug testing, manufacturing and sales in order to prevent harm to the public and promote the development of effective drugs. In the US, the Food and Drug Administration (FDA) regulates drug testing, manufacturing and sales (Brody 1995). Although this duty is fairly obvious, its application is usually complex and controversial, as societies must consider benefits, harm, justice and basic liberties in deciding questions about approving the sale of new drugs (Schüklenk 1998).

Many writers have argued that pharmaceutical companies should promote access to medications as a way of promoting justice. According to Brody (1996), pharmaceutical prices should not be so high that they make important medications inaccessible. Spinello (1992) applies egalitarian principles to pharmaceutical pricing and argues that medication prices should promote social justice. Both authors acknowledge that the duty of justice must be balanced against the practical need to make a reasonable return on investment. A 'reasonable price' is a price that allows the company to earn its money but also promotes accessibility and equity (Brody 1996).

Other writers have argued that companies should distribute the benefits and burdens of research participation equitably. For example, if a company sponsors a study using a specific population, then members of the population that participate in the study should derive some benefits from their participation. In particular, the drug should be made available to members of the population at a reasonable price. It is not fair to place members of the population at risk without a reasonable expectation of a benefit to that population. Research protocols that recruit subjects from a population without a reasonable expectation of some benefit to that population are exploitative (Crouch & Annas 1998, Resnik 2003).

How do the above considerations apply to developing drugs for the developing world? In general, these considerations imply that pharmaceutical companies have moral responsibilities to develop drugs that benefit society and to make those drugs available to participant populations at a reasonable price. Some pharmaceutical companies, such as Bayer Corporation, have adopted ethics and values statements that mention responsibilities to the community, customers and the environment. Ciba-Geigy, a chemical company that merged with Sandoz (a pharmaceutical company) in 1997, adopted a vision and values statement that includes responsibilities to the environment and society (Murphy 1998). However, merely recognising that pharmaceutical companies should be socially responsible provides little guidance in determining how companies should exercise that responsibility. It does not provide specific guidance as to what a company should do, how much it should do, how many resources it should devote to a project, or even where it should focus its attention.

To get some insight into these questions, consider how an individual might decide how to act socially responsible. Most major moral theories, including Kantianism, utilitarianism and virtue ethics, hold that individuals have duties relating to beneficence and justice. However, there is also strong theoretical support for the idea that many moral duties, including the duty of beneficence, are not absolute: there are morally acceptable and desirable limits on the amount of good one may do for others. Although we should all do our part for society, we are not required to be moral saints. Since most individuals cannot completely sacrifice themselves for the good of society, they must weigh and consider other moral obligations and commitments in the light of their circumstances and conditions in order to decide how to be socially responsible. Social responsibilities, such as the duty of beneficence, are Kantian imperfect duties (Pojman 1995).

Companies, like individuals, have obligations to be socially responsible, but these obligations are not absolute.

These points apply to social responsibility at the corporate level. Companies, like individuals, have obligations to be socially responsible, but these obligations are not absolute. Companies should not act like moral scoundrels, but they do not need to act like moral saints. To meet their social responsibilities, corporations must weigh and consider many factors, such as their talents, abilities, resources, interests, commitments and obligations. As far as pharmaceutical companies are concerned, the goals of developing medications for populations and promoting access to those medications would seem to be a natural fit, given their interests, talents, and so on. But this still leaves open the question of how far a company should go in meeting this responsibility. Corporations, like individuals, must consider their resources, such as time and money, as well as other obligations and commitments, when deciding how to act responsibly. Most pharmaceutical companies will have little trouble fulfilling some minimal responsibilities if they develop drugs that benefit people and make those drugs accessible.

The harder question to answer is *how far* companies should go in exercising this responsibility. Companies also have commitments to their stockholders and employees. They have obligations to make a profit and to use their economic resources effectively. For example, Bayer's values statement also mentions duties to capital investment and resource allocation. Ciba-Geigy's statement mentions commitments to financial performance and improved market shares (Murphy 1998). If one agrees that profit should play a key role in business decisions, then it is morally legitimate (and perhaps even morally responsible) for a company to weigh and consider financial factors when making a decision to be socially responsible (DeGeorge 1995).

Money is not the only factor in deciding how to exercise social responsibility. Companies may also consider social, economic, legal or political conditions, since these factors may impact on the effectiveness of a particular programme aimed at meeting social responsibilities. These factors may provide significant barriers to implementing social responsibility. For example, a company might decide that it is not worth the effort to supply free medications to a country if that country is in such political turmoil that distribution is futile or impossible. A company might also decide that it is not worth selling a medication at a discounted price in a country that does not honour the company's pharmaceutical patents. On the other hand, a company might decide to initiate a research programme aimed at developing a vaccine for an infectious disease, if the company obtains financial and political support from a country that would like to have such a vaccine.

Finally, companies also need to consider geography in deciding how to exercise their social responsibility. I think there are several reasons why pharmaceutical companies have social responsibilities to the developing world. First, if a company conducts business in a country, then it has duties to act responsibly in that country. This type of social responsibility can be justified in terms of reciprocity and should not be especially controversial: if you make money in a country, you have an obligation to give something back to that country over and above taxes, goods and services. But companies can avoid this responsibility by simply not doing business in developing nations. A pharmaceutical company could market its products in the developed world in order to avoid the economic, social, political and legal challenges of conducting business in the developing world.

This brings us to a second, perhaps more important reason why pharmaceutical companies have social obligations to the developing world: companies should promote the welfare of humankind. This implies duties of beneficence and justice to all people, not just to people living in the US or Europe. Obviously, it may be difficult for small, local corporations to promote the welfare of humankind, but large, global corporations, such as Merck, Glaxo-Wellcome or Pfizer, should be concerned with the welfare of humankind and they should therefore conduct business in developing nations and attempt to meet social responsibilities to developing nations (Simpson 1982). However, even global companies may decide to avoid doing business in some countries in the developing world owing to adverse financial, political, legal or other conditions.

Many pharmaceutical companies have taken important steps to act on their social responsibilities to the developing world. First, companies are now sponsoring research on diseases that affect people in the developing world, such as tuberculosis, HIV/AIDS and malaria. Second, some companies have decided to provide free medications to people in developing nations. For example, Merck and the Gates Foundation have pledged to give $100 million worth of medicine and money to Botswana. Bristol-Myers Squibb is providing $100 million over five years to train doctors and develop community outreach programmes in sub-Saharan Africa (Sternberg 2000). Pfizer recently agreed to donate $50 million worth of Fluconazole to be distributed in South Africa, a nation where 20 percent of adults are infected with HIV (Swarns 2000). Although these offers have been met with a degree of skepticism and cynicism, they do represent a step on the path of social responsibility.

Thus, one can conclude that global pharmaceutical companies have social responsibilities to developing nations. How much should they do to help? These are complex issues that depend, in part, on how developing nations respond to pharmaceutical companies. If we think of exercising social responsibility as an attempt to make a gift to a society (or societies), and we understand giving as a relationship (or agreement) between the giver and recipient, then we need to say a bit more about the recipient of the gift. Exercising social responsibility in the developing world depends, in part, on social, economic, political and legal conditions in the developing world, since these conditions can either assist or impede a company's attempt to exercise social responsibility or its business practices. Most companies, I believe, will resist doing business in the developing world if 1) they have no guarantee of a reasonable profit, and 2) they must overcome an unproductive business climate. But what is a reasonable profit and what is an unproductive business climate? We need to address these issues before returning to the topic of social responsibility.

Exercising social responsibility in the developing world depends, in part, on social, economic, political and legal conditions in the developing world.

Reasonable profits, drug prices and patents

Determining what counts as 'reasonable' profit is a complex issue in business ethics. According to some commentators, there should be no limits on profit other than the free market. If a company can make a 30 percent profit, then this is 'fair' in the market sense of 'fairness'. Moreover, profits are morally justifiable in that they contribute to the overall social welfare. Businesses that make profits can use those funds to compensate employees or stockholders or make investments in new equipment, buildings or other resources (Jacobsen 1991). Furthermore, according to this argument, attempts to control or regulate profit margins could have drastic economic consequences for businesses that would restrict their ability to contribute to society. First, investors might avoid an industry where the government regulates profits. Second, companies will have a more difficult time with financial planning and resource allocation if there are some legal limits on profits. Third, since profits depend in part on prices, profit regulation must involve some form of price regulation which could lead to market inefficiencies because prices need to change quickly in response to market demands but government agencies often act slowly. Fourth, if companies face limitations on profits or prices, they may cut back on their investments in R&D and focus more on marketing.

For these as well as many other reasons, government regulation of profits under normal, free market conditions is morally and economically questionable. However, when free markets cannot set fair prices owing to monopolies, exclusive dealing, price discrimination or collusion, the government may regulate or scrutinise prices in order to buffer or counteract these restrictions on trade. For example, there are good reasons to regulate the prices charged by public utilities and other corporations that have a monopoly. There may also be good reasons to investigate pricing practices when one suspects that different companies have adopted agreements designed to inflate prices (Ferrell and Frederick 1991).

There is nothing inherently wrong with being wealthy (or having a high profit margin) but greater wealth implies greater responsibility.

One might accept the thrust of this argument yet maintain that companies that make healthy profits have strong moral obligations to return more of those profits to society because they are better equipped to meet obligations of beneficence and justice. Consider the analogy with an individual. One might argue that a person making a high salary has an obligation to give more money to charity than a person making a low salary because he can afford to give more to charity. There is nothing inherently wrong with being wealthy (or having a high profit margin) but greater wealth implies greater responsibility.

Now there are many ways that a profitable company could return some wealth to society. The company could offer price discounts, it could give away some of its products, it could invest funds in developing drugs to treat orphan diseases, or it could invest in other social programmes. In any case, all decisions concerning the exercise of social responsibilities have an effect on profit margins because these choices incur additional costs or expenses. Thus, a morally reasonable profit (the profit a company should be allowed to realise) might be lower than an economically reasonable profit (the profit a company can realise). If a company decides to return some wealth to society through pricing practices, then its 'morally reasonable' prices (the prices it ought to charge) could be lower than its 'economically reasonable' prices (the prices it can charge).

How does all of this apply to the pharmaceutical industry? The argument implies that companies with high profit margins should consider taking additional steps to be socially responsible, such as discounts on prices, product give-aways, etc. If a company decides to fulfil its social responsibilities through pricing policies, then the company should be willing to lower its drug prices (and therefore perhaps lower its profits) in order to make those drugs more accessible. Since it is probably not very efficient to lower the prices of all drugs in all markets, a company should probably be selective in its socially responsible pricing policies, focusing its discounts on specific drugs in specific markets. If we focus our attention on the developing world, this argument implies that global companies with high profit margins, such as Pfizer, Merck and Glaxo-Wellcome, should be willing to forego some profits in the developing world in order to fulfil social responsibilities to the developing world. They can accomplish this task through many different ways, including price discounts or drug give-aways.

But how much money should a pharmaceutical company devote toward socially responsible projects? The answer to this question depends in part on the company's current and projected profits. Global pharmaceutical companies can (and should) be able to devote hundreds of millions of dollars toward projects designed to benefit developing nations without losing a great deal of profit. However, their ability to continue realising these profits depends on strong patent protection. Patents play a key role in profitability in the pharmaceutical industry since patents allow companies to obtain returns on their R&D investments (Goldhammer 2001). Without this protection, companies would not make these risky investments. Pharmaceutical R&D investing is a high-risk proposition for several reasons. First, the new drug may not prove to be safe and effective and the company may decide to abandon the drug in the middle of clinical testing. Second, if the company completes its clinical trials, there is no guarantee that the FDA (or other relevant agency) will approve the new drug. Third, if the agency approves the new drug, it may not have a strong market because of competition from other drugs or lack of consumer demand. Fourth, once the drug is on the market, the agency could take it off the market to protect public health and safety. Finally, there is always the possibility that the company will face lawsuits from consumers that are harmed by the drug. Without adequate patent protection, a company might take these risks and develop its product only to have a competing company manufacture the product at a lower price. According to the pharmaceutical industry, only 30 percent of new drugs are profitable (Goldhammer 2001).

Although patents offer pharmaceutical companies control over their inventions, this control is not absolute. First, in the US (and most other countries), a patent lasts 20 years from the time of the application, which gives a drug company an approximately ten-year window to make a return on its R&D investment (Goldhammer 2001). Once the patent expires, a generic drug company can make the drug without infringing the patent. Second, most patent laws allow for some degree of 'copycat' inventions. A copycat invention is an invention that is very similar to a previous invention but it represents a useful innovation or improvement. In the US, companies can patent new copycat drugs by making slight changes to the original patented drugs. The possibility of copycat drugs creates a potential limit on a company's ability to control the market for a drug. For example, the company could invent a new blood pressure medication and dominate the market for this product until other companies develop copycat versions of the medication (Goldhammer 2001). However, it is important to realise that the US Patent and Trade Office (PTO) does not accept all copycat drugs; it only accepts those drugs that are useful improvements (Miller and Davis 2000).

We should also note that patents provide legal protection only in the country in which they are issued: a US patent provides no legal protection in Britain. Thus, when a drug company develops a new drug, it usually applies for patent protection in the countries where it plans to sell the drug. If a country does not provide the company with patent protection, then it may lose business in that country and perhaps in others. If we think of the whole world as a potential market, a company that invents a new drug and patents it in many countries may still lose a significant portion of its potential market volume if several countries do not honour the patent and export the drug around the world. This is why the pharmaceutical companies find India's patent policies so troubling: the companies lose out on the market in India as well as markets in other countries that import drugs from India.

Drug companies can still make a profit when their patents are not honoured around the world, but they have to make their profits in countries that honour those patents. It is hard to say exactly how much money pharmaceutical companies lose as a result of the failure to recognise patents globally. Industry representatives claim that they lose as much as ten percent of their profits this way, and it is likely that drug prices would be lower if the companies could take advantage of a larger market (Reich 2000).

So what does pharmaceutical patenting have to do with reasonable profits, prices and social responsibility? A great deal, I think. Briefly, companies can afford to do business in a country and exercise social responsibility insofar as they have a guarantee of reasonable profits. But obtaining these profits depends, in large part, on patent laws. When companies have strong patent protection, they can expect to profit from their R&D investments, and they can afford to devote more resources to socially responsible programmes. If they fail to realise profits, they have less money to devote to programmes designed to enhance social welfare.

Drug companies can still make a profit when their patents are not honoured around the world, but they have to make their profits in countries that honour those patents.

Thus, developing nations that fail to honour pharmaceutical patents may ultimately be harming themselves. In the short run, a developing country might obtain some benefit by not honouring pharmaceutical patents because it could acquire inexpensive drugs or attract generic drug companies or distributors. This strategy could backfire in the long run, however, since larger, global pharmaceutical companies may decide to not do business in countries that do not honour their patents, and they may decide to not invest money in R&D for developing drugs for the developing world. Why invest several billion dollars in developing a malaria vaccine if generic drug companies will reverse engineer the vaccine and sell it at a very low price? If companies lack sufficient patent protection in the developing world, many patients in the developing world will remain therapeutic orphans.

One might attempt to undercut this argument by pointing out that pharmaceutical companies make very little money from sales to the developing world, and that over 95 percent of their sales revenues come from the developed world (Sterckx 2004). Even so, this economic reality is not a good reason for nullifying patent protection in the developing world. Pharmaceutical markets are global in scale and scope. A drug invented and tested in the US may be manufactured in India, imported to Canada or Mexico, and then imported to the US. If companies lose control of their patent rights in any nation, there is a chance that the global pharmaceutical trade could undermine the profits that they make in the developed world. Pharmaceutical companies vigorously defend their patent rights around the world to maintain maximum control of these different markets.

Productive business environment

This section will address briefly another important factor in conducting business in the developing world and exercising social responsibility: the business environment. There are many different social, economic, political and legal characteristics that contribute to a good business environment. A few of these are (Samuelson 1980):

- a coherent and effective legal system;
- ethical business practices;
- a stable currency;
- a reliable banking system;
- free and open markets;
- a well-educated public;
- a middle class or consumer class;
- a physical and social infrastructure;
- democratic institutions.

These characteristics played a key role in the rise of capitalism, and they can be found to a great degree in developed nations such as the US, Germany and Britain. Very often, developing nations lack the characteristics that define a good business environment. Moreover, it may take many years for developing nations to develop some of these characteristics, such as a well-educated public, a physical and social infrastructure, or democratic institutions. It simply takes time to build bridges, roads, power lines and telephone networks, acquire education, develop a middle class, establish democracy, and so on. A company that refuses to do business in the developing world because its business environment is less than ideal would be acting foolishly and unfairly: in order to expand their markets and their influence, companies need to take some risks and conduct business in undeveloped nations.

A company that refuses to do business in the developing world because its business environment is less than ideal would be acting foolishly and unfairly.

However, there are some acceptable limits on what a company should be willing to do to expand into a developing nation. Some business environments can be so adverse that doing business in that country is impossible or highly inefficient. Consider the difficulties involved in selling products in a society that uses the barter system, investing funds in a society where the banks do not insure savings or checking accounts, hiring employees in a society where employee theft is common, or signing contracts in a society where bribery is expected. In order to do business in the developing world and exercise their social responsibility, companies need to have a reasonable expectation that those nations are taking steps to promote the rule of law, ethical business practices, a stable currency and banking system, free and open markets, etc. Doing business in a country with an extremely poor business climate is going above and beyond the call of corporate duty. Developing nations can attract businesses by demonstrating that they are making progress towards developing a good business environment.

Conclusions

I began by arguing that large, global pharmaceutical companies have social responsibilities (or duties of beneficence and justice) to the developing world. There are a variety of ways that companies can exercise these responsibilities, including investing in R&D related to diseases that affect developing nations, offering discounts on drug prices and initiating drug give-aways. However, I also argued that these social responsibilities are not absolute requirements and may be balanced against other obligations and commitments in the light of economic, social, legal and other conditions.

In the second and third sections of this chapter, I argued that the degree to which a company may exercise social responsibility in a society depends on two major factors: 1) the prospects for a reasonable profit and 2) the prospects for a good business environment. Developing nations can either help or hinder the pharmaceutical industry's efforts to exercise social responsibility through various policies and practices. To ensure that companies can make a reasonable profit, developing nations should honour pharmaceutical patents. If they do not honour those patents, this will lower the industry's profits and take away money that could be devoted to projects designed to promote access to medications. To ensure the companies have a good business environment, developing nations should try to promote the rule of law, ethical business practices, stable currencies, reliable banking systems, free and open markets, democracy, and other social, economic, legal and political conditions conducive to business.

Pharmaceutical companies and developing nations need to work together to develop affordable medications for the developing world. Companies can do their part by investing in R&D for the developing world's diseases, offering drug discounts, or establishing drug give-away programmes. In return, developing nations should also take steps to promote a sound legal, ethical, financial and social environment for business. Developing nations should provide strong patent protection and take steps to establish productive business environments. Developing nations should adhere to international agreements on intellectual property, such as the TRIPS agreement. The TRIPS agreement sets minimum standards for patent protection and requires that signatory countries do not undermine one another's intellectual property rights. TRIPS allows nations to engage in compulsory licensing and importation to address public safety or public health crises.

I do not oppose measures consistent with the TRIPS agreement that governments may use to respond to public health emergencies, such as the HIV/AIDS pandemic. It is very important for nations, especially developing nations, to have the ability to override intellectual property rights (IPRs) to deal with national emergencies. Overriding intellectual property rights should be regarded as a last resort, however. A country should take this drastic measure only after negotiating in good faith with the party who holds the IPRs. In some countries, such as the US, constitutional due process rules also require that governments compensate IPR-holders for their losses when they override these rights (Resnik & De Ville 2002). To prevent nations from abusing their authority to override IPRs under the TRIPS agreement, it is also important to define clearly the concept of a national emergency. There has been a great deal of dispute about what counts as a 'national emergency'. For a public health crisis to count as a national emergency, it would have to be so severe that it interferes with basic functions of government, society or the economy. For example, HIV/AIDS in sub-Saharan Africa may fit this definition of a national emergency, but HIV/AIDS in North America does not.

In pursuing this cooperative approach, developing nations may use a variety of other strategies to encourage pharmaceutical companies to act responsibly. For example, a nation could help reduce the cost of R&D and marketing by subsidising R&D funding and by providing a company with a guaranteed market. If developing nations lower these costs to the company, the company will be able to develop a drug, sell it at a low price and still make a reasonable profit. A developing nation could also help a drug company design research protocols and help the company with recruitment of subjects, informed consent, data monitoring, and other important aspects of human subjects research. A nation could also help a company develop a drug give-away programme by providing an efficient, reliable and fair system for distributing these medications. Finally, developing nations can also buy drugs in large quantities directly from pharmaceutical companies in order to take advantage of bulk buying. Nations could sell these drugs at a discounted price or give them away. Many countries have already pursued some of these strategies and there are many more constructive solutions than those mentioned in this chapter (Reich 2000).

Although I believe strongly in the importance of reciprocal arrangements between pharmaceutical companies and developing nations, I also recognise that these agreements may not always work and that an atmosphere of animosity can easily develop. If a developing nation starts making concessions to the pharmaceutical industry and the industry does not respond through socially responsible policies and programmes, then it would be reasonable for that nation to take retaliatory measures, such as compulsory licensing or importing drugs from countries that do not honour pharmaceutical patents. On the other hand, if a pharmaceutical company offers to aid a developing nation and that nation does not respond in kind, then that company would also have reasons to not make good on its commitment to that nation. I can foresee that these situations will arise and I would not admonish either side for retaliatory conduct. However, I would still strongly urge developing nations and pharmaceutical companies to work together in addressing the urgent economic and moral dilemma of developing drugs for the developing world.

I am not a naïve defender of the pharmaceutical industry. I recognise that industry decisions are based on profit and greed, and that most companies engage in socially responsible activities only as a means of enhancing their public relations activities, which tend to have a positive impact on profits. While I remain firm in my conviction that pharmaceutical companies have social responsibilities, I recognise that many companies ignore these responsibilities or do not take them seriously. Elsewhere, I have discussed many different ethical problems related to pharmaceutical research, such as suppression of research results, bias and conflicts of interest (Shamoo & Resnik 2003). My defence of intellectual property rights for pharmaceuticals stems from a pragmatic approach to the justification of intellectual property, not from an ideological commitment to big business (Resnik 2003b). It would be wonderful if knowledge could always be shared freely at no cost to anyone. But we do not live in such a world. Knowledge is power and often costs much money to produce. In this less than ideal world, intellectual property rights are a necessary evil.

This chapter is based on Resnik, D. Developing Drugs for the Developing World: an Economic, Legal, Moral, and Political Dilemma. *Developing World Bioethics* 2001, 1, 1: 11–32.

References

Angell, M. (2000). 'The pharmaceutical industry – to whom is it accountable?' *New England Journal of Medicine* 342: 1902–4.

Angell, M. (2004). *The Truth about Drug Companies*. New York: Random House.

Benatar, S. (2000). 'Avoiding exploitation in clinical research', *Cambridge Quarterly of Healthcare Ethics* 9: 562–65.

Brody, B. (1995). *Ethical Issues in Drug Testing, Approval and Pricing*. New York: Oxford University Press.

Brody, B. (1996). 'Public good and fair prices: balancing technological innovation with social well-being.' *Hastings Center Report* 26, 2: 5–11.

Chetley, A. (1990). *A Healthy Business? World Health and the Pharmaceutical Industry*. Zed Books, London.
Crouch, R. and Arras, J. (1998). 'AZT trials and tribulations', *Hastings Center Report* 28, 6: 26–34.
Daniels, N. (2001). 'Social responsibility and global pharmaceutical companies' *Developing World Bioethics* 1: 38–41.
DeGeorge, R. (1995). *Business Ethics* 4th ed. Englewood Cliffs, NJ: Prentice-Hall.
Ferrell, O. and Fraedrick, J. (1991). *Business Ethics*. Boston: Houghton Mifflin.
Friedman, M. (1970). 'The social responsibility of business is to increase its profits', *New York Times Magazine* (13th September 1970): 1.
Gerth, J. and Stolberg, S. (2000). 'Drug firms reap profits on tax-backed research', *New York Times* (23 April 2000): A1, A20–21.
Goldhammer, A. (2001). 'Current issues in clinical research and the development of new pharmaceuticals'. *Accountability in Research* 8: 283–92.
Jacobsen, R. (1991). 'Economic efficiency and the quality of life' *Journal of Business Ethics* 10: 201–209.
McNeil, D. (2000a). 'As devastating epidemics increase, nations take on drug companies'. *New York Times* (9th July 2000): A1.
McNeil, D. (2000b). 'Selling cheap generic drugs, India's copycats irks industry'. *New York Times* (1st December 2000): F1.
Miller, A. and Davis, M. (2000). *Intellectual Property*, 3rd ed. St. Paul, MN: West Group.
Murphy, P. (1998). *Eighty Exemplary Ethics Statements*. Notre Dame, Indiana: University of Notre Dame Press.
Pharmaceutical Research and Manufacturing Association (PHRMA). (2004). Research and Development. Available at: http://www.phrma.org/issues/researchdev/. Accessed: 20th December 2004.
Pojman, L. (1995). *Ethics*. Belmont, CA: Belmont, CA.
Reich, M. (2000). 'The global drug gap,' *Science* 287: 1979–1981.
Resnik, D. (2003a). 'Exploitation in biomedical research,' *Theoretical Medicine and Bioethics* 24: 233–259.
Resnik, D. (2003b). 'A pluralistic account of intellectual property,' *The Journal of Business Ethics* 46: 319–35.
Resnik, D. (2004). 'The distribution of biomedical research resources and international justice,' *Developing World Bioethics* 4: 42–57.
Samuelson, P. (1980). *Economics*. New York: McGraw Hill.
Schüklenk, U. (1998). *Access to Experimental Drugs in Terminal Illness*. New York: Pharmaceutical Products Press.
Shamoo, A. and Resnik, D. (2003). *Responsible Conduct of Research*. New York: Oxford University Press.
Simpson, J. (1982). 'Ethics and multinational corporations *vis-à-vis* developing nations,' *Journal of Business Ethics* 1: 227–37.
Spinello, R. (1992). 'Ethics, pricing, and the pharmaceutical industry', *Journal of Business Ethics* 11: 617–626.
Sterckx, S. (2004). 'Patents and access to drugs in developing countries: an ethical analysis', *Developing World Bioethics* 4: 58–75.
Sternberg, S. (2000). 'AIDS activists discount big drugmakers' gifts,' *US Today* (11th July 2000): 9D.
Stolberg, G. and Gerth, J. (2000). 'Medicine merchants: holding down the competition,' *New York Times* (23rd April 2000): A1.
Swarns, R. (2000). 'South Africa to distribute $50 Million in donated AIDS drugs,' *New York Times* (2nd December 2000): D1.

Chapter 8

Affordable access to essential medication in developing countries: conflicts between ethical and economic imperatives[1]

The vast majority of HIV/AIDS patients in developing countries have no access to life-saving drugs. In this chapter **Udo Schüklenk** *and* **Richard Ashcroft** *argue on broadly consequentialist grounds that compulsory licensing is preferable, both morally and pragmatically, to the alternatives, notably price cuts and drug donation schemes.*

The scope of the epidemic and its likely devastating consequences for socio-economic development has made the issue of access to essential medications a particularly urgent one. Edwin Cameron, an openly HIV-positive South African Appellate Court judge, sums up the problem:

> Nearly 34 million people in our world are at this moment dying [of AIDS]. And they are dying because they don't have the privilege that I have, of purchasing my health and life . . . Now why should I have the privilege of purchasing my life and health when 34 million people in the resource-poor world are falling ill, feeling sick to death, and dying? That to me . . . seems a moral inequity of such fundamental proportions that no one can look at it and fail to be spurred to thought and action about it. That is something which we in Africa cannot accept. It is something that the developed world also cannot accept (Cameron 2000).

In South Africa, of an estimated more than four million HIV-infected individuals, only 10 000 are able at current prices to afford access to life-sustaining essential AIDS medication. In Malawi the reported figure is 30 out of one million infected Malawians. In Uganda about 1.2 percent of the estimated 820 000 people living with AIDS can afford any of the drugs used to treat the illness (AFP 2001). The same picture is repeated all over the developing world, except in a few countries that do not have restrictive patent laws. Brazil is one such country. It started producing generic copies of essential AIDS medications in the mid-1990s. The result is that the country's AIDS mortality rate declined by about 50 percent (Chequer, Sudo & Vitfria 2000). What this suggests is that the pricing of essential AIDS medication is one of the key factors in bringing the AIDS mortality rate down in societies with functioning health care delivery infrastructures. This is not disputed even by the pharmaceutical industry's lobby organisation, International Federation of Pharmaceutical Manufacturers' Associations (IFPMA 2000).

Our objective in this chapter is to analyse problems related to the pricing of essential AIDS medications and the economic reasons why the vast majority of patients in developing countries have no access to such life-saving drugs. We then develop a substantive argument in favour of compulsory licensing of essential AIDS medications in the current conditions of public health emergency.

The regulatory frameworks

What factors control the level of availability of medications in a country? A product is available in a market if there is a manufacturer who is prepared to make the product and willing to sell it in that market and a purchaser who is able to pay for that product. These factors are variables that are relevant to the access to HIV/AIDS medications in Africa. In many situations, for instance, the health care infrastructure needed to make use of these medications effectively is lacking. But for the most part, and with most reason, critics have concentrated on supply factors that influence the availability of HIV/AIDS drugs, rather than on demand factors.

The two principle features on the supply side are the price of HIV/AIDS drugs in developing world markets and the maintenance of barriers to entry into the manufacture of such drugs. Prices in markets are normally fixed by two factors – the willingness of suppliers to supply goods at varying price levels and the willingness of purchasers to buy the goods at varying price levels. However, where there are few suppliers or only one supplier of a good, purchasers have relatively little influence over the price set, and the manufacturer will choose whatever level of price best reflects the ability to manufacture the goods in question and the level of profit that can be expected at that price. In non-competitive markets, suppliers have the freedom to choose the level of profit they take. And the level of manufacture they choose will vary according to the alternative markets they can enter, the other goods they can manufacture and the overall business requirement to maximise profits (or shareholder value).

In these conditions, buyers have little *economic* power to vary the price, beyond threatening to withdraw from the market altogether or to dramatically cut the quantity of goods they purchase. Where a good is 'essential', and where the purchaser is a state, acting as a proxy for a group of end-users, whose interests are in purchasing the good if at all possible, this threat is more formal than actual.

States can vary the quantity of drugs they purchase only within certain hard constraints, set by national income (taxes, trade and loan capital), and other claims on government expenditure. In many states in Africa, assuming the prices remain at current levels, making HIV/AIDS medication the highest budgetary priority would make some progress into universal coverage, but would still not get close to achieving that aim. An important factor influencing price and purchase of drugs is therefore the chosen level of profit of the drug companies, and the barriers to entry to drug manufacture. Amongst these are international regulatory standards on quality and purity of manufacture (which can be met as the examples of India and Brazil demonstrate) and the enforcement of intellectual property rights.

There are three issues to consider relating to the latter. Firstly, even if companies' intellectual property rights are honoured and enforced, this does not address whether the price they charge is fair, and what their responsibilities to set a fair price might be. We will return to this point below. Secondly, are there recognised exceptions or limits to intellectual property rights? Thirdly, if there are, why are these not in fact applied in the current international arena?

The division on Trade Related Aspects of Intellectual Property Rights (TRIPS) of the World Trade Organisation (WTO) oversees the national patent laws of the WTO national member nations. A great deal of criticism has been levelled by treatment access activists against the WTO and the TRIPS agreement (Pollock and Price 2000). They are seen as the reason why developing world governments have refused to simply issue compulsory licenses in order to facilitate the local production of essential AIDS drugs (i.e. to producers of high-quality generic drugs, such as India's CIPLA). On paper, however, it seems as if TRIPS does not actually prevent developing countries from issuing compulsory licenses. Article 31(b) provides that:

> Such use may only be permitted if, prior to such use, the proposed user has made efforts to obtain authorisation from the right holder on reasonable commercial terms and conditions and that such efforts have not been successful within a reasonable period of time. This requirement may be waived by a Member in the case of a national emergency or other circumstances of extreme urgency or in cases of public non-commercial use (World Trade Organisation).

Speculation that the US government or the European Commission, succumbing to lobbyists sponsored, for instance, by IFPMA, would declare a trade war against developing countries that used TRIPS Article 31(b) does not seem to be true either. The European Commissions Trade Commissioner, Pascale Lamy, stated in September 2000 during a Round Table on Communicable Diseases:

> . . . in the trade area, I am committed to do whatever is necessary in order to shape the right conditions so that the poorest of the poor will have access to the medicines they deserve at affordable prices . . . In the area of intellectual property rights, it is acknowledged that TRIPS provides for the necessary flexibility to address public health concerns and emergency situations (European Commission 2000).

On 27 January 2000, the US government wrote, as follows, to the Thai government through its Assistant Trade Representative for Services, Investment and Intellectual Property:

> If the Thai government determines that issuing a compulsory license is required to address its health crisis, the United States will raise no objection, provided the compulsory license is issued in a manner fully consistent with the WTO Agreement on TRIPS (IPI 2000: 17).

It can be seen, thus, that there are recognised exceptions to intellectual property rights in situations of national emergency.

The question we now turn to is why developing countries do not make use of the TRIPS provision to issue compulsory local licenses of essential AIDS drugs and begin local production. There seem to be various reasons for this, not all of which are 'hard' reasons in the sense that they are technically plausible. Most, but not all, are related to perceived economic types of punishment that could be meted out by various players against developing countries. Pharmaceutical companies have threatened to close down operations in countries that decide to issue such licenses (PhRMA 1999). Invariably, the threat of job losses makes a substantial impact in countries with high unemployment rates. Indeed, various attempts by developing world governments to pass legislation designed to permit compulsory licensing have been met by vigorous legal responses by the pharmaceutical industry. For instance, in South Africa the government passed a new law on 23 November 1997 – the Medicines and Related Substances Control Act Amendments – that, if implemented, would allow the issuing of compulsory local licenses for essential AIDS medications. Specifically, Article 15(c) of the new law states:

> The Minister may prescribe conditions for the supply of more affordable medicines in certain circumstances so as to protect the health of the public, and in particular may – (a) notwithstanding anything to the contrary contained in the Patents Act, 1978 (Act No. 57 of 1978), determine that the rights with regard to any medicine under a patent granted in the Republic shall not extend to act in respect of such medicine which has been put onto the market by the owner of the medicine, or with his or her consent.

A coalition of 39 pharmaceutical multinationals took, and then dropped, court action against the South African government in order to prevent this law from coming into effect. Largely due to outrage voiced internationally across all ideological divides, the multinationals withdrew the case. However, the US-based pharmaceutical industry lobby organisation, Pharmaceutical Research and Manufacturers of America (PhRMA), asked the United States Trade Representative (USTR) to put South Africa on the watch list of countries suspected of breaching TRIPS (PhRMA 2001). In another incident, the *Wall Street Journal* reported:

> In letters to a drug distributor in Ghana and an Indian generic-drug maker, Glaxo said sales of generic versions of its drug, Combivir, in Ghana would be illegal because they would be violating company patents. As a result, the Indian company, Cipla Ltd. of Bombay, has stopped selling its low-cost version in Ghana, a small country in West Africa. However, officials at the multilateral African agency that issued the Glaxo patents in question said they are either invalid in Ghana or don't apply (Schoofs 2000).

It is not the objective of this chapter to analyse these legal battles exhaustively. Yet even this brief survey indicates how the pharmaceutical industry and its lobbyists inside and outside the US government and the European Commission threaten the ability of governments of developing countries to facilitate local, cheap production of essential AIDS drugs or the importation of drugs from producer countries of high-quality generics. The international Red Cross organisation is sufficiently alarmed to issue a statement on the legal case in South Africa and a related one in Brazil. Its president, Astrid Heiberg, states unequivocally that the current drug pricing for developing countries is 'unacceptable', and that 'the public health emergency provisions of the World Trade Organisation framework would be rendered useless if the (legal) cases against Brazil and South Africa succeeded' (IFRC 2001). At the time of writing the Brazil case is still pursued by the manufacturing industry. To sum it up in the words of Peter Piot, executive director of UNAIDS:

> In the north, in return for innovation, intellectual property is protected and profits are made. This has benefited both northern shareholders and society. But it doesn't work for the south, where 95 percent of the world's population of 36.1 million with HIV/AIDS lives (Collins 2001).

There is another possible reason why developing world governments have embarked on a major publicity campaign against pharmaceutical companies. This reason is related to the fact that even if drug prices came down dramatically and local production began as a consequence of compulsory licensing, developing the necessary delivery infrastructure and financial resources to deliver the drugs would come at a high price tag. It is possible that developing countries may engage in high-profile campaigns against pharmaceutical companies in order to deflect from their own failure to put the necessary infrastructure in place to deliver the medication. Countries such as South Africa would be able to provide this infrastructure, if the political will existed to foot the bill. The South African government, for instance, did nothing to prepare its health care system for a possible court victory, thereby giving rise to the question of whether it is seriously intent on delivering essential AIDS medication to its people. Companies have complained about the difficulty they face in getting access to governments in order to negotiate. In other words, although high drug prices are a major hindrance in attempts to deliver essential medication to the poor, they are not the only reason. It would be wrong to paint a simplistic picture of the evil industry versus the brave governments of developing countries trying to save the lives of their suffering peoples.

Proposed solutions to the access problem

Given that access to medications is a real problem and that the price of such medications and the barriers to entry constructed by international policy decisions and pharmaceutical industry business decisions are, in part, the basis of this, what solutions exist?

Arguably both pharmaceutical companies and developed world governments recognise that they have a *moral* responsibility to act to prevent the AIDS holocaust from happening. They do not seem to think that because they have not caused the HIV infection rates in developing countries, they are not responsible for preventing (some of the) preventable deaths from happening.[2] We shall describe in the following brief and incomplete survey how both industry and other developed country donors have responded to the moral challenges posed by AIDS. In essence, we see three types of responses: donation of drugs, price discounts, and compulsory licensing to bypass patent protection and permit production of generic versions of HIV/AIDS drugs.

1. Private donations by pharmaceutical companies

Individual pharmaceutical companies have pledged by means of a panoply of schemes to donate essential AIDS medication free of charge to developing countries. Among these donations was Boehringer-Ingelheim's offer to provide Nevirapene, a drug proven to reduce drastically the mother-to-child transmission of HIV, for free for a limited period of time. Pfizer has agreed to provide free Fluconazole to South Africans affected by cryptococcal meningitis. The problem with these handouts is, of course, that such offers are fraught with conditions, time and quantity-based limitations and a continuing dependence of the developing country's health care planning on the generosity of commercial organisations. It is probably not unfair to suggest that this generosity could cease in an instant should the public interest move on to the latest CNN-provided coverage of yet another worldwide catastrophe, or should some commercial contingency arise.

Other organisations have donated funds to developing countries. Merck provided US$3 million to the Harvard AIDS Institute to develop and implement a care programme in Senegal and Brazil, and Bristol-Myers Squibb provided US$100 million to its own 'Secure the Future' programme, which involves setting up a large number of programmes in African countries, and training of African health care professionals at US tertiary institutions. While these initiatives are commendable, questions over the role of the pharmaceutical industry in sponsoring academic departments exist, particularly in the light of the recent scandals in Canada (Spurgeon 1999, Boseley 2001).

The philanthropic approaches discussed here are very important morally, in two opposed ways. On the one hand, they represent a recognition by corporations that they do have the capacity to act morally and, possibly, have a duty to aid those affected by disaster. To the extent that these donations link charity with a drive for a good public reputation and a strong negotiating position in regulatory or pricing discussions, we can grumble about their intentions. The positive features of such donations are that they occur, they are not coerced and they represent an assumption of moral agency and moral responsibility by corporations. On the other hand, there is a moral distinction between charitable giving as voluntary and honorable and acting on duty. Duty – in this case, the duty to prevent preventable deaths where one can – is not optional but required. Charity involves the liberty to divert one's giving elsewhere if it suits one, and to arrogate to oneself the right to desist if the recipient is 'ungrateful' or 'undeserving' (Chapter 6 explores this issue in more detail).

A second argument against charity is that it morally degrades the individual by fostering dependence, promoting an attitude of humility toward the giver, and depriving the recipient of the ability to set terms and negotiate the terms of receipt. This argument is difficult to use because it may imply that aid *per se* is wrong, rather than the specific form of aid, namely supererogatory, discretionary, conditional charity. One might develop instead a theory of charity that appeals to principles of mutual aid, solidarity and reciprocity, and that overcomes the 19th century paternalism hinted at in charitable donation. More radically, one might argue that the donation of drugs is a partial fulfilment of a duty to the disaster-struck or of a more general historical debt owed by the developed world to the developing. We have no space to develop these suggestions here, but they are familiar arguments in development studies (Unger 1996, Rodney 1972).

Donation of drugs is thus an ad hoc solution, which may go part way to solving the problem, but is morally problematic.

Donation of drugs is thus an ad hoc solution, which may go part way to solving the problem, but is morally problematic. The reasons for this are aretaic (to do with the motives and character of donor and recipient) and consequentialist (the solution is not sustainable and overlooks the sense in which companies and states have an obligation to prevent avoidable deaths when they have the power to do so).

2. Price reductions

Pharmaceutical companies have also begun to reduce the prices of their patented essential drugs in order to make them available to more people in need. Bristol-Myers Squibb announced the price reduction of two widely used AIDS drugs, ddI and d4T to about US$500 in Senegal. Mark Harrington of New York-based Treatment Action Group analysed this offer as follows:

> Senegal has 79 900 people living with HIV. If one quarter of them need antiretroviral therapy this would mean that about 20 000 Senegalese would need anti-HIV therapy. The BMS discount, when added to one by Merck, would bring the cost of one year's triple therapy to between US$950–1,850. The median income in Senegal is US$510 per year (Harrington 2000).

Merck is providing a US$50 million donation, primarily in the form of a price reduction (matched by another US$50 million by the Gates Foundation) to Botswana. The money is primarily given to develop a comprehensive infrastructure for dealing with HIV/AIDS. An unspecified percentage of the Merck donation comes in the form of drug subsidies (i.e. subsidies for Merck drugs). Harrington comments, 'If Merck and Gates together are giving US$10 million per year, this means that 50 000 (of 290 000) could be treated per year if the cost of antiretroviral therapy was US$200 per year. There would be no money left over for prevention, testing and counselling, health care clinics, treatment and prevention of opportunistic infections and palliative care (Harrington 2000). Other companies, such as Hoffmann-LaRoche, have promised steep discounts that are yet to transpire.

Effectively, the companies are moving towards a solution that encompasses differential prices in developed and developing countries. Strange as it may sound to the uninitiated observer, many patented drugs are substantially *higher* priced in developing countries than they are in some developed countries. Much of this has to do with the fact that many developed countries (such as, for instance, Australia, Norway and others) put price caps on patented drugs. Manufacturers are not permitted to sell drugs at a higher price or else governments withdraw the approval for the drug to be sold in the particular market (Brody 1995).

The problem with the discount-based approach is, as in the case of donations, that such offers are fraught with conditions, time- and quantity-based limitations and a continuing dependence of developing country's health care planning on the goodwill of commercial organisations. Moreover, this is a solution that corporations are quick to criticise in other circumstances: parallel pricing is the classic revenue profit maximisation method for monopolists and oligopolists, yet it is always at risk of being undermined by market entrants and through 'arbitrage'. Arbitrage is the buying of a good 'G' at price 'p' in one market 'M', and selling it at price 'q' ($q > p$) in another market 'N' where good G is priced at price r ($r > q$), so as to capture part or all of the market N for good G. The arbitrageur does not produce good G, but 'steals' from the producer of G a good proportion of the producer's profits. The social efficiency of the markets M and N is increased by bringing the price in N closer to that in M, so everyone except the producer is happier.

The price reduction solution is therefore limited in its utility, in the form in which it has been applied to date, because formally it is similar to the donation solution.

A classical way of blocking arbitrage is to enforce patent rights over G, use them to construct barriers to entry to markets, and to issue manufacture or sales licences that ban arbitrage or make it uneconomic. It is precisely this strategy that pharmaceutical manufacturers use to ban parallel importing (as far as possible) in the developed world, and to block competition by generics manufacturers. The market mechanism is blocked from generating competitive prices. Note also that parallel pricing is 'good' if the patent-holder does it, but 'bad' if someone else tries to do so. And further, parallel pricing is not primarily about goodwill, but about revenue maximisation. Even in low-price markets, price is still in excess of marginal cost. So the seller is making a sale it would not otherwise have made and makes no loss on that sale.

The price reduction solution is therefore limited in its utility, in the form in which it has been applied to date, because formally it is similar to the donation solution. Like that, it represents as charitable what is actually sound business policy, and from a consequentialist point of view is suboptimal in both the avoidance of avoidable death and in terms of the sustainability of the policy and the recognition of the social responsibilities of companies and states.

3. Public-private partnerships

The latest buzzword amongst international UN agencies, governments such as the UK and pharmaceutical companies is 'public-private partnership' (Price, Pollock and Shaoul 1998, Gaffney et al. 1999). This concept, too, does not question the industry's control over prices through patents. Instead it proposes to work together with pharmaceutical companies and developing world governments to secure sustainable price reductions. The idea is, partly, to purchase huge quantities of essential drugs and thereby to achieve price reductions caused by the combined purchasing power of various countries and agencies. All countries in a UNAIDS pilot programme (Chile, Côte d'Ivoire, Uganda and Vietnam) established non-profit organisations designated to distribute the purchased drugs. This UNAIDS-sponsored programme was anything but successful. Dr Peter Mguyenyi of the Joint Clinical Research Centre in Kampala, Uganda commented during the International AIDS Conference in Durban in a paper entitled 'Market Failure in Uganda':

> The UNAIDS pilot treatment access initiative which has been carried out for the last two years in Côte d'Ivoire and Uganda has not been a success. It has resulted in no appreciable reduction in the cost of drugs. In some cases prices went up. It's been a miserable failure. The UNAIDS/pharmaceutical company announcement this spring about 'massive' price reductions was more political than practical; it was done for the media.

Overall, at the end of 2000 it seems that about 4 000 people in developing countries received access to essential medication through the programme. Considering that it took years to get to that stage, and considering the overall number of people worldwide who need access to such medications and do not have it, this strategy does not exactly constitute an overwhelming success. Arguably, however, 4 000 more people with access to essential drugs is better than none. In October 2000 WHO, UNICEF and UNAIDS put out a public tender to provide essential AIDS medications at a preferential price to developing countries. These organisations' strategy clearly is to not question the industry's patents and to use the market mechanism to achieve the desirable lower prices. Yet the role of patents is precisely to prevent the market mechanism from operating to reduce prices in the short run, and it is not clear why this strategy is supposed to work.

David Resnik defends a different idea of public-private partnerships in biomedical research (Resnik 2001, Brock 2001, Daniels 2001). He believes that developing countries have a moral obligation to contribute to research efforts just as much as commercial organisations do. That would then entitle them to a seat at the table, so to speak. In his paper Resnik uncritically repeats claims of the pharmaceutical manufacturers, such as 'the plain truth is that a great deal of research would simply not be done without money from this industry' (Resnik 2001: 14). It seems quite conceivable that non-profit operators such as universities, charities and indeed governments would step in to fill this breach.

One might argue that non-commercial actors would be less efficient in seeking new treatments or less able to bear the financial risk of developing new drugs. If this is so, we might question why so much primary research in highly applied disciplines such as biotechnology is actually based in the largely public university sector (but also why that sector is being privatised piecemeal as a means of raising money for universities). Some authors, in fact, have questioned whether it is acceptable that taxpayer-funded research is exploited by pharmaceutical companies. These companies often buy such results for a paltry fee, patent them and effectively re-sell the product to the very same taxpayers that financed their development (Arno and Davis, in press). Resnik's argument appeals to an evidential claim about industrial policy, which requires him to produce evidence for it.

Decency and common humanity require agents capable of preventing a death to do so, where possible, as a prima facie *duty.*

In any case, Resnik bases his arguments for patent protection and recognition on the industry's need to make money. He ignores, however, that the profits necessary to sustain sufficient investment in research have never been made in developing countries. The pharmaceutical industry, by any standards amongst one of the most profitable industries (Gerth and Stolnick 2001, Resnik 2001: 13) makes its profits *not* in developing countries where the vast majority of people are unable to purchase its products, but in developed countries.

Analytically, we can also question the 'need' to make money. The 'essence' of firms, in some Aristotelian sense, might be the attempt to make money, although micro-economists such as Herbert Simon have been questioning whether real corporations are actually profit-maximisers in their behaviour for a generation. They have legal obligations to their shareholders, and tough-minded 'business ethicists' agree that the morality of business requires them to promote 'shareholder value'. But these same thinkers require businesses and business people to act with common human decency (Sternberg 2000). Decency and common humanity require agents capable of preventing a death to do so, where possible, as a *prima facie* duty. So, arguably, Resnik's appeal to business norms as prior to common norms for corporations is misplaced or at least incomplete.

In their respective replies to Resnik's paper, both Dan Brock and Norman Daniels point out that even if African countries ignored patents, either by breaking international trade agreements such as TRIPS, or by compulsory licensing, or by parallel importation of the required generic drugs, it would not make a significant difference to these organisations' financial bottom lines (Brock 2001, Daniels 2001). In Brock's words:

> When developing countries choose not to respect product patents as their only effective means of making available pharmaceuticals necessary to save lives and protect the health of their citizens, doing so is arguably a step forward to greater justice between the developed and developing world; this may be a case where two wrongs make a right, that is where existing global injustices make not respecting product patents, which in the absence of those injustices would be wrong, all things considered, morally justified (Brock 2001: 37).

Public-private partnerships have as yet not yielded the desired effect, i.e. to provide essential drugs (and we should not limit this unduly to the fashionable AIDS issue) to poor patients whose life is at stake. Arguably then, making use of the above-mentioned TRIPS provision or even breaking international trade agreements might be a given developing country's most effective means of providing life-saving medication time-efficiently to its people. What the description of the status quo above has shown, in our view, that appeals to a given pharmaceutical company's moral responsibilities, ethical corporate citizenship and so on and so forth, lead nowhere. There is a quite considerable amount of window-dressing, but no action has been forthcoming as yet that would bring us even close to what is required to save the millions of lives that are at stake.

4. Compulsory licensing

Compulsory licensing, to permit the manufacture of generic equivalents of patented drugs for HIV/AIDS at prices set in a competitive market, is lawful (with respect to TRIPS) in situations of national emergency and when negotiations have failed to ensure a fair price that would enable parties to satisfy their objectives – of recouping investment costs and of maximally preventing avoidable deaths from HIV/AIDS. We note that there is an obligation on states to define 'emergency' responsibly, and to take all reasonable steps to prevent such emergencies.

Prima facie, the validity of this approach is established by elimination of the other alternatives – donation, ad hoc price reduction, and public-private partnership – on moral and pragmatic grounds. However, we believe that there are good intrinsic reasons to support the compulsory licensing approach. Firstly, intellectual property rights are designed to promote innovation in the public interest. However, where they contravene the public interest, the justification for their enforcement in that context is removed. Secondly, intellectual property rights have been used in this debate as a diversion from the real issue here, which is the unaffordability of essential medications in the situations where they are most needed.

Thirdly, while intellectual property rights are important, and should be defended, and while parallel importing into high-price markets in the resource-rich world is a matter for legitimate concern in the industry, companies have been too quick to make airy allegations about the destruction of shareholder value and their ability to recover costs and pursue a full R&D programme without setting out their evidence in the public domain. Their appeal to intellectual property rights is consequentialist in character, but few serious attempts have been made to give these arguments a foundation in evidence. In the absence of this, we argue that the effective prevention of avoidable deaths, the operation of efficient competitive markets through lowering of artificial barriers to entry, and the assertion of legitimate national sovereignty in the international arena are conclusive *prima facie* justifications of compulsory licensing.

Prices set in a competitive market could still be unaffordable by states and citizens.

Of course, prices set in a competitive market could still be unaffordable by states and citizens. Marginal costs could still be too high for sustainable purchase in many countries. Our argument here does not establish a duty on generic manufacturers to sell at below cost. There is still a major role for international aid, state investment and, especially, primary prevention of infection and the construction of sustainable infrastructure. State parties to the various UN declarations and charters on human rights are obliged to develop health infrastructure (Andreopoulos 2000).

As good consequentialists, we should note that the compulsory licensing approach is not without risk. Corporations may feel less able to assume research and development (R&D) risks if their right to sell goods at a profit to regain investment costs is compromised by the risk of compulsory licensing. And this may also affect their choice of products to develop – for instance, they may concentrate on 'luxury' high-cost drugs for lifestyle conditions, rather than 'essential' medications for life-threatening and chronic disease. However, we note that corporations are still at liberty to derive monopoly profits in markets where poverty and epidemics do not combine to create large-scale health and development disasters, as with AIDS (and other endemic diseases) in Africa and elsewhere in the developing world. Parallel importing is still open to regulatory control. Even with the current liberal approach to trade, investment in diseases endemic in the developing world is low, so the argument from a need to maintain liberalism to continue such investment appears to rest on a false premise. Moreover, much R&D is actually public sector work, or supported in partnership with the public sector.

Conclusions

We have established the compelling need to address the HIV/AIDS health and development crisis in the resource-poor countries of the world. We have also examined the commonly accepted approaches to addressing this need through charitable donation, price reduction and public-private partnership, and the current evidence for their (lack of) effectiveness. We have seen that the WTO's TRIPS regulations permit states, in national emergencies, to compulsorily license the production-patented goods. We hold that for efficiency and moral reasons the conditions for using this clause exist, and that the alternatives, whatever their intrinsic moral merits, are less effective and less morally acceptable than compulsory licensing. Our arguments have aimed to show firstly that there is an emergency; secondly, that corporations and states, no less than individuals, have a moral duty to maximise the prevention of preventable deaths by making AIDS drugs cheaply available; thirdly, that this is a matter of need and duty, rather than want and supererogatory charity, and fourthly, that evaluation of corporations' motives, while an enjoyable pastime, is actually irrelevant from the points of view of law, economics and ethics.

Endnotes

[1] The authors wish to thank the anonymous referees of this journal, as well as Loretta M Kopelman and Anton A van Niekerk for constructive criticism of earlier drafts of this paper. Joanna Taylor provided invaluable research assistance to Udo Schüklenk.

[2] The moral reasons for this have, of course, much to do with a rejection of the acts and omissions doctrine (Glover, 1977).

References

AFP Report. (2001). Price cuts have little impact on access to AIDS drugs in Uganda. March 23rd, 2001 http://sg.news.yahoo.com/010323/1/kz9m.html (accessed 03-24-2001).

Andreopoulos, G. (2000). Declarations and covenants on human rights and international codes of research ethics. In Levine, R.J., Gorovitz, S., Gallagher J. (eds.) *Biomedical research ethics: updating international guidelines – a consultation* Geneva: CIOMS.

Arno, P.S. & Davis, M.H. (in press). Why don't we enforce existing price controls? The unrecognised and unenforced reasonable pricing requirements imposed upon patents deriving in whole or in part from federally-funded research. *Tulane Law Review*.

Boseley, S. (2001). Bitter pill. *The Guardian* 7th May 2001 http://www.guardian.co.uk/Archive/Article/0,4273,4181987,00.html (accessed 05-08-2001).

Brock, D.W. (2001). Some questions about the moral responsibilities of drug companies. *Developing World Bioethics*. 1:33–37.

Brody, B. (1995). *Ethical issues in drug testing, approval and pricing: The clot dissolving drugs*. New York: Oxford University Press.

Cameron, E. (2000). Press conference, XII International AIDS Conference, Durban, South Africa, July 10, 2000 (as quoted in Harrington, M. (2000)).

Chequer P., Sudo, E.C. & Vitfria, M.A.A. (2000). The impact of anti-retroviral therapy in Brazil. Paper presented at International AIDS Conference in Durban, paper no. MoPpE1066.

Collins, H. (2001). UN Agency calls on drug firms to do more in AIDS fight. *Philadelphia Inquirer* 15th February.

Daniels, N. (2001). Social responsibility and global pharmaceutical companies. *Developing World Bioethics*. 1:38–41.

European Commission (2000). Press release: Commissioner Lamy pledges action on access to medicines. http://europa.eu.int/comm/trade/whats_new/medic.html. Accessed on 03-17-2001.

Gaffney, D., Pollock, A.M., Price, D. & Shaoul, J. (1999). The private finance initiative: The politics of the private finance initiative and the new NHS. *British Medical Journal* 319: 249–253.

Gerth, J. & Stolberg S. (2001). Drug firms reap profits on tax-backed research. *New York Times* 04–23–2001:A1, 20–21.

Glover, J. (1977). *Causing Deaths and Saving Lives*. London: Penguin Books.

Harrington, M. (2000). *Brazil: What went right? The global challenge of access to treatment and the issue of compulsory licensing*. Address to the 10th national Brazilian meeting of people living with HIV and AIDS. http://www.aidsinfonyc.org/tag/activism.brazil.html. Accessed on 11-07-2001.

IFPMA (2000). *Increasing Access to Health Care in Developing Countries: The Need for Public-Private Partnerships*. Geneva: IFPMA.

IFRC (2001). Press release: Drug pricing for developing countries unacceptable. http://www.ifrc.org/Docs/News/01/031201/. Accessed 03-12-2001.

IMS Health (2000). Market report: five years forecast of the global pharmaceutical markets. http://www.ims-global.com/insight/report/global/report.htm. Accessed on 01–10–2001.

Intellectual Property Institute (2000). *Patent Protection and Access to HIV/AIDS Pharmaceuticals in Sub-Saharan Africa* Washington, DC: IPI.

PhRMA (1999). http://www.cptech.org/ip/health/phrma/301–99/safrica.html. Accessed 28-05/2001.

PhRMA (2001). http://www.phrma.org/intnatl/news/2001-02–20.40.pdf. Accessed on 03-12-2001.

Pollock, A.M. & Price, D. (2000). Rewriting the regulations: How the World Trade Organisation could accelerate privatisation in health systems. *Lancet* 356: 1995–2000.

Price, D., Pollock, A.M. & Shaoul, J. (1998). How the World Trade Organisation is shaping domestic policies in health care. *Lancet* 354: 1889–1892.

Rachels, J. (1986). *The End of Life*. New York: Oxford University Press.

Resnik, D. (2001). Developing drugs for the developing world: An economic, legal, moral and political dilemma. *Developing World Bioethics*. 1:11–32.

Rodney W (1972). *How Europe Underdeveloped Africa*. London: Bogle L'Ouverture Publications.

Schoofs, M. (2000). Glaxo attempts to block access to generic AIDS drugs in Ghana. *Wall Street Journal*. 12-01-2000.

Spurgeon, D. (1999). Toronto research funding dispute. *British Medical Journal*. 318:351.

Sternberg, E. (2000). *Just Business: Business ethics in action* (2nd Edition) New York: Oxford University Press.

Unger, P. (1996). *Living High and Letting Die*. New York: Oxford University Press.

World Trade Organisation. TRIPS: Agreement on Trade-related Aspects of Intellectual Property Rights. http://www.wto.org/english/tratop_e/trips_e/t_agm1_e.htm. Accessed on 03–12–2001.

Chapter 9

Mother-to-child transmission of HIV/AIDS in Africa: ethical problems and perspectives

The morality of placebo-controlled trials for drugs to prevent mother-to-child transmission (MTCT) of HIV/AIDS in Africa and the lack of political leadership and responsibility to implement proven programmes that combat MTCT are two major ethical issues. In this chapter **Anton A van Niekerk** *explores the relevant facts of MTCT before discussing the ethical issues and, in conclusion, presents some of the insights that these issues yield.*

It is commonplace to identify and bewail a plethora of problems in the developing world generally, and in Africa in particular. Poverty, illiteracy, famine, political instability, natural disasters and many more misfortunes dominate the history of this part of the world over the past 50 years. It was therefore adding uncalled (undeserved?) insult to already overwhelming injury when HIV/AIDS visibly[1] struck the (also developing) world in the mid-1980s. Despite all the other calamities that Africa has to deal with, it is no exaggeration to claim that HIV/AIDS now constitutes the most serious health and social crisis and challenge that has ever befallen that continent.

There are a range of ethical problems raised by the phenomenon of HIV/AIDS on the continent of Africa, and a large literature exists about many of these problems. In the course of this chapter, I shall occasionally refer to this literature. I have dealt elsewhere (cf. Van Niekerk 2002a and 2002b) with problems evoked by poverty as the social context for HIV/AIDS in Africa, the lack of political will to address the issue, the challenges surrounding the need for changes in people's sexual behaviour, issues of women's vulnerability to the epidemic, the disenchantment of intimacy as a result of the discourse on AIDS, and whether issues of privacy or publicness ought to take centre stage in the moral debate about HIV/AIDS. In this chapter, I shall focus on the ethical problem raised by the issue of mother-to-child transmission (MTCT) of HIV in Africa.

In what follows I describe relevant facts on MTCT before discussing the major ethical issues in this regard. In conclusion, I shall discuss a number of insights that these issues yield for our understanding of our power over disease in the contemporary world, the implications of these issues for our understanding of scientific methodology in medicine, the dangers of politicising a health problem such as HIV/AIDS, the need for renewed reflection on the global disparities in the provision of health care, and the need for imaginative and responsible political leadership and co-operation between the developed countries, Africa and the pharmaceutical corporations to address and combat a catastrophe of unprecedented global proportions.

Relevant facts on MTCT of HIV/AIDS in Africa

MTCT of HIV/AIDS in Africa represents one of the most contentious issues in the current debate about ethical problems related to HIV infection and management. HIV/AIDS, as is well known, is, as yet, an incurable viral infection. There also is, as yet, no available vaccine; at the time of writing, there are reports in the press about the results of clinical trials of the world's first systematic attempt at a vaccine, the so-called AidsVax. Researchers ascertained that this vaccine, based on the B and E strains of the virus (which are not prevalent in Africa), is safe, but that it protected only 3.8 percent of people injected with it (Altenroxel 2003: 1). Many other trials, some of them also based on the C strain of the virus that is affecting Africa, are currently researched and planned and will probably get underway soon, but the trials are set to last for many years. Normally a vaccine would have to be proven at least 70 percent effective to be considered for registration; however, given the severity of the problem in Africa, a 30 percent success rate might well be considered efficacious. In a country such as South Africa, where 1 500 people are infected daily, such a vaccine could then theoretically prevent 450 infections per day (Ibid.).

HIV is transmitted through the exchange of bodily fluids during homo- and heterosexual intercourse as well as by the sharing of needles by (ab-)users of drugs administered intravenously. This is known as 'horizontal' transmission, i.e. transmission from one person to another. The most significant other mechanism for infection is the so-called 'vertical' transmission from a pregnant woman to her unborn child. In the absence of both a cure and/or a vaccine, MCTC of HIV, however, does represent the one area where a significant reduction in the infection rate, and the concomitant saving of lives and relief of suffering, can be achieved. It is a well-established fact that the use of antiretroviral treatment during pregnancy can prevent the transmission of the virus from mother to child; the success rate with certain drugs is in the order of 50 percent (with highly active antiretroviral therapy in the US, the transmission rate is one percent – a 30-fold reduction).

It is therefore doubly ironic and tragic that this very possibility – one of the few potential areas of 'success' in combating this deadly epidemic – has become the arena of so much controversy, both as regards the legitimacy of the research methodology on which the trials to establish the efficacy of these drugs were concerned, as well as the utilisation by authorities, particularly in South Africa, of the opportunity to implement programmes for MTCT prevention. In what follows, I shall use the South African situation as a case study of how tragically a pertinent opportunity was and still is being forfeited in this regard.

HIV seroprevalence in pregnant women in South Africa, where statistics[2] are based on the attendance of country-wide antenatal clinics (and where anonymous testing is done regularly and systematically), averages 23 percent, rising up to 33 percent in the worst-hit provinces (MacIntyre & Gray 2000: 30–31). The UNAIDS figures of December 2002 show a decrease – about 15 percent – in the infection rate for women under the age of 20. However, for women in the age range of 20 to 29, the infection rate is still around 30 percent (UNAIDS Epidemic Update December 2002). Transmission figures can reach 35 percent when breastfeeding (which exacerbates the possibility of transmission) occurs, as some studies have shown. 'With a conservative estimate of 800 000 births per year in South Africa, this suggests that 70 000 infants are affected annually' (MacIntyre & Gray 2000: 30). Children that are born uninfected can become infected with HIV as a result of being breastfed by HIV-positive mothers.

HIV seroprevalence in pregnant women in South Africa averages 23 percent, rising up to 33 percent in the worst-hit provinces.

The possibility of a significant reduction of MTCT was first proven in 1994 when the Paediatric AIDS Clinical Trial Group (PACTG) did a comprehensive clinical trial in the US with the antiretroviral drug Zudovudine (AZT)[3]. It was conclusively shown that a regime – the so-called (and now famous) 076 regime – of this drug reduced vertical transmission of HIV from 25 percent to eight percent, i.e. by two thirds (De Zulueta, 2001: 290–291). These findings have repeatedly been confirmed, and have even been improved upon. A study in France, for example, showed that HIV-positive women who received the 076 regimen had a transmission rate of only 0.8 percent (Mandelbrot, Chenadec et al. 1998).

Is this regimen then not the answer to the serious MTCT problem that we are seeing in developing countries? In theory possibly, but not in practice. For this there are two main reasons. The first is a simple matter of cost; the 076 regimen is prohibitively expensive. Up until quite recently, a single treatment programme cost more than US$800, a sum that is several hundred times the annual per capita health care allocation in many developing countries (Resnik 1998: 289), particularly in Africa. Schüklenk points out that the producer of Zudovudine, Glaxo-Wellcome, offered the drug to women in developing countries at a price of between US$50–150 – something that might be affordable in a country such as Taiwan, but is still way beyond the financial capacity of most African countries (Schüklenk 1998: 317). In 2003, three milligrams of Zudovudine in South Africa cost R1 989.00 (US$331 at the February 2005 exchange rate) plus dispensing fees per prescription.

The second reason is that the 076 protocol is a very complex regimen that *inter alia* requires a great deal of labour, takes a long time to be administered effectively, and requires careful surveillance in order to address possible side-effects (Resnik 1998: 289). Given the short supply of qualified health care workers, particularly in the rural parts of most African countries, these represent almost insuperable barriers.

There was, consequently, an urgent need to investigate the efficacy of antiretroviral therapies that could be administered by means of short courses to HIV-positive women late in their pregnancies. Several trials were conducted in Thailand, Côte d'Ivoire, Burkina Faso and South Africa in which significantly shortened regimens of AZT were tested. The drug was administered in oral form from the 36th week of pregnancy for four weeks, followed by a single loading dose at the onset of labour, and twice daily for seven days after delivery. Significant reductions of MTCT – up to 38 percent in many cases – were noted in comparison with control groups, even in cases where breastfeeding continued (MacIntyre & Gray 2000). On the score of both problems identified above with the conventional 076 protocol, these regimens seemed better suited to the needs of developing countries. The cost of a single treatment programme was significantly cut; the alternative treatment regimen uses US$80 worth of AZT as compared to the US$800 worth of the drug in the 076 protocol (Resnik 2001: 289–290). Because patients are treated for much shorter periods of time, the complexity of administering the drug was also significantly reduced.

The drug regimen that has been the cause of the most controversy and debate in South Africa, however, is Nevirapine[4]. It is a 'fast-acting and potent antiretroviral with a long half-life' (MacIntyre & Gray 2000). It was originally tested in a trial called the 'HIVNET 012 trial' in Uganda. The trial investigated the use of a single 200mg dose administered orally to women at the onset of labour, followed by a single dose of 2mg/kg administered to infants within 72 hours of birth. This regimen was then compared to one in which 'intrapartum ZDV [i.e. AZT] and one week of infant ZDV treatment' (Ibid.) were administered. Almost all babies were breastfed. It was found that, in the Nevirapine group, the transmission rate, at the time when the newborns were 14 to 16 weeks of age, was 13.1 percent, contrary to 25.1 percent in the group with which they were compared (i.e. the group that received AZT as indicated above). The efficacy of Nevirapine was thus found to be 47 percent. The side effects of the two regimens were similar, and both were well tolerated (Ibid.). The wholesale cost of this regime is quoted as being US$4 per mother/child – almost incomparably cheaper than the original AZT regimens used in the developed worlds (De Zulueta 2001: 298).

The ethics of randomised placebo-controlled trials for shortened drug regimens to prevent MTCT of HIV

The results of trials for shortened, affordable and manageable drug regimens to prevent MTCT in developing nations were seemingly quite positive and provided laudable opportunities to set in place arrangements that could significantly reduce MTCT in (South) Africa. Yet the whole enterprise was steeped in serious controversy from the beginning, and until now has hardly been translated into a comprehensive programme of MTCT prevention in South Africa. For this apparent anomaly, there are two reasons of moral import, the first associated with the research process leading to the development of these drugs, and the second with the political impediments to the implementation of the knowledge yielded by these developments. I will deal with each in turn.

The first ethical issue that dominated discussion of the moral management of MTCT in the previous decade was whether double-blinded, randomised placebo-controlled trials (RPCT) for the shortened regimens of antiretroviral drugs in the developing world were at all ethical. The use of RPCT in the assessment of drugs is accepted worldwide. RPCT, as is well known, amounts to a procedure where the research subjects are divided into two groups. Over a fixed period of time one group receives the new drug, and the other a 'placebo', i.e. the equivalent of no relevant drug at all (or the so-called 'sugar pill'). Neither the research subjects nor the health care professionals administering the drugs are aware of which patients belong to which group; that information is only available to the managers of the trial, who are not in contact with the patients. Full written informed consent has to be given by all participants. The rationale for the procedure is to assess whether the drug in question makes any notifiable difference to the condition for which it is administered by comparing its outcome in patients who use it and those who do not.

The use of placebo in drug trials is morally justifiable only when the researchers are in a state of equipoise at the outset of a trial.

The controversy over the use of RPCT in the case of the shortened regimens of antiretrovirals in Africa was sparked by an article by Lurie and Wolfe (Lurie & Wolfe 1997) in which it was claimed that these trials were unethical since they violated an important moral rule that has been accepted for RCPT all over the developed world: if a new drug is tested for a condition for which there is a known, established and effective treatment, the patients in the control group have to, at least, receive this treatment, and not a mere placebo. Put differently, the use of placebo in drug trials is morally justifiable only when the researchers are in a state of equipoise at the outset of a trial. That means simply that a placebo may be used only when there exists no evidence that a treatment is more effective than a placebo (Resnik 1998: 290). If an effective drug for the condition is available and a new drug has to be tested, the drug trial ought, accordingly, not to be a randomised double-blind placebo-controlled trial, but rather a so-called 'equivalency' trial. Paquita de Zulueta explains this as follows:

> The use of a placebo is not a necessary or specific feature of the RCT (i.e. the randomised controlled trial), but it is required for answering the research question 'Is this treatment better than nothing?' An alternative question might be 'Is this treatment as good as, or nearly as good as, the accepted effective treatment?' The latter question would call for an equivalency trial (preferably a double-blind trial to eliminate bias) as recommended by Lurie and Wolfe' (De Zulueta 2001: 293).

Marcia Angell, executive editor of the *New England Journal of Medicine* (NEJM – arguably the most prestigious journal for medical science in the world), wrote an editorial (Angell 1997) in which she compared the RPCT in Africa with the infamous Tuskegee syphilis study that ran in the USA from the 1930s to the 1970s, in which poor, uneducated men continued to be used as a 'control group' in a syphilis drug study long after it was clear that penicillin was an effective drug for their disease. The Africa trials were, in turn, defended by Harold Varmus, Director of the National Institutes of Health (NIH) and David Satcher, Director of the Centre for Disease Control and Prevention in the United States (CDC). They argued that the critics of these trials were unfair and did not fully grasp the scientific, social and economic complexities of the research.[5] As a result of this controversy David Ho (*Time* Magazine's Man of the Year in 1996 because of his landmark research on antiretroviral 'cocktails') and Catherine Wilfert resigned from the board of the NEJM in protest at the editorial by Angell. (Marc Lallemant has, in the meantime, successfully conducted a ZDV equivalence study in Thailand.)[6]

An analysis of this debate shows a clear conflict between a deontological and a consequentialist approach to the problem. In a deontological approach, the moral argument takes one or more moral 'principles' or 'rules' as point of departure and applies them to the situation at hand. The position defended by Lurie, Wolfe and Angell is a deontological approach wherein the rule governing RPCT and equivalency trials is clearly formulated and stuck to at all costs and at all times. The idea of 'double standards' for research on human subjects in the first and third world respectively, is rejected out of hand. Such double standards, it is argued, will result in nothing but the exploitation of the third by the first world. Respect for human subjects and beneficence requires us to, at all costs, maintain the ethical standards for research on humans that are prevalent in the West and that are formulated in codes of research ethics such as the Helsinki Declaration and the Code of the Nuffield Council on Bioethics. In fact, in a spirited defence of this position, where she addresses the issue of cost and applicability of Western standards in Africa, De Zulueta even makes the following statement: 'The revised version of the Helsinki Declaration [which the author endorses] reinforces the deontological or 'clinical care' ethic, as opposed to the utilitarian ethic. Some might argue that the revised guidelines will create serious obstacles to carrying out research that could benefit poorer nations. Others would argue that this is the price that has to be paid if the moral responsibilities of researchers to individual participants are maintained' (De Zulueta 2001: 307–308).

Respect for human subjects and beneficence requires us to, at all costs, maintain the ethical standards for research on humans that are prevalent in the West.

What would the implication of this statement be? Is the author seriously arguing that, if the standards that govern the research on drug trials in the first world cannot be maintained *at all times* when doing research in the developing world, the latter research should simply *not ever be attempted*, even if arrangements are made by local people who conduct the research that are adapted to local circumstances and possibilities? This is a position that could hardly be taken seriously by people who are the actual victims of such a deadly pandemic as HIV/AIDS, and for whom participation in a drug trial often constitutes the only opportunity of accessing drugs that might relieve their suffering.

The argument in favour of placebo-controlled trials is normally developed along broad consequentialist lines. Consequentialism as an approach to moral reasoning requires that only the consequences of an act be considered when deciding on the moral status of the act. Utilitarianism, as the best known variety of consequentialism, requires that the greatest good for the most people involved be sought when assessing the moral status of an act. The consequentialist argument in this regard contains these three aspects[7]:

1. The recognised regimens of antiretrovirals that do quite successfully prevent MTCT in the developed nations, such as the AZT 076 regime, are prohibitively expensive and entirely unaffordable for women living with AIDS in Africa. In a country such as South Africa, the bulk of HIV-positive women (estimated at about two and a half million) are dependent on public sector medicine and have no form of health insurance. That means that they are entirely dependent on the state for health care. A simple calculation shows that, if we take the number of pregnant women that would require treatment in a single year to be 1.5 million, and the 076 regimen is assumed to cost US$800 per person (1998 figures), it would cost the South African government US$1.2 billion (i.e. ZAR7.2 billion). The entire budget for AIDS support in the most recent[8] (February 2003) budget of the South African Parliament, however, is ZAR3.3 billion, a third of the amount required. Note also that South Africa is one of sub-Saharan Africa's richest countries. There is, therefore, no realistic chance that something approaching the 076 AZT regimen can be utilised in most other sub-Saharan states. The only hope for HIV-positive mothers wishing to prevent MTCT to their newborns is significantly shortened (and hopefully more affordable) drug regimens. The development of such regimens is therefore absolutely essential if we want to assure that, at least in the one area where infection can be contained, such containment occurs.

   It can therefore generally be argued that placebo trials promote concerns such as social utility and justice for the most people possible under the dire constraints of the African context in which the effort is being made to improve the lives of HIV/AIDS victims, particularly children. The clear aim of the trials is to develop safe, cheap and effective treatments for, if not all, then at least for considerably more Africans than would have been the case without the knowledge yielded by these trials. The aim of social utility, understood as meeting urgent social and medical needs, is thus served. Resnik also points out that 'the trials promote justice by providing a fair distribution of the benefits and burdens of research ... The studies provide physicians and public health administrators in developing nations with practical answers about preventing perinatal transmission of HIV. Another way of putting this point is that the research satisfies the Declaration of Helsinki's requirement of reasonable availability' (Resnik 2001: 300).

2. Placebo controls are required for the sake of scientific rigour. They are the best way to ensure the safety and efficacy of the new drugs. Equivalency trials are not called for when testing the shortened regimens of antiretrovirals in Africa. Specifically, it cannot be simplistically assumed that the 076 AZT protocol has been sufficiently established to require that all research subjects be treated with AZT as the minimum required standard of care. The research questions underlying the two regimens are different. What was now being investigated in Africa was not a safe way of preventing MTCT in the developed world, but a safe way of preventing MTCT in Africa. Resnik points out that the research question has changed in two respects. First, what was pertinent was whether the shorter and cheaper regimens were as effective as no treatment at all. The standard level of care for HIV-positive women in Africa is, unfortunately, mostly no treatment at all. Second, the disputed studies operate in a population of research subjects that differ considerably from the ones targeted when the 076 regimen was tested. For example, children were used in the Nevirapine study, and children, in medicine, represent a completely different set of variables to deal with. The general condition and health risks of pregnant women in developing countries differ markedly from those in developed countries (cf. the high incidence of malaria and tuberculosis in the former). According to authors such as Varmus, Satcher and Resnik, all of these factors require a placebo control group in order to establish the safety and efficacy of the new drugs that were tested for the shortened regimens (Resnik 2001: 295–296).
3. It has been argued that the use of placebos is desirable in situations where the prescribed doses of AZT or other drugs required for equivalence trials are unaffordable. The argument in this regard is that, if the trials are performed by Africans and adapted to local conditions and to the capacity of the researchers performing them, and if sufficient informed consent is attained from the research subjects, it is paternalistic, if not downright imperialistic and maleficent to oppose such trials. This sentiment is expressed by David Ho, referred to above, in an article in *Time* from which I quote the following passage: 'These clinical trials ... were created for Africans by Africans with the good of their people in mind and with their informed consent. The studies were designed to be responsive to local needs and to the constraints of each study site. African scientists have argued that it is not in their best interest to include a complicated and costly AZT regimen for the sake of comparison when such a regimen is not only unaffordable but logistically infeasible. They have, instead, opted for a study design that is achievable in

practice and is likely to provide lifesaving answers expeditiously, even though it includes a group of women receiving a placebo. While the inclusion of this placebo group would not be acceptable in the US, the sad truth is that giving nothing is the current standard of care in Africa' (Ho 1997: 59).

I agree with Resnik (2001: 300) that this consequentialist argument suffers from the crassness often attached to arguments where the end justifies just about any means. It is dubious to argue that economic considerations should dictate experimental designs. Placebo controls should, preferably, only be used when required in terms of scientific rigour, otherwise people (i.e. those receiving placebos) are clearly and exclusively used to benefit others without any identifiable benefit to themselves. If placebos are not used for the sake of scientific rigour, and only for the sake of getting the trials funded, they are used for the wrong reasons. Over and against this, the consequentialists argue that, without funding, procured in this (possibly morally dubious) way, the trials would never take place and no one would benefit. It is clear that the large pharmaceutical companies can, in this respect, come to the aid and provide funding in such a manner that the use of placebos are limited to situations where the canons of scientific method, and nothing else, require them.

If placebos are not used for the sake of scientific rigour, and only for the sake of getting the trials funded, they are used for the wrong reasons.

An area of major concern in the literature is the legitimacy of the informed consent acquired from participants in these trials in Africa. Udo Schüklenk, for example, remarks that 'the voluntariness of the HIV women's consent is ... questionable. Is it not a coercive offer to force terminally ill pregnant women to choose between joining a placebo-controlled trial which gives them a shot at an established HIV intervention, and no treatment at all?' (Schüklenk 1998: 315). The counter-question, of course, is: what is the alternative? If this trial really is her only chance of 'getting a shot', at least, at attempting to assure the survival of her unborn child, and every attempt is made (which of course does not always happen) to help her to make an informed, competent and voluntary choice, are we to forfeit her the opportunity purely because we have doubts about the voluntariness of her act?

De Zulueta, in turn, has misgivings about Western criteria for informed consent, but then continues to argue that 'if you cannot obtain consent that fulfils "Western" criteria, there is a *stronger* case for absolute stringency in fulfilling article 1.10 of the Helsinki Declaration (1996 version) which states: "The researcher should be particularly cautious if the subject is in a dependent relationship to him or her or may consent under duress"' (De Zulueta 2001: 303). Marcia Angell also doubts whether informed consent does give sufficient protection from exploitation 'because of the asymmetry of knowledge and authority between researchers and their subjects' (Angell 1997: 847).

I have already raised the issue of what alternatives are available to try to acquire as much informed consent as possible from people who are, admittedly, often illiterate, frightened, quite ill and dependent on the researcher. Another factor is the question whether all these concerns about informed consent are not indicative of an unjustified paternalism as regards the practice of informed consent in Africa. Why does it have to be assumed that people in developing countries are necessarily so gullible and without understanding that their oral or written consent cannot be taken seriously? Resnik rightfully argues in this regard that we will be well advised not to over-emphasise Western models and procedures of informed consent when dealing with people in Africa. He writes: 'One method that researchers have used to improve informed consent in HIV research in the third world is to employ trusted community leaders to convey information to people in local populations' (Resnik 2001: 301). This idea has, in turn and by implication, been sharply criticised by Ijsselmuiden & Faden (1992: 830–833) and Ekunwe (1984: 23) who are very doubtful of the assumed bona fides of such community leaders in countries with poor human rights records.

This is a difficult problem, although I am convinced that it is also problematic to simply apply Western standards of informed consent to indigenous Africans. The African's idea of personhood is much less related to Western ideas of individual autonomy, and is much more closely related to family ties and community. Decisions are therefore seldom made by people as entirely independent individuals, as is assumed in most Western models of informed consent. A broader understanding of this phenomenon is required whenever reflecting on informed consent in Africa.[9]

For example, in a recent Masters dissertation for the M.Phil (Bioethics) degree at the University of Cape Town, Paul Roux argues persuasively for the thesis 'that the process of informed consent, although appropriate in Africa as an exercise in the recognition of autonomy, when applied in the case of African women may have the unexpected and deleterious effect of isolating her from a traditional support base and enhance the likelihood of non-disclosure of HIV status, and should therefore be adapted to meet the needs of this special situation' (Roux 2001). This 'adaptation', according to the author, mainly entails involving the family much more in the process of obtaining consent. Roux argues that his research has shown that this approach greatly contributes to a lesser risk of stigmatisation when these women reveal their HIV status in their communities.

The following conclusions can be drawn from this discussion:

- There is, particularly in view of the prohibitive costs associated with conventional regimens for antiretroviral treatment, a serious need for cheaper and simplified (preferably shorter) regimens of these drugs to prevent MTCT in Africa.
- Randomised placebo-controlled trials for shortened drug regimens to manage

MTCT in Africa are justified *if the research question is of such a nature that scientific rigour requires it.*

- If scientific needs justify equivalency trials rather than placebo trials and the latter are prohibited because of expense, special appeals ought to be made to foreign governments and pharmaceutical companies to provide the standard level of care required by equivalency trials.
- It is a mistake – and overly paternalistic – to judge the quality of informed consent in Africa merely by the standards applied in the West. Models of informed consent appropriate for Africans ought to be researched much more intensively. Steps ought at all times to be taken to ensure that the beneficial results of drug trials in the third world be made available to the people in whose communities this research was done.

Denial of the problem and lack of political will to prevent MTCT in South Africa

The debates referred to in the previous section are intriguing, and although the ethical issues have not been settled, they did not prevent the actual research for shortened drug regimens to prevent MTCT – placebo based or not – from taking place. As I have indicated, a number of new drugs (of which Nevirapine is the best known) or shortened regimens of existing drugs (e.g. Zudovudine) have been developed and have been proved to be highly efficient in preventing MTCT.

This then leaves the question as to why the development of a comprehensive programme of providing these drugs to pregnant women and newborns has been so slow in coming (theoretically it has only been introduced in 2004; some would argue at least ten years too late!), and, once the programme was introduced, why it has been so slowly and seemingly reluctantly implemented. Benatar writes in this regard about the situation in South Africa:

> While government's recent commitment to providing antiretroviral treatment is welcome relief from long-standing vaccilation, the rollout programme, like implementation of the strategic plan, is far too slow (only about 65 000 of the 500 000 who require antiretroviral treatment are currently receiving it). Many lives have been sacrificed through denial and delay. There is urgent need to correct these shortcomings (Benatar, 2005: 9).

This reluctance to get on with what is so obviously required constitutes one of the most serious moral issues associated with the pandemic in South Africa, and will in all probability be acknowledged by future generations as one of the really tragic (if not outrageous) eventualities that accompanied the epidemic in current times. A golden opportunity has thus been lost to relieve the suffering of thousands in a situation where millions are, in any case, suffering and dying, as the figures in this book clearly indicate.

Why is the South African government so hesitant to address the problem and provide the antiretrovirals to prevent MTCT? Firstly, the current Minister of Health has consistently expressed fears that Nevirapine – the drug with clearly the best potential, particularly because of its low cost (US$4 per regimen) and the relative simplicity of its administration – is dangerous because of its possible toxicity. In addition, the argument has often been made by the Minister in the press that Nevirapine has not been approved by the American Medicines Control Board and is thus not being used in the US. Why should it then be 'dumped', with all its alleged 'dangers', on the South African populace?

These concerns are not at all justified. Firstly, there are no indications that Nevirapine is unacceptably toxic. McIntyre and Gray, two eminent scientists in the field whose work I have already referred to extensively, state explicitly: 'These trials of antiretroviral interventions [they refer, in particular, to Nevirapine] have included several thousand African mother-infant pairs. To date, none of these trials has demonstrated significant toxicity or serious side-effects in mothers or infants' (2000: 31). This finding about toxicity was also confirmed by all the relevant scientific literature, and has also been confirmed by research done by South Africa's Medicines Control Board in 2003, which officially, following a request for such research by the Minister, found the drug to be 'safe and efficient' (as has also been found by the National Institutes of Health in the United States) (Brümmer 2003: 2).

While it is unrealistic to expect the 'perfect' drug, the point about Nevirapine . . . is in fact that it does not seem to be toxic at all.

Secondly, even if the drug had a level of toxicity, would that necessarily rule out its use, given the gravity of the ailment that it might prevent in newborns? If we only were to use entirely non-toxic drugs in medicine, most of the currently worldwide utilised regimens of chemotherapy for diseases such as leukemia and lymphoma – regimens that, particularly in the case of children, have dramatically improved the prognoses for these life-threatening diseases – must have been ruled out, since they all are, to a greater or lesser extent, toxic and require careful surveillance when administered. Surely the seriousness of the MTCT of HIV would justify a level of toxicity in a drug if the drug can prevent such transmission? While it is unrealistic to expect the 'perfect' drug, the point about Nevirapine, to refer to the last quotation again, is in fact that it does not seem to be toxic at all.

What has been found about Nevirapine is that there is a possibility that HIV-positive women who use it in a second or further pregnancy might develop resistance to the drug (it works quite well in first pregnancies). However, there is uncertainty about whether all the information on this issue is yet available. What is clear is that there were some (though not major) violations of Good Clinical Practice Guidelines (GCPG) when the original trials on Nevirapine were done in Uganda (the so-called HIVNET 012 trial). This has caused South Africa's Medicines Control Council to express reservations about Nevirapine. The issue in this regard, however, is resistance and not toxicity. There seems to be general consensus in the medical fraternity that Nevirapine is safe to use when not administered in isolation, but in combination with other antiretroviral drugs. As has been argued by Nattrass in Chapter 3 of this book, the cost issue of these combined drugs is rapidly becoming less of a problem because of the significant lowering of drug prices in recent times.

The Minister's second concern is the issue of cost. Is antiretroviral treatment to prevent MTCT affordable? Current estimates are that these treatments will cost the current tax payers in the vicinity of R90 million (US$15 million) per annum – literally a drop in the ocean of the government's current health budget. In addition, large pharmaceutical companies have gone to great lengths to cheapen the drugs or to make them available free of cost. (Note the figures provided in Chapter 3 about the greatly reduced costs of antiretroviral drugs in South Africa.)

Even more significantly, the popular government-endorsed theory that the provision of antiretroviral drugs (not only to pregnant women and newborns, but to all South Africans living with AIDS) is totally unaffordable, has increasingly been challenged. The economists Nattrass, Geffen and Raubenheimer have, in a recent study (2003; cf. also Nattrass 2004), shown that highly active antiretroviral therapy (HAART) is indeed affordable for the government, and much more advantageous for society than non-treatment. They added their set of cost-estimates to those of Johnson and Dorrington, and came to the conclusion that to provide HAART to people in the fourth stage of AIDS will cost less than ZAR1 billion (approximately US$117.6 million) and will reach a peak of R18.2 billion by 2015, when 2.3 million people in South Africa will be needing these drugs. If services such as counselling, prevention of MTCT and the treatment of other sexually transmitted diseases are added to this, the entire cost of the intervention, including infrastructure, will be R20.3 billion (about US$2.3 billion) in 2015. This represents the highest limit of the costs. If we assume that the South African economy will grow by two percent (inflation adapted) in the Gross National Product (GNP) between now and 2015, it means that a full-fledged prevention and treatment programme for HIV/AIDS will cost the public sector about 1.7 percent of GNP at the height of the epidemic. According to the World Health Organisation's Commission on Macroeconomics and Health, it is attainable for countries with a low and middle income to increase budget allocations for health to one percent of GNP by 2007, and to two percent of GNP by 2015. The cost projections by Nattrass and colleagues are within these limits (cf. Nattrass 2003). This means that not only is the prevention of MTCT affordable to the South African government, but also the wholesale provision of antiretroviral drugs to the entire population in need of it.

Should a country such as South Africa be 'tough' and sacrifice the HIV/AIDS generation for the sake of social utility?

Should a country such as South Africa be 'tough' and sacrifice the HIV/AIDS generation for the sake of social utility? Innuendos of concern about 'what will happen to the AIDS orphans if we save their lives' are also, from time to time, heard from the ranks of government and the ruling ANC party spokespeople. Nattrass rightly has a twofold response that I fully agree with. The first is that treatment programmes (with antiretrovirals) turn out to be prevention programmes and might therefore contribute greatly to lowering the general infection rate in the population. But, as Nattrass remarks, there is an even bigger ethical problem: 'What does it mean for us as a society to opt for the route of sacrificing a whole generation? Do we really want to sacrifice other people who can be treated for less than two percent of the GNP at the peak of the epidemic, thus restoring life and hope for them?' (Nattrass 2003; my translation).

A third reason for the government's hesitance to embark on a full-scale programme of (even) MTCT prevention is, in all probability, of a deeper nature. It has to do with a deep-seated scepticism of the scientific facts about the nature of the epidemic, fuelled by the influence of dissident scientists like Rasnick, Geshekter and Duesberg who question whether HIV causes AIDS at all (cf. Duesberg 1996; Rasnick 2000 and Geshekter 2000). It has become clear that the South African President has been under the influence of the dissidents for a long time – he even appointed some of them to a 'task group' to 'do research' to establish the relationship between HIV and AIDS – and has been exerting a very strong influence on the official position taken on these matters by the Minister of Health and other prominent members of the government and the ANC. The reader is, in this regard, referred to citations from an article that President Mbeki wrote on this matter as well as a speech that he made at the University of Fort Hare in 2001, provided in footnote 2 of Chapter 2 of this book. From these statements, the extent of his denial of the seriousness of the AIDS pandemic seems indisputable.

Given the almost cataclysmic nature of the AIDS epidemic in (South) Africa, this kind of denial can only be judged as morally dubious. Space will not allow me to explore fully the ethics of denial.[10] Denial is an acknowledged and even accepted psychological disposition in situations where people are struck by very bad news that they find difficult to accept. It represents one of the 'phases' that Elisabeth Kübler-Ross (1975) identified in typical reactions of people who discover that they are terminally ill. As such it is well known and can even evoke our sympathy. There is, however, no justification for the head of a state and/or government of a country with such a serious problem as our AIDS pandemic to become stuck in the first phase of people's typical response to bad news. AIDS is indeed bad news, and we would all have loved it if there were no AIDS. However, it is intolerable that the leadership of a country experiencing such a crisis creates the impression that it almost does not exist, or is not at all a priority. This behaviour must be morally condemned; it indeed creates the impression of irresponsibility. It is no wonder that, in recent times, it has increasingly become a serious question whether the denial and subsequent delayed action of the South African government in respect of the AIDS epidemic in the country does not amount to a form of deplorable negligence. Stephen Lewis, the current United Nations envoy for AIDS in Southern Africa is the latest international figure who has accused the South African government of 'criminal negligence'

(Hooper-Box & Battersby 2003: 2) in its handling of the epidemic, particularly concerning its reluctance to rollout a programme of MCTC prevention, in spite of having been ordered to do so by the highest court in the land.

Conclusions

The following short conclusions seem appropriate in view of the previous discussion:

- The phenomenon of HIV/AIDS has, probably more than anything else, proved our vulnerability to disaster, in spite of the unprecedented advances in medical science at the beginning of the 21st century. I have elaborated on this point at the end of Chapter 4 of this volume, and will not repeat those remarks here, valid though they remain.
- The dispute about the ethics of randomised placebo-controlled trials for the development of drugs to combat MTCT in Africa reiterates Stephen Toulmin's long-standing insight that 'science is not an intellectual computing machine, but a slice of life' (Toulmin 1961). Science is no value-free enterprise with methods, procedures and assumptions that are in no way influenced by the social contexts within which it operates and for which it becomes functional. As a 'slice of life', science participates in the uncertainties and instabilities of our historical life as human beings. For a legitimate, accountable and adequate understanding of science we are compelled to reflect on the variety of relationships within which science can be practised, ranging from its relation to labour and technology, to the relations to society and politics, as well as the relations to views of life and religious belief (Rossouw 1980: 14–15).

  This is well illustrated by the following observation by Ranaan Gillon: ' . . . clinical research . . . always has two components: a component of pure research intended to produce generalisable medical knowledge, and a component of therapy, where the intention is to benefit the particular patient/subject's own health . . . The less a trial shares in that Hippocratic commitment, i.e. the less it is intended and likely to benefit the individual patient subject, the more it should be treated as non-therapeutic research aimed at benefiting others, and not the participant subjects, and therefore the more such a trial should incorporate the safeguards appropriate to non-therapeutic research, including the need for extensively informed consent' (Gillon 2001: 263). This judgement makes clear that the nature of the science practised cannot be divorced from the moral concern about the extent to which the investigated subjects will, eventually, benefit from the knowledge gained in the process. The issue of drug trials for the sake of reducing MTCT makes us aware of both the possibilities and the social responsibility of science, the tragedy of scarce and depleted resources, the need to act for people's benefit in spite of these impediments, and the possibility of hope that scientific innovation might incur in situations that otherwise seem hopeless.

- The tragedy of the South African government's neglect to act in accordance with people's real needs as far as MTCT in that country is concerned, unequivocally proves the dangers of an unjustified politicisation of the discourse about HIV/AIDS and the concomitant problem of MTCT in Africa. Such politicisation holds the potential of exacerbating an already occurring catastrophe. HIV/AIDS is primarily a health problem and not a political problem, although we may recognise that socio-political factors, such as chronic poverty and illiteracy, can negatively impact on the pandemic. What is required in South Africa and other African countries is what was undertaken in Uganda, where the impact of the disease has been significantly curbed by a national, co-ordinated and comprehensive treatment and prevention campaign that had the prevention of MTCT as a core component.
- Once the previous point has been made in its own right, it is as important to acknowledge that the catastrophe compels us to reflect critically on the massive imbalances between the wealth of Africa and the West, and thereby to rethink the requirements for human well-being on a global scale. No other health phenomenon has in recent years more emphatically demonstrated the need for the development of a global bioethics. The reader is invited to read what has been argued in this respect in Chapters 5 and 6.
- MTCT of HIV in Africa is a serious problem, but it can be managed in an affordable way. The most serious impediment to its humane and effective management is not a lack of knowledge, the unavailability of drugs, the infrastructure to make them available or their unaffordability. It is the lack of political will and the denial of the seriousness of the problem on the part of the political leadership, particularly in South Africa. Once this leadership assumes its rightful responsibility, all the indications are that aid from the rest of the world, be it governments or pharmaceutical companies, will be forthcoming, and a very significant reduction in MTCT can be expected. Opportunities and goodwill in this regard abound. It is for the leadership in African countries to seize the day: co-operate with both countries and pharmaceutical companies who are willing to come to our aid, accept their offers, make the infrastructure available for the distribution of these drugs and do what is now possible to prevent an almost unspeakable tragedy.

Endnotes

[1] Whether the disease was prevalent in earlier times, and not as such known or visible, is still a matter of considerable contention and speculation. The anthropologist Virginia van der Vliet argues that AIDS is probably a fairly recent phenomenon, and might have lingered unobtrusively in small African villages over a period of time, only emerging in its visible manifestation and spreading rapidly since because of modernising influences such as urbanisation and its accompanying altered sexual mores. Cf. Van der Vliet 1996: 10–51.

[2] For an analysis of the problems related to reliable statistics about HIV in Africa, cf. Chapter 2.

[3] Zudovudine is marketed under the brand name of Retrovir (formerly called azidothymidine [AZT]). It is made available in tablets, capsules and a syrup. Each film-coated tablet contains 300 mg of Zudovudine and the inactive ingredients hypromellose, magnesium stearate, microcrystalline cellulose, polyethylene glycol, sodium starch glycolate and titanium dioxide.

[4] The name 'Nevirapine' is currently commonly in use in South Africa. The drug is in fact marketed by Boehringer Ingelheim under the brand name Viramune. It is structurally a member of the dipyridodiazepinone chemical class of compounds. It is available in tablets for oral administration. Each tablet contains 200 mg of nevirapine and the inactive ingredients microcrystalline cellulose, lactose monohydrate, povidone, sodium starch glycolate, colloidal silicon dioxide and magnesium stearate.

[5] See discussion by Resnik 2001: 287.

[6] Personal communication by Mark Cotton.

[7] I broadly draw on the discussion of Resnik 2001: 293–304 for these arguments.

[8] At time of original writing.

[9] Cf. for this argument Moodley 2002: 209–213

[10] On the topic of denial, cf. Garvey 2001: 3–20.

References

Altenroxel, L. (2003). World's first AIDS vaccine is a failure. *Pretoria News*, 25 February.

Angell, M. (1997). The ethics of clinical research in the third world. *New England Journal of Medicine, 337* (1997), 847–849.

Benatar, S.R. (2001). Commentary: Justice and Medical Research: A Global Perspective. *Bioethics, 15* (4), 333–340.

Benatar, S.R. (2005). The Lost Potential of our Health System. *The Cape Times*, 14th January 2005, 9.

Brümmer, W. (2003). Teenvigsmiddel veilig, sê MBR. *Die Burger*, 28th April.

De Zulueta, P. (2001). Randomised placebo-controlled trials and HIV-infected pregnant women in developing countries. Ethical imperialism or unethical exploitation? *Bioethics, 15* (4), 289–311.

Duesberg, P.H. (1996). *Inventing the AIDS Virus*. Washington D.C.: Regnery.

Ekunwe, E.O. (1984). Commentary: Informed Consent in the Developing World. *Hastings Center Report, 14* (3), 22–24.

Forrest, D. & Streek, B. (2001). Mbeki in bizarre Aids outburst. *Mail & Guardian*, 26th October–1st November.

Garvey, B. (2001). Simon Browne and the Paradaox of 'Being in Denial'. *Inquiry, 44*(1), 3–20.

Geffen, N., Nattrass, N. & Raubenheimer, C. (2003). The Cost of HIV Prevention and Treatment Interventions in South Africa. *Centre for Social Science Research*, University of Cape Town, Working Paper no. 28 *www.uct.ac.za/depts/cssr.*

Geshekter, C. (2000). The Plague that Isn't: Poverty is Killing Africans, not an alleged AIDS Pandemic, says U.S. Policy Adviser. *http://www.virusmyth.com/aids/data/cgpoverty.htm.*

Gillon, R. (2001). *'Fully' Informed Consent, Clinical Trials and the Boundaries of Therapeutic Discretion*, in: Doyal, L. & Tobias, J.S. (eds.): *Informed Consent in Medical Research.* London: BMJ Books.

Ho, D. (1997). It's AIDS, not Tuskegee. *Time*, 29th September.

Hooper-Box, C. & Battersby, J. (2003). Health Minister lashes out at UN Envoy. *The Sunday Independent*, 23rd February.

Ijsselmuiden, C. & Faden, R.R. (1992). Research and Informed Consent in Africa – Another Look. *NEJM, 326*, 830–833.

Kindra, J. (2003). What's so special about AIDS? *Mail & Guardian*, 21st–27th February.

Kübler-Ross, E. (1975). *Death: the final stage of growth.* New Jersey: Englewood Cliffs.

Lurie, P. & Wolfe, S. (1997). Unethical trials of interventions to reproduce perinatal transmission of the human immunodeficiency virus in developing countries. *New England Journal of Medicine, 337* (1997), 853–856.

MacIntyre, J. & Gray, G. (2000). Preventing mother-to-child transmission of HIV – African Solutions for an African Crisis. *Southern African Journal of HIV Medicine (Launch Issue), 1* (1), 30–31.

Makgoba, M.W. (Ed.) (1999). *African Renaissance: The New Struggle.* Cape Town: Mafube & Tafelberg.

Mandelbrot, L., Chenadec, J. et al. (1998). Perinatal HIV-1 transmission: interaction between zidovudine prophylaxis and mode of delivery in the French Perinatal Cohort. *JAMA, 280* (1), 55–60.

Mbeki, T. (1998). *Africa: The Time has Come: Selected Speeches.* Cape Town: Tafelberg & Mafube.

Mbeki, T. (2000). Reciting comfortable catechisms on AIDS is not good enough. *The Sunday Times*, 23rd April.

Moodley, K. (2002). HIV vaccine trial participation in South Africa – an Ethical Assessment. *The Journal of Medicine and Philosophy, 27*(2), 209–213.

Nattrass, N. (2003). Die Koste van 'n Lewe – Suid-Afrika kán Vigsepidemie hokslaan. *Die Burger*, 13th February.

Nattrass, N. (2004). *The Moral Economy of AIDS in South Africa.* Cambridge: Cambridge University Press.

Rasnick, D. (2000). Talked with President Thabo Mbeki. *http://www.virusmyth.com/aids/news/drtalkmbeki.htm.* 2nd March 2000.

Resnik, D. (2001). The Ethics of HIV Research in Developing Nations. *Bioethics, 12* (4), 286–306.

Rossouw, H.W. (1980): *Wetenskap, Interpretasie, Wysheid,* Port Elizabeth, Universiteit van Port Elizabeth Seminare, Simposia en Lesings B7, 14–15.

Roux, P. (2001). Informed Consent for Voluntary Counselling and Testing for HIV Infection in South African Mothers and Children: An Assessment of Burdens and Consequences and an Argument for a Modification in the Process of Informed Consent. *Unpublished M.Phil. (Bioethics) Dissertation*, University of Cape Town.

Schüklenk, U. (1998). Unethical Perinatal HIV Transmission Trials establish Bad Precedent. *Bioethics, 12* (4), 312–319.

Smith, J.W. (1991): *AIDS, Philosophy and Beyond.* Aldershot: Avebury.

Steyn, P. (2001). VSA-Firma sal nie patente afdwing in Suid-Afrika. *Die Burger*, 16th March.

Toulmin, S. (1961). *Foresight and Understanding: An Enquiry into the Aims of Science.* London: Hutchinson.

UNAIDS Epidemic Update December. (2002). http://www.unaids.org (author not mentioned).

United Nations AIDS (UNAIDS). (2002). AIDS Epidemic Update. *http://www.unaids.org.*

Van der Vliet, V. (1996). *The politics of AIDS.* London: Bowerdean Publishing Company Limited.

Van Niekerk, A.A. (2002a). Moral and social complexities of AIDS in Africa. *Journal of Medicine and Philosophy, 27* (2), 143–162; also, in revised form, Chapter 4 of this volume.

Van Niekerk, A.A. (2002b). Etiese en sosio-politieke kwessies betreffende VIGS: openbaarheid, ontkenning, kwesbaarheid en armoede. *Die Joernaal vir Etiese Medisyne, 3* (1), 41–49.

Watney, S. (1989). Missionary Positions: AIDS, 'Africa' and Race. *Critical Quarterly, 31* (3), 46–62.

Whiteside, A., Barnett, A., George, G. & Van Niekerk, A.A. (2003). Through a glass, darkly . . . data and uncertainty in the AIDS debate. *Developing World Bioethics, 3* (1), 49–76, also, in revised form, Chapter 2 of this volume.

http:/www.lovelife.org.za (author not mentioned).

Chapter 10

HIV vaccine trial participation in South Africa: an ethical assessment

When first world countries sponsor research in sub-Saharan Africa, inevitable tensions arise. In this chapter **Keymanthri Moodley** *looks at the first world individualistic focus, which may fail to accommodate the communalism prevalent in rural African regions and may create a lack of co-operation and the authorisation needed for research in Africa today.*

With more than 14 000 people newly infected daily throughout the world, HIV/AIDS is increasingly being recognised as an illness of global importance and a major priority for the world community. It is generally accepted that an effective preventive HIV vaccine could be a powerful tool in the struggle against the pandemic. However, in the absence of a suitable animal model, such a vaccine would have to be tested in clinical trials using human subjects. HIV vaccine trials began ten years ago in the United States and Europe and are now increasingly being planned and implemented in developing countries (Guenter 2000: 37).

Developing communities around the world are seen as excellent candidates for medical research, largely because of the unfortunate but typical characteristics of these communities – they tend to be over-populated, poor, malnourished, illiterate and desperate. Under these conditions, together with a fragile health-care infrastructure, diseases thrive, especially infectious diseases. In this scenario empirical scientific research also thrives – statistically significant data can be obtained from large-scale clinical trials on thousands of human 'volunteers'.

As a result, some measure of protection has become necessary: 'Residents of impoverished, post-colonial countries, the majority of whom are people of colour, must be protected from potential exploitation in research. Otherwise, the abominable state of health care in these countries can be used to justify studies that could never pass ethical muster in the sponsoring country' (Lurie and Wolfe 1997: Public Citizen's Health Research Group). In the aftermath of the controversial HIV vertical transmission trials, HIV vaccine trials are emerging as the next major ethical challenge in South African research circles.

Recruiting volunteers for such trials is critical to the success of the endeavour, but is fraught with scientific, social, political and ethical concerns – especially when the target communities live in the third world. Possible host community responses range from 'opposition and obstruction, to indifference, support or active participation' (Hodel 1994: 255). For individual participants, a wide range of factors might influence a decision to participate. Thus, to achieve truly informed consent, it is critical to determine what information is to be given to potential volunteers in order for them to make an informed decision. A vital component of such patient information is the risk-benefit ratio that determines the ethical acceptability of clinical research. In AIDS vaccine research, however, the half of the equation that deals with risk is 'virtually unknown'. There is no data about the potential for risks such as 'vaccine-induced immunotoxicity or antibody-induced enhancement of infection' (Tacket and Edelman 1990: 356).

In anticipation of the launch of HIV vaccine trials worldwide, guidelines have been developed to ensure that 'ethical issues do not impede the development of a new vaccine' (United Nations Programme on AIDS). These ethical guidelines are designed to protect the rights of those participating in international vaccine trials and are based on the Helsinki Declaration of 1975, which mandates that 'concern for the interest of the individual must always prevail over the interests of science and society'. As such the issues central to this endeavour include, *inter alia*, individual informed consent, obligations of trial sponsors to host countries to provide vaccines if they prove to be effective, and the use of expensive antiretroviral treatment for participants in developing countries who become infected during the trials.

In keeping with the ethos of the sponsor country - the United States - the ideal of liberal individualism reigns supreme. Informed consent is detailed as follows - participants must be given a subject information sheet, a third party advisor must be accessible, participants should have time to reflect on their decisions and then give written informed consent. The paradox inherent in this endeavour involves the high priority placed on *the individual* and the rights of the individual to ultimately achieve not only societal good but *global good.*

The ethical dilemma central to this chapter revolves around individual good as opposed to societal good. Many of the principles of African 'communitarianism' or Ubuntu, which exists in various forms especially in rural, traditional South African communities, are in stark contrast to the individualistic principles of the West yet are beginning to be influenced by Western individualism. This change in emphasis from the community to the individual has started to influence research opportunities and possibilities in the third world; fulfilling all the criteria of international guidelines for the performance of ethical research in the third world is starting to become problematic. How will the West respond? Will ethical relativism become a viable option and a convenient solution?

To explore ethical concerns central to the HIV vaccine trials, I examine the classical 'Four Principles' approach and discuss its relevance in the African context. It might be that an appeal to Ubuntu is our only hope of conducting ethical HIV vaccine trials in South Africa. However, will this retreat to ethical relativism be acceptable to the people of Africa?

HIV vaccine trials in the third world – the Four Principles approach?

The Belmont Report of 1979 requires that biomedical research be conducted in a manner consistent with four ethical principles: autonomy, beneficence, non-maleficence and justice (Loue 1996: 49). The applicability of these basic ethical principles within different cultural settings is increasingly being questioned. This is especially so because the international bodies that originally formulated these principles were unfamiliar with the different settings in which they would have to be applied (Barry 1988: 1083).

While the Declaration of Helsinki was the result of a medical professional body attempting to regulate itself, it was not without shortcomings. Many concepts are not clear; in particular, there is no guidance on how to resolve conflicts resulting from an attempt to maximise more than one principle simultaneously (Kunstadter 1980: 289–96).

In spite of this, the Declaration of Helsinki has become the benchmark for ethical practice in research (London 1999: 812). As such, it is important to establish whether this Western standard based on the Four Principles approach may be appropriately applied to biomedical research in developing countries.

PRINCIPLE ONE: Respect for autonomy and informed consent

Western society emphasises autonomy in its conception of personhood. It has been charged that individual informed consent is a Western construct based on the Western notion of personhood. In particular, the American notion of personhood is 'markedly rational, and also legalistic – prototypically expressed in the language of rights' (De Craemer 1983: 19–34). The Nuremberg Code and its progeny require that participation in biomedical research be based on 'freedom of individual choice, with no element of coercion or constraint. It dictates further that a person should understand the subject matter of the research sufficiently to make an enlightened decision' (Barry 1988: 1083). Hence all the details of the trial must be made known to the participant. Such a conception of autonomy reflects the 'basic premise of individual sovereignty' (Loue 1996: 49).

Applying this concept of autonomy and the requirements of informed consent can prove to be problematic in many cultures in the third world where personal choice is extremely limited. In many African cultures, the concept of personhood differs substantially from that in Western cultures. Personhood is defined by one's tribe, village or social group. However, in certain African societies, selfhood cannot be extricated from a dynamic system of social relationships, both of kinship and of community as defined by the village (Barry 1988: 1083). This African concept of personhood is further elaborated by South African philosopher, Augustine Shutte in his work on Ubuntu: persons exist only in relation to other persons. According to him, in all African languages, there is the local variant of the Nguni saying *umuntu ngumuntu ngabantu* – a person is a person through persons (unpublished data).

This view is supported by Nhlanhla Mkize, a South African clinical psychologist based at the University of KwaZulu-Natal and contributing author of the book *Critical Psychology*. According to him, unlike the Western concept of personhood that defines a person as rational, autonomous, individual and separate from others, the traditional African notion of personhood is relational, communitarian and extended. Reciprocity and interdependence are reflected in the Nguni notion of Ubuntu. The family or community are regarded as the moral agent as a result of the family being the most important aspect of identity. A horizontal and vertical dimension of being is described where a person is connected to the living, the ancestors and those yet to be born. A deep respect for elders is cultivated and the authority of these elders is vested in a socio-moral responsibility to promote community and familial interests (Mkhize 2004: 46).

. . . in certain African societies, selfhood cannot be extricated from a dynamic system of social relationships, both of kinship and of community as defined by the village.

Similarly, in Ugandan culture, the wishes of the individual are often subordinate to those of the immediate or extended family. As such, participation of an individual in biomedical research may depend on the acquiescence or consent of another family member (Loue 1996: 49). The concept of family consent is not peculiar to Africa. It is an important concept in Japanese culture as well, and the principle of autonomy, as it exists in its traditional North American paradigm, is not entirely applicable to Japanese culture. Instead, Edmund Pellegrino refers to 'something close to autonomy' that is respected in the context of Japanese society (Akabayashi 1999: 296–301). In the same way, ancient Chinese medical ethics, established on the foundations of Confucian ethics, emphasise a respectful attitude towards one's patients based on an unconditional value for human life, but do not include respecting their autonomous choices (Tsai 1999: 315–321). It is thus clear that where the notion of persons as individuals is not dominant, the consent process may shift from the individual to the family or community (Christakis 1988: 34).

An investigator seeking informed consent from individual persons in such settings may need to approach community elders for their consent before attempting to obtain informed consent from individual persons (Barry 1988: 1083). The person acknowledged to be a 'community leader' will vary from one culture to another and from one investigator to another. What is established, though, is that proxy consent is not acceptable in the absence of consent from the individual trial subject.

In order to acknowledge the need for family consent in biomedical research, a waiting period would be necessary before an informed consent form is signed, should the potential participant desire this option. This waiting period will, however, often be problematic – transport to outlying areas is costly and time-consuming and, as a result, potential participants may abandon the trial altogether. Furthermore, the nature of the information regarding the trial may have been misunderstood and in subsequent transmission to a family member or significant other, may undergo further modification. Under such circumstances, truly informed consent will not be obtained. However, with no suitable alternatives, a waiting period remains an option when obtaining informed consent in Africa (Mugerwa 2002: 226–229).

Having established 'who' will consent to participation in a research trial, it is essential to present the 'information element' of the trial to the prospective participant. Coupled to this disclosure is the element of understanding on the part of the patient (Beauchamp & Childress 1994: 145). During a workshop held in South Africa to discuss ethical issues in HIV vaccine trials in September 1998, Oliver Ransome, the medical ombudsman, outlined the prerequisites for obtaining informed consent – a subject information sheet, third party adviser, time to reflect, and the actual written consent. The details on the information sheet should include the overall purpose of the research 'in comprehensible language'. Confidentiality should be stressed and it should be clear that the subject is free to decline or withdraw. Questions should be invited and time should be allowed for reflection. He highlights essential and crucial components of a subject information sheet. However, in South Africa, with very high rates of illiteracy (MacFarlane 2000: 18), such a sheet may be inappropriate to use. In a similar workshop in Uganda, it was established that with their currently 'high rate of illiteracy, many prospective research participants would be unable to read a form and understand it' (Loue 1996: 50). This would also have serious implications for obtaining the 'written consent' referred to by Ransome.

Illiteracy coupled with language barriers in Africa make the description of AIDS-related studies difficult. When concepts like germ theory, viruses and vaccines are alien, it is indeed challenging to respond to the question posed by Mark Heywood (AIDS Law Project, University of the Witwatersrand): What *is* sufficient information for informed consent? Ron Bayer (HIV Centre, New York) also expresses concern regarding the explanation of 'complicated scientific methods such as randomisation, placebos, vaccine inefficiency, the fact that participation in one trial may exclude future participation in trials of more effective vaccines and discrimination linked to participation'.

An interesting problem related to language arose in the HIV Vertical Transmission Trials conducted on pregnant women in South Africa in 1997. The placebo drug used in these trials was translated as being a 'spaza' drug or a 'chuff-chuff' drug. While a 'chuff-chuff' drug is understood to be a 'pretend' drug, the word 'spaza' is a colloquial term generally meaning 'half the real thing' or a pretence of the real thing. In no way are they associated with the concept of inertness inherent in a placebo. As such, the use of the term 'spaza' to describe a placebo is clearly misleading. In 1998, attention was drawn to the informed consent documents used in Thailand. Discrepancies were noted in the Thai and English versions of the documents. The Thai version described the placebo as a 'comparison drug that does not contain Zudovudine' while the English version described the placebo as an 'inactive substance' which was 'like a sugar pill'. The Thai critics charged that the words 'inactive substance', 'placebo' and 'sugar pill' did not appear in the Thai documents even though Thai words or concepts did exist for these words (Achrekar 1998: 1331–32).

In their description of informed consent, Beauchamp and Childress describe two preconditions or threshold elements – competence (to understand and decide) and voluntariness (in deciding). In the third world, where research participants are usually poor, desperate and dependent, voluntariness is a significant precondition for obtaining truly informed consent. Research participants should be able to choose freely amongst alternatives and have the right to refuse to participate. In a research setting, manipulation tends to occur rather than coercion or persuasion. In the context of decision-making in health care, manipulation of information tends to be the key form of manipulation employed. Misleading research participants, as in the use of the word 'spaza' to describe a placebo, is a form of deception that is clearly inconsistent with autonomous choice.

In the third world, where research participants are usually poor, desperate and dependent, voluntariness is a significant precondition for obtaining truly informed consent.

Attractive offers such as free medication or extra money can leave persons without any meaningful choice apart from accepting the offer, largely because such persons are trapped in a desperate situation. Whatever we may decide to call this, it is widely held that offers of this magnitude to a person in desperate need are inherently exploitative and are not consistent with autonomous choice.

In South Africa, it has been general research practice that trial participants be paid R50 ($8) per trial visit to cover costs for transport and meals for the day. In 2004, this amount was increased to R150 ($26) per study visit by the Medicines Control Council (MCC). It is also a requirement that this amount be included in the patient information leaflet (Moodley 2003: 677–678). Including this amount in the informed consent document is problematic in poor communities where people would consent to such research for half this amount of money. Research methodology and statistical validity may also be adversely influenced by follow-up visits if patients are offered payment for these visits. The development of 'side-effects' might be very attractive if one is aware that one will be paid for all 'illness visits' to a trial site.

Looking specifically at the ethical design of an AIDS vaccine trial in Africa, Christakis (1988: 35) warns researchers that:

> . . . it is difficult to avoid coercing subjects in most settings where clinical investigation in the developing world is conducted. African subjects with relatively little understanding of medical aspects of research participation, indisposed toward resisting the suggestions of Western doctors, perhaps operating under the mistaken notion that they are being treated, and possibly receiving some ancillary benefits from participation in the research, are very susceptible to coercion. Their vulnerability warrants greater care in procuring consent and necessitates greater sensitivity to protect this class of research subjects.

Research conducted in Thailand amongst potential volunteers in a phase 1 HIV vaccine trial to explore their motivations for participation in these trials found that personal benefit as opposed to altruistic motives was important (Jenkins 1995: 36–42). Another Thai study found that 'the principal inducement to join a trial was health insurance' (Celentano 1995: 1079–1083). Undoubtedly, the search for incentives has begun!

Research conducted in Durban, South Africa, to assess whether informed consent for HIV testing in a South African hospital was truly informed and truly voluntary, yielded interesting results. Of the 56 women studied, 88 percent felt compelled to participate, even though they were assured that their participation was entirely voluntary. Twenty-eight percent of the women 'perceived the research to be integral with the service at the hospital and agreed to the HIV test because they thought that refusal would compromise their care. This subtle coercive element may stem from the social context of a hospital where the health professionals are held in high regard'. When patients have little recourse to alternative medical care, they may have no choice but to participate in a research study conducted at the only tertiary hospital at their disposal. It is highly probable that informed consent sought under such circumstances might be 'less than voluntary'. This study concludes that 'subtle and unexpected elements of coercion can reside in the perceptions (real or imagined) held by patients recruited into a research project in a medical care setting' (Abdool Karrim 1998: 640).

Too little protection of these subjects risks their exploitation; too much protection risks unjustified paternalism.

A discussion on informed consent would be incomplete without examining the important precondition of competence. In biomedical contexts a person has been viewed as competent if able to understand a therapy or research procedure, to deliberate regarding major risks and benefits, and to make a decision in light of this deliberation (Beauchamp & Childress 1994: 136). The label of 'incompetence' has traditionally been applied to children, the mentally retarded, people with major psychiatric illnesses and those with delirium or dementia. Such people are regarded as vulnerable research subjects because they lack capacity to give informed consent and because they depend on others to protect them (Kopelman 1994: 2291). Little attention has been paid to the millions of people in developing countries, like South Africa, who due to poverty, malnutrition and lack of opportunities for education are either illiterate or uneducated. Coupled to this are the constraints of cultural belief systems, especially where causation in illness is concerned.

To these people, many concepts in science and medicine are alien and they often have to undergo an enormous paradigm shift in order to understand and deliberate about the complexities of Western biomedical research. Empirical research from South Africa has found that only 20 percent of participants on an influenza vaccine trial were able to understand the concept of randomisation, while only 19 percent had a clear understanding of the use of placebos (Moodley

2004). Participants who do not understand research design and procedures, yet provide consent, also fall into the category of 'vulnerable research subjects' because fear, ignorance, pressure or trust may account for their agreement to participate. Too little protection of these subjects risks their exploitation; too much protection risks unjustified paternalism (Kopelman 1994: 2292). At the risk of the latter charge, I believe that it is highly probable that in many cases of biomedical research in the developing world, subjects, although adult and not mentally impaired or retarded, do not fulfil all the criteria for competence outlined above.

Often, subjects do not understand what they have been told about a complicated and foreign research protocol, and when they do not understand they are not competent to decide whether to accept or reject their involvement in such a setting. The capacity necesssary for such understanding includes 'a memory for words, phrases, ideas and sequences of information'. Furthermore, the 'chance nature of the occurrence of risks and benefits highlights the importance of the ability to understand causal relations and the likelihood of various outcomes. Finally, it may be important for patients to be able to understand not only what they are told, but also that they have a critical part to play in the decision-making process. Deficits in attention span, intelligence and memory may detract from these abilities' (Appelbaum 1988: 1636).

It is not my intention to suggest that all people from developing communities are incompetent and hence cannot give informed consent to participate in research conducted in the third world. This would deprive such subjects of their decision-making rights and would represent a serious infringement of liberty. Rather, it is possible that a position of 'limited competence' exists in many instances.

In the aftermath of the apartheid era in South Africa, many people who are completely competent still relinquish their decision-making rights to authority figures, be they doctors or researchers or both. This is accentuated when researchers and study participants belong to different racial groups and where asymmetrical power relationships, based on the previous apartheid system, exist. Enormous efforts are required on the part of the medical profession and researchers to create the level of understanding necessary to meet the criteria of competence. Coupled with this is a need for empowerment of many patients, who, as a result of decades of oppression, have never learnt how to exercise their decision-making rights.

It is evident from this discussion on the procurement of informed consent from prospective participants in HIV vaccine trials that the concept is riddled with intricacies. The precise demands of the principle of autonomy are largely unsettled and remain 'open to interpretation and specification'.

PRINCIPLES TWO AND THREE: Non-maleficence and beneficence

Researchers need to make an effort to secure the well-being of research participants. This entails achieving a favourable balance between the risks and benefits of the proposed research (Loue 1996: 50).

To begin with, adverse effects of the vaccine itself may occur as with other vaccines in current use, such as pain or infection at the injection site, fever or allergic reactions. A study conducted in Thailand among high-risk populations to assess willingness to participate in AIDS vaccine trials found that vaccine side-effects were considered important barriers to trial participation (Celentano 1995: 1079).

More specifically in the case of an HIV vaccine, participants are likely to be concerned about actually developing HIV disease from the vaccine. With the current use of genetically altered or killed viruses, this risk is unlikely. The current subunit vaccine candidates, which employ genetically engineered proteins from the HIV envelope (using a piece of the viruses), are likely to allay much anxiety. However, participants' fears are likely to magnify as vaccine developers incorporate the use of a whole killed or live attenuated virus. Scientists are already becoming impatient to test live attenuated virus vaccines, but leading clinicians are still hesitant regarding the safety of such vaccines. The majority opinion at present is that 'there is just not enough evidence that a live-attenuated HIV-1 vaccine is safe or effective' (McCarthy 1997: 1082).

Even with current genetically engineered vaccines, while it is possible that disease will be prevented, infection might still occur. Few of the candidate HIV vaccines appear promising for preventing infection, and the expectation that HIV vaccines will in fact prevent infection is yielding, in the scientific community, to the hope that they may prevent disease' (Bloom 1998: 186). In reality, when the first AIDS vaccine trials were launched in the United States and Thailand in 1998, using the HIV envelope protein, gp120, in a vaccine called AIDSVAX, two outcome measures were to be assessed – 'infection by HIV and viral load in those infected'. These trials were actually conducted in 2003: one in the United States testing a clade B vaccine on 5 400 men who have sex with men (MSM) and one in Thailand testing a clade B/E vaccine on 2 500 injecting drug users (IDUs). The results of the Thai study conducted over 36 months unfortunately yielded vaccine efficacy of 0.1 percent with a confidence interval of –31.2 percent to 23.6 percent. One hundred and five participants in the placebo group became HIV positive and 106 participants in the vaccine group demonstrated seroconversion. In these trials, the candidate vaccines tested did not demonstrate efficacy (Choopanya 2004).

Hence the possibility of vaccine failure is a very real one, and the occurrence of 'breakthrough HIV infections' or disease cannot be excluded. This particular risk to the subject needs to be assessed in the context of the different types of trials that are performed. It is reasonable to assume that the risk of developing HIV infection during the course of phase 1 or 2 trials by low-risk participants will be far greater than the risk taken by people entering phase 3 trials, already at high risk by virtue of lifestyle or other predisposing factors. Where the HIV vaccine is concerned, in South Africa, phase 1 and 2 trials will have to be conducted here as these vaccines are specifically directed against the clade C virus.

In South Africa, will researchers have an obligation to provide antiretroviral treatment to subjects who become infected during the course of the trials? Scientists and researchers are concerned that treatment with antiretroviral drugs will compromise the ability of the trial to measure the efficacy of the vaccine in preventing disease (Bloom 1998: 186). A critical measure of the success of an AIDS vaccine trial would be whether the vaccine lowers the 'viral load' in people who get infected. Antiretroviral treatment will also lower the viral load. If many of the participants who become infected begin taking potent antiretroviral drugs, reduction in viral loads due to the vaccine cannot be assessed. Scientists fear that it will become impossible to design a 'scientifically valid' trial if there is widespread use of antiretroviral drugs. However, the head of the biotech company VaxGen, which launched the first efficacy trials of an AIDS vaccine in the United States, argued that not everyone would start treatment immediately, and because researchers would be taking blood from participants every 24 weeks or so they should be able to make at least one viral load measurement in many untreated people who become infected (Cohen 1998: 22).

In South Africa, will researchers have an obligation to provide antiretroviral treatment to subjects who become infected during the course of the trials?

However, delaying drug treatment until viral loads can be measured, as is implicit in VaxGen's trial design, only adds to the complex ethical problems already inherent in treating participants who develop HIV infection during the trials. This delay in treatment will pose problems in the developed world where it will be ethically required that individuals in vaccine trials who have acquired HIV infection will be offered antiretroviral therapy. It is also expected that a delay in treatment will not be tolerated in the West. While the standard of care in the developing world was 'no treatment for HIV/AIDS', the ethical dilemma of delaying treatment to measure viral load was obviated. However, the implementation of government-sponsored antiretroviral programmes since 2003 has rendered treatment delays unacceptable. The recent development of 'surrogate endpoints' in the design of HIV vaccine trials has made it possible to treat seroconverters and to continue to monitor the viral markers.

The question of treating trial participants with antiretroviral drugs if they develop infection during the trials has raised considerable controversy in South Africa. While the issue was skirted in 1998 by stating that this issue would be left up to the host country to decide, by 2003 it was clarified that all seroconverters on HIV vaccine trials would have to be treated. Exactly how the treatment is to be operationalised remains unresolved (Tucker 2003: 995).

Various 'social harms' may burden participants in a vaccine trial. Participants might be identified as high risk for AIDS, or might be mistakenly assumed to have AIDS. A Thai study has shown that 24 to 49 percent of participants believed that their partners would refuse to have sex with them after immunisation (Celentano 1995: 1079). Discrimination based on HIV-antibody status may occur in a number of settings – acceptance into the military, the job corps, the peace corps or the foreign service; the purchase of insurance; permission to immigrate or travel abroad or incarceration (Hodel 1994: 256). While it is possible to distinguish between HIV-positive results from a vaccine as opposed to natural infection using different laboratory tests, many potential participants might be unaware of this; hence this will be perceived as a significant risk.

The possibility of being included in a control group in the trial, where a placebo will be used instead of the HIV vaccine, will also shift the risk-benefit ratio in a rather negative direction. Researchers in Philadelphia have already reported that interest in participating in a vaccine trial dropped from 47 percent to 24 percent when the possibility of using a placebo was mentioned (Jenkins 1995: 37).

Finally, a further risk inherent in an HIV vaccine trial is the possibility of increased risk-taking behaviour by participants who mistakenly believe that they have been protected by the vaccine.

What are the benefits, if any, of trial participation?

As scientists weigh the potential benefits of conducting a trial against the potential risks, so too will individual participants and target communities weigh relevant data before deciding to participate. This risk-benefit calculus will ultimately be informed by social values. This is of special relevance to the third world where in communities already 'burdened by violence, drugs, alcohol, unemployment, urban decay and the like, the AIDS epidemic has merely exacerbated an already arduous burden of day-to-day survival. For many inner-city residents, the threat of random gunfire easily exceeds the somewhat less immediate threat of HIV infection, a risk profile that is difficult for outsiders to appreciate' (Hodel 1994: 255). This sentiment is echoed by South African social anthropologist, Virginia van der Vliet, in her book *The Politics of AIDS*, in a chapter entitled 'The Savagery of Life: Powerlessness and Vulnerability':

> Increasingly, those affected are the poor in urban ghettos, illegal migrants, drug users, street children, prostitutes, or the impoverished people in third world countries. They are not unacquainted with the savagery of life. For them, AIDS is just an additional problem, often faced with their customary fatalism. Fatalism is no protection against AIDS (Van der Vliet 1996: 77–78).

It is against this backdrop of fatalism that one needs to assess whether the development of a protective vaccine against AIDS will be *perceived to be* of overwhelming benefit to the third world.

Thus far the benefits cited have been located at two extremes of a narrow range of limited possibilities. Subjects may be motivated to join a trial either on altruistic grounds or on grounds of personal benefit. A few studies have been conducted to date to assess the motivation of people to participate in trials. In one such study in Thailand, purely altruistic motives were unrelated to willingness to participate (Jenkins 1995: 40–41).

Where HIV vaccine trials are concerned, the risk-benefit ratio is situated in a rather precarious position.

Similarly, in another survey of 2 180 Thai people, 62 percent found that the principle inducement to join a trial was health insurance (Celentano 1995: 1079–1082).

Where HIV vaccine trials are concerned, the risk-benefit ratio is situated in a rather precarious position. It is clear to see that participants have little to benefit personally from such trials and potentially much to lose. In a French vaccine trial, only 57 of 645 persons who had expressed initial interest by mail actually enrolled in the trial. Other surveys have found that under the relatively hypothetical condition of being asked to join a phase 2 or 3 HIV vaccine trial, levels of willingness have ranged from 37 percent to 84 percent.

Studies that have gone beyond asking the simple question of whether participants would be willing to join a trial have found that interest dropped dramatically when specific trial features or procedures were explained. Research on intravenous drug users in the New York City area found that the percentage of 'very interested' potential volunteers dropped from 50 percent to 17 percent after they received information normally contained in a consent form. Another study found that 73 percent of those approached in Baltimore were interested in participation, although this figure dropped to 49 percent after the issue of testing HIV antibody-positive as a consequence of immunologic response to the vaccine was discussed (Jenkins 1995: 37). Both studies were conducted on people at high risk to develop HIV infection.

Interestingly, studies are also finding that willingness to participate in vaccine trials is associated with lower levels of education. In a Thailand study of 255 participants, high school-educated respondents were more willing to participate than university graduates (Jenkins 1995: 39). One wonders whether this choice not to participate by more educated respondents is not the result of a more accurate appreciation of the risk-benefit ratio inherent in these trials, namely the high risk-low benefit scenario.

Given full details of the risks and benefits of an HIV vaccine trial, participants will either exercise their right of refusal to participate or will agree to participate only if the benefit is maximised in terms of personal incentives, in particular, health care, in the developing world. A crucial factor to be considered is that in order for the benefits to outweigh the risks in the trial of an HIV vaccine, an individual would have to be at some risk of HIV infection. The necessity of being at risk, therefore, has scientific and ethical import.

THE FOURTH PRINCIPLE: Justice

The principle of justice or fairness requires that the benefits and the burdens of research be equitably distributed among individuals or communities. No single group can be required to bear a disproportionate share of the risk or be favoured with a disproportionate share of the benefits (Loue 1996: 51).

Under the principle of justice, research subjects should be chosen 'for reasons directly related to the problem being studied', and not 'because of their easy availability, their compromised position, or their manipulability'. As a result, the 'practical concerns that make an AIDS vaccine trial easier to conduct in Africa do not alone constitute sufficient justification to use Africans as subjects. Only the scientific concerns related directly to the problem of establishing the ability of a vaccine to prevent HIV infection are relevant' (Christakis 1988: 36).

Where HIV/AIDS is concerned, it is evident that this disease is rampant in Africa. As a result, it may be unavoidable that a higher degree of research risk is tolerated in order to deal with the problem and this may even be socially sanctioned. However, this does not mean that Westerners should 'indiscriminately benefit from research conducted in Africa if Africans are systematically subjected to excess research risks with the prospect of deriving but little benefit' (Christakis 1988: 36).

Where an AIDS vaccine is concerned, much of the world stands to gain from the development of an effective vaccine. In keeping with the principle of justice, those who stand to benefit from the vaccine should also bear the burden. Hence, the research risks should be fairly distributed, as should the benefits. Vaccine development trials need not be restricted to the African continent.

In Africa, economic constraints may prevent adequate distribution of such a vaccine. The benefits to Africans are thus 'only hypothetical unless there is a financial commitment by the developed world to provide the vaccine. In this light, it would be frankly unethical to subject Africans to a disproportionate share of the research risks' (Christakis 1988: 36).

The Council for the International Organisations of Medical Sciences (CIOMS) Guideline 15 on Externally Sponsored Research requires that any trial 'must be responsive to the health needs of the host country. Any product developed through such research (should) be made reasonably available to the inhabitants of the host community or country at completion of successful testing' (Bloom 1998: 186–187). This is also a requirement of the latest version of the Declaration of Helsinki (October 2000). A contingency of any trial of an AIDS vaccine in Africa by Western scientists should thus be to provide access to the technology once it is developed – possibly in the form of free or subsidised vaccine (Christakis 1988: 36).

In South Africa, the HIV Vertical Transmission Trials are an excellent example of the violation of the principle of justice in a research setting. By 2001, four years after the completion of these trials to find shorter courses of antiretroviral treatment for HIV-infected pregnant women, millions of eligible women had not received treatment. It had clearly been shown that these shorter regimes of treatment are effective. Yet, there was no funding forthcoming from the South African government or from the developed world, in particular the

United States, who were involved in these research trials. It was only in 2002, five years after the trials were completed, that pregnant women in South Africa were given Nevirapine to prevent vertical transmission of HIV.

In a paper published in the *American Journal of Public Health*, this issue is discussed openly. The outcome of the trials performed on impoverished populations around the world was clearly not the delivery of the necessary drugs to these developing countries. Instead, the purpose was 'to provide information that the host country can use to make a sound judgement about the appropriateness and financial feasibility of providing the intervention' (Annas 1998: 561). Good intent in the absence of a sound plan to provide the intervention, once proven to be effective, is no justification for the performance of such research. Annas goes on to say:

> Unless the intervention being tested will actually be made available to the impoverished populations that are being used as research subjects, developed countries are simply exploiting them in order to quickly use the knowledge gained from the clinical trials for the developed countries' own benefit. If the research reveals regimens of equal efficacy at less cost, these regimens will surely be implemented in the developed world. If the research reveals the regimens to be less efficacious, these results will be added to the scientific literature, and the developed world will not conduct these studies (1998: 561).

Once again, with the proposed vaccine trials, South Africa has not clarified that it will conduct these trials on condition that a definite plan is in place to acquire the vaccine for widespread use, if it proves to be effective. Of note, however, is the fact that South Africa has decided not to conduct trials using a clade B vaccine that has already been developed in the United States. This viral subtype is not common in sub-Saharan Africa but it is the predominant clade in North America where homosexual transmission of HIV is common. In South Africa, with a predominantly heterosexual transmission of disease, the predominant subtype is clade C. South African researchers have opted to rather develop an appropriate clade C vaccine for experimentation here.

Yet another way in which the principle of justice can be violated involves the counselling of trial participants to continue practising other preventative measures after the vaccine has been administered. With the promotion of these measures, it will be difficult to assess vaccine efficacy. These interventions could diminish the ability of the study to detect a difference between true vaccine recipients and controls by decreasing the incidence of HIV infection in all participants for reasons unrelated to vaccine status (Christakis 1988: 34). On the other hand, failing to stress these measures could result in a greater risk of contracting HIV infection, especially if the vaccine proves to be ineffective. To circumvent this problem, a larger study group would be required to detect the relatively smaller measured influence of the vaccine. As a result, more individuals will be exposed to the experimental vaccine and the cost of the trials will be higher. It will also take longer to get statistically significant results. To prevent this potential harm to participants and in all fairness to them, it is imperative that researchers continue to promote preventative measures other than the vaccine.

Relevance of the Four Principles in Africa

It is obvious from the preceding discussion that the principles are 'far from comprehensive and lack extensive guidance on issues of major importance, including the simultaneous maximisation of principles or the prioritising of conflicting principles. Moreover, they are Western constructs and, as such, do not take into account local customs and traditions that should be respected and incorporated into the research process to the extent possible' (Loue 1996: 51).

It is increasingly being realised that in:

> . . . most settings in Africa, informed consent will be problematic and difficult, and it may even preclude ethical research. This is because, in the absence of health care, virtually any offer of medical assistance (even in the guise of research) will be accepted as 'better than nothing' and research will almost inevitably be confused with treatment, making informed consent difficult (Annas 1998: 562).

Support for this conclusion was elicited in interviews with trial participants in the Côte d'Ivoire where it was found that 'many of the participants did not understand the implications of the trial, even though they gave their consent'. In the words of an African researcher:

> . . . in an environment where the majority can neither read nor write and is wallowing in poverty and sickness, hunger and homelessness, and where the educated, the powerful, the rich, or the expatriate is a semi-god, how can you talk of informed consent? (Zion 1998: 1330).

In the context of third world settings in Africa, balancing the principles of beneficence and non-maleficence in the form of the risk-benefit ratio has already been shown to be problematic. The odds are leaning heavily in the direction of high risk-low benefit, especially if the intervention being tested is not made available to the third world after the trials. It appears as though only those at high risk of developing HIV/AIDS will derive benefit. The risk-benefit ratio can also be viewed in terms of the Belmont Report which requires that 'risks to subjects be outweighed by the sum of both the anticipated benefit to the subject, if any, and the anticipated benefit to society' (Christakis 1988: 35). Any principles that prevent harm to research subjects and demand their beneficient treatment are particularly relevant in a third world setting where vulnerable subjects need more protection than usual.

It is increasingly being realised that in most settings in Africa, informed consent will be problematic and difficult, and it may even preclude ethical research.

The basic ethical principles that guide human investigation, as defined by the

Helsinki Declaration and the Nuremberg Code, need to be interpreted and applied within different cultural settings. In Africa,

> . . . making respect for autonomy a trump moral principle, rather than one moral principle in a system of principles, gives it an excessive value. In many clinical circumstances the weight of respect for autonomy is minimal, and the weight of non-maleficence or beneficence is maximal. Similarly, in public policy, the demands of justice can easily outweigh the demands of respect for autonomy (Beauchamp and Childress 1994: 181).

In the third world it appears as though the principles of beneficence, non-maleficence and justice should be maximised relative to the principle of autonomy. It is obvious that by using material inducements to shift the risk-benefit ratio in a positive direction, voluntariness of informed consent is compromised. However, fair distribution of the benefits of the research, in the form of an effective vaccine, would justify some of the research risk taken by impoverished third world populations. At the same time, sincere efforts to obtain truly informed consent should not be abandoned.

Trial participation – the tension between liberalism and communitarianism

In South Africa, as we emerge from a history where the rights of the vulnerable and poor have been negated in the service of apartheid, the preference for a subject-oriented view, where research is concerned, is a logical choice. Our new democratic order, our Constitution and Bill of Rights, bear testimony to this. Liberal individualism has reached South Africa also. Unlike a subject-oriented approach, a balancing approach is more closely aligned to a sense of society or community – medical research is seen as one of the essential goods in society and is therefore vital to the survival of such a society (Ackerman and Strong 1989: 166–179). Christakis comments that an African might find it 'difficult to see how the interests of the subject conflict with the interests of the society except, of course, if the society is not his own'. In traditional Africa, the interests of the subject and of society are necessarily congruent. People see themselves as 'potential persons' who become fully human to the extent that they are included in relationships with others (Shutte, unpublished data).

South Africa is an ideal site for HIV vaccine research. The HIV vaccine trials pose a grave and significant risk to the individual who may subsequently have little to gain. Under such circumstances, statistically significant trial participation can only be ensured by an appeal to altruism – in the African context, Ubuntu. In this regard, the interests of science and society are seen as one with the interests of the individual. Interdependence and connectedness are prominent features of traditional African society. In such a setting, trial participation and hence medical research will be possible.

However, with the influence of Western liberalism, an appeal to Ubuntu will be difficult. The principle of autonomy is becoming slowly but firmly entrenched in Africa. A retreat to Ubuntu will be seen for what it is – a convenient retreat to a comfort zone for Western researchers. It would appear that the West has realised that the very concept of liberal individualism, which has generally worked well so far, is becoming problematic as a result of its spread to Africa. Having developed a strong sense of self-preservation in keeping with the ethos of liberal individualism, it appears as if a retreat from the universal principles of equality and liberty to 'different', local standards of care is being favoured. This can only be achieved if some of the 'rules' are changed and the World Medical Association takes the lead in attempting to amend the Declaration of Helsinki in 2000. These attempted revisions tended towards ethical relativism. Such relativism would threaten to 'institutionalise global injustice in the application of ethical standards' (London 1999: 812).

In rural Africa, an appeal to Ubuntu could succeed in harnessing trial participation. However, in the developed areas of Africa, where individualism is spreading, this will not be possible (Leach 1999: 139–148).

Conclusions

If the principles that underpin the Declaration of Helsinki are strictly adhered to, constraints on the rights of the individual will not be permissible and in the third world, this would render research unethical and hence, impossible. Conversely, many of the world's dominant cultures allow infringements on the rights of the individual to produce societal good. Hence, it is evident that it is problematic to pursue an individualistic view, perhaps in general, but especially where research in the third world is concerned.

This does not imply that the ethical guidelines which already exist and which protect the interests of research subjects should be abandoned. Nor should one aim for universality of existing Western principles because the global population is not homogenous and universality 'obscures and obliterates the particularity and specificity of morality which is grounded in communal traditions' (Bernstein 1982). For example, if autonomy is to be viewed as a truly universal principle, is it not possible that the 'North American paradigm is only one version of it'? It is therefore unnecessary for 'every country to follow the practice of autonomy in all of its details in a fashion identical to that found in North America' (Akabayashi 1999: 299).

The Four Principles approach provides a valid framework in which to consider the various ethical issues but, as a Western construct, does not 'take into account local customs and traditions that should be respected and incorporated into the research process' as far as is possible (Loue 1996: 51). So, although incomplete, it is not incompatible with values in other cultures. As such, culturally relevant ethical issues need to be incorporated into existing frameworks to augment them with cultural sensitivity. However, changing the rules from time to time and from place to place to achieve the research aims of the West will be both unjustifiable and morally reprehensible.

Undoubtedly, the HIV vaccine trials in South Africa will pose a major ethical challenge to all involved. We must, however, be wary that in our haste to develop and test an HIV vaccine, we do not cause an ethical catastrophe that we will never be able to justify. It has taken a long time for the research community to recover from Tuskegee. May we never tread along that path again!

References

Abdool Karim, Q., Abdool Karim, S.S. et al. (1998). Informed Consent for HIV Testing in a South African Hospital: Is It Truly Informed and Truly Voluntary? *American Journal of Public Health*, 88(4): 637–640.

Achrekar, A., Gupta, R. (1998). Informed Consent for a Clinical Trial in Thailand. NEJM 339: 1331–32.

Ackerman, T.F., Strong, C. (1989). *A Casebook of Medical Ethics*. New York: Oxford University Press.

Akabayashi, A. et al. (1999). Family consent, communication, and advance directives for cancer disclosure: a Japanese case and discussion. *Journal of Medical Ethics*, 25: 296–301.

Annas, G.J., Grodin, M.A. (1998). Human Rights and Maternal-Fetal HIV Transmission Prevention Trials in Africa. *American Journal of Public Health*, 88(4): 560–562.

Appelbaum, P.S., Grisso, T. (1988). Assessing Patients' Capacities To Consent To Treatment. *The New England Journal of Medicine*, 319(25): 1635–1636.

Barry, M., Ethical Considerations of Human Investigation in Developing Countries - The AIDS Dilemma. *The New England Journal of Medicine*, 319(16): 1083–1085.

Beauchamp, T.L., Childress, J.F. (1994). *Principles of Biomedical Ethics*. 4th edition. New York: Oxford University Press.

Bernstein, R.J. (1982). Nietzsche or Aristotle? Reflections on Alasdair MacIntyre's After Virtue. *Philosophical Profiles. Essays in a Pragmatic Mode*. Cambridge: Polity Press.

Bloom, B.R. (1998). The Highest Attainable Standard: Ethical Issues in AIDS Vaccines. *Science*, 279: 186–187.

Celentano, D.D., Beyrer, C., Natpratan, C., Eiumtrakul, S., Sussman, L., Renzullo, P.O., Khamboonruang & Nelson, K.E. (1995). Willingness to participate in AIDS vaccine trials among high-risk populations in northern Thailand. *AIDS*, 9: 1079–1083.

Choopanya, K., Tappero, J.W., Pitisuttithum, P., Suntharasamai, P., Kaewkungwal, J. et al. (2004). Preliminary results of a phase 3 HIV vaccine efficacy trial among injecting drug users in Thailand. Oral presentation. 15th International AIDS conference, Bangkok 15th July 2004.

Christakis, N.A. (1988). The Ethical Design of an AIDS Vaccine Trial in Africa. *Hastings Centre Report*, (June/July): 31–37.

Cohen, J. (1998). No Consensus on Rules for AIDS Vaccine Trials. *Science*, 281: 22–23.

De Craemer, W. (1983). A cross-cultural perspective on personhood. Milbank Memorial Fund Quarterly 61: 19–34.

Guenter, D., Esparza, J., Macklin, R. (2000). Ethical considerations in international HIV vaccine trials: summary of a consultative process conducted by the Joint United Nations Programme on HIV/AIDS (UNAIDS) *J of Med Ethics*. 26: 37–43.

Heywood, M. (1998). What is Informed Consent? *Workshop on ethical issues in the conduct of HIV vaccine trials*. Durban, South Africa.

Hodel, D. (1994). HIV Preventive Vaccine Efficacy Trials in the United States: An Overview of Target Communities' Concerns. *AIDS Research and Human Retroviruses*. 10(2): 255.

Jenkins, R.A., Temoshok, L.R., Virochsiri, K. (1995). Incentives and Disincentives to participate in Prophylactic HIV Vaccine Research. *Journal of Acquired Immune Deficiency Syndromes and Human Retrovirology*, 9: 36–42.

Kopelman, L.M. (1994). 'Research Policy/ III. Risk and Vulnerable Groups.' *Encyclopaedia of Bioethics*. 2nd edition. New York: Macmillan Free Press.

Kunstadter, P. (1980). Medical ethics in cross-cultural and multi-cultural perspectives. Social Science & Medicine 4: 289–296.

Leach, A., Hilton, S., Greenwood, B.M., Manneh, E., Dibba, B. et al. (1999). An evaluation of the informed consent procedure used during a trial of a Heamophilus influenzae type B conjugate vaccine undertaken in The Gambia, West Africa *Social Science & Medicine* 48: 139–148.

London, L. et al (1999). Revision of the Helsinki Declaration – Ethical standards at risk? *South African Medical Journal*, 89(8): 812–813.

Loue, S. et al. (1996). Research Bioethics in the Ugandan Context: A Program summary. *Journal of Law, Medicine & Ethics*, 24: 47–53.

Lurie, P., Wolfe, S.M. (1997). Unethical Trials of Interventions to Reduce Perinatal Transmission of the Human Immunodeficiency Virus in Developing Countries. *The New England Journal of Medicine*, 337(12): 853–855.

Macfarlane, D. (2000). Almost half of SA is illiterate. *Mail & Guardian*, 1st–7th December 2000:18.

McCarthy, M. (1997). AIDS doctors push for live-virus vaccine trials. *The Lancet*, 350: 1082.

Mkize, N. (2004). Psychology: An African Perspective. *Critical Psychology*. Ed. D. Hook. Cape Town: UCT Press: 24–52.

Moodley, K., Myer, L. (2003) Participant Remuneration for Research – How Much Is Enough? *South African Medical Journal*, 93.9: 677–78.

Moodley, K., Pather, M., Myer, L. (2004) Informed Consent: Participants' Knowledge and Perceptions of Influenza Vaccine Trial Involvement in South Africa.

Mugerwa, R.D., Kaleebu, P., Mugyenyi, P., Katongole-Mbidde, E., Hom, D.L. (2002). First trial of the HIV-1 vaccine in Africa: Ugandan experience.*BMJ* 324: 226–229.

Prabhakaran, S. (1997). Mothers give support to placebo trials. *Mail & Guardian* (3rd–9th October 1997): 5.

Ransome, O. (1998). What is Informed Consent? *Workshop on the ethical issues in the conduct of HIV vaccine trials*. Durban, South Africa.

Shutte, A. *Ubuntu. The African Vision*. Chapter Two. Unpublished book.

Tacket, C.O., Edelman R. (1990). Ethical Issues Involving Volunteers in AIDS Vaccine Trials. *The Journal of Infectious Diseases*, 161: 356.

Tsai, D.F. (1999). Ancient Chinese medical ethics and the four principles of biomedical ethics. *Journal of Medical Ethics*, 25: 315–321.

Tucker, T., Slack, C. (2003). Not If but How? Caring for HIV-1 Vaccine Trial Participants in South Africa. *The Lancet* 362: 995.

Van der Vliet, V. (1996). *The Politics of AIDS*. London: Bowerdean Publishing Company Limited.

Zion, D. (1998). The Ethics of AIDS Vaccine Trials. Letter. *Science*, 280: 1329–1330.

Chapter 11

The HIV/AIDS pandemic, African traditional values and the search for a vaccine in Africa

Traditional African values have a lot to offer in an approach towards fighting HIV/AIDS. In this chapter **Godfrey B. Tangwa** *argues that values such as empathy and unpaid assistance for those in genuine need will do more to curb the pandemic than the first world's market-driven, profit-oriented practices have done. He also outlines what he believes to be some encouraging research done in Africa towards an AIDS vaccine.*

The response to the AIDS pandemic in Africa should take into account traditional African outlooks and attitudes to commerce and disease. My central claim here is that some of the international responses to the AIDS pandemic probably show the limitations of the 'Western approach' to medical problem-solving. This situation also creates a unique opportunity to re-appraise and re-evaluate traditional African communitarian values, knowledge systems and practices, which, though in danger of being abandoned in preference for borrowed ones, could be of help in the search for a solution to the scourge of AIDS.

What are these 'African outlooks, values and attitudes to commerce and disease'? They are succinctly captured in a remark made by my mother a few years ago, to the effect that medicine and commerce are bad companions (Tangwa 2001: S37). In traditional Africa, curative medicine particularly, but also diagnostic and prophylactic medicine to some extent, were divorced from commerce. The resources of the immediate community were always mobilised on behalf of a seriously ill person and, especially in face of an epidemic, no traditional healer worthy of the name could charge a direct fee for his/her services without being considered a quack or even a con person or losing his/her God-given special skills and endowments (Tangwa 1999a: 277).

Any typical African market, and the system of haggling that goes on there, is highly indicative of an attitude based on a deeply ingrained value system and worldview. In a typical African market, the prices of goods are never fixed. Today there are, of course, modern shops all over Africa, especially in the big cities and urban centres, where the prices of goods and products are fixed. But 'fixed prices' are a borrowed practice in Africa, which has not yet been fully accepted and integrated into the culture and everyday practice. It is not at all uncommon today to witness an African trying to beat down the fixed price of an article in a shop, even in one of the big Western cities, if s/he needs or wants it badly but does not have enough money to pay for it.

In traditional Africa and in any typically African market today, the price quoted to a prospective buyer by a seller usually depends on who the buyer happens to be. In any case, the quoted price is always an invitation for an animated and lively dialogue in which both buyer and seller reveal and learn information about each other and the particular situation and circumstances of the other. (In the last ten years or so, successive batches of my American students from Dickinson College, on a six-month exchange programme here in Yaounde, Cameroon, have found this one of the most difficult aspects of African culture and practices to adapt to or deal with, as can be witnessed from their course essays describing aspects of African culture and practices most at variance, in their opinion, with their expectations or from what obtains in their own country.)

I once witnessed a scene in an African market (the weekly Mbvë Market of Kumbo Town in Cameroon) where, on being told the price of an article, the buyer, without any further ado and without saying anything, immediately removed the amount of money quoted, threw it in front of the seller, took the article and started walking hurriedly away. The seller was sufficiently worried by such behaviour to run after him, give him back his money and retrieve the article, under the pretext that it was, after all, not for sale. The real reason for such a reaction was that he was worried that the buyer may not be a genuine human being and that his money and manner were liable to 'bring misfortune'.

In the course of haggling over an article, the seller and buyer sometimes discover that they are kinsfolk or blood relations, in which case the latter could end up obtaining the said article for free or with a generous addition or other gift. And whenever the product needed is for a patient or is an ingredient for preparing the medicine of a patient, then, more often than not, it is given either free or very cheaply. On the other hand, the situation of the seller and the reason for which s/he is selling the article could cause the buyer voluntarily to pay much more for it than the quoted price. The poverty or otherwise of both buyer and seller as well as his/her situation and need are always a factor to be considered in reaching the final price of any product or article in any typical African market. The same attitude underlies traditional practice within my own natal culture, Nso' culture, whereby it was permissible for anybody to pick fruits fallen from any orchard, no matter to whom the trees belonged, or to harvest enough of a directly edible crop to stem hunger for the moment. As long as you did not climb up the fruit tree or harvest the crop to store or resale (both of which were strictly taboo), you were considered to be well within the narrow bounds of morally permissible action (Tangwa 2000: 13).

The general underlying idea is that no one should die from sheer need or want in a situation where the remedy is readily available. This can be considered as the antithesis of the Western economic idea and practice, now more or less successfully globalised, where the more desperately you need a product or a service, the more you are required to pay for it under the so-called law of demand and supply. For sure, the African traditional practices and the worldview and attitudes that sustained them had their negative aspects and disadvantages, such as their tendency to encourage complacency and individual laziness, let alone a generally stagnant and unprogressive society. Moreover, they now seem to be receding out of history irretrievably under the combined onslaught of colonialism, modernism and globalisation. Many of the younger generation of Africans have been born, raised and live in the melting pot of urbanised cities and towns with a highly syncretistic culture whose underpinnings are Western influences. Some among this category of modern-day Africans know little or nothing about unadulterated traditional African ways of life and cultural practices.

Nevertheless, the spirit and moral imperatives that imbued some of the traditional African customs and practices could still be salvaged, modernised and even globalised (Tangwa 2001: S37). It would be a good idea to attempt confronting, in a more sustained and systematic way, the antithetical moral intuitions and attitudes of traditional Africa with those of modern Western society, which have been exported and imported or simply imposed all over the globe. This, however, is not the time or place to attempt such a task. My rather modest aim here is to search in the 'junk bag', so to speak, of abandoned or about to be abandoned traditional African values and practices to see whether there may not be elements therein that might be more helpful in the face of the AIDS crisis in Africa than has so far been considered.

Although there are dangers of over-generalising, Western countries seem to place greater emphasis on individual rights (over community needs), libertarian philosophy and market-driven economies. The central importance of commerce in Western thought and practice and the linkage of medicine and health care to the market in the system has its positive side and advantages, such as the very rapid development of medicine in general and of new drugs and treatments in particular. However, it is attended by the understandable tendency of industries and business companies to be driven by morally blind, purely economic logic and the lure of profit. This tendency is often on the lookout for and sees economic opportunities and advantages in even the most distressing of human situations. Such a situation will not be changed by wishful thinking or, under any circumstances, in the short run; many Westerners who are themselves unhappy with this state of affairs are quite powerless to do anything about it. In Africa, where traditional attitudes to both commerce and to disease and treatment suggest an alternative approach, self-reliance initiatives that are supported by genuine humanitarian international help would seem to be the surer way forward against the AIDS epidemic.

The African scene

The lethal nature of the HIV/AIDS pandemic, its causal connection with sexual activity, its non-respect for geographical or cultural boundaries, and its implications for human reproduction, clearly conjure the spectre of the annihilation of the human species. But, while HIV/AIDS has the poise and posture of a global pandemic, there is no doubt that it is particularly an African problem. According to recent statistics (March 2001), of the 53 million people infected with HIV/AIDS worldwide, about two-thirds are in sub-Saharan Africa. Some of the latest estimates from UNAIDS sources put the number of new HIV infections in 2000 at 5.3 million of which 45 000 occurred in North America, 60 000 in the Caribbean, 150 000 in Latin America, 30 000 in Western Europe, 80 000 in North Africa and the Middle East, 500 in Australia and New Zealand, and 3.8 million in sub-Saharan Africa (*Kenya Times*, Vol. 2, No. 32732, Tuesday 5th December 2000). In my own country, Cameroon, the rate of HIV infection amongst the sexually active population has rapidly progressed from 0.5 percent in 1987 to 11 percent in 2000. At the time of writing (May 2001), nearly a million Cameroonians, including 5 000 infants, out of a population of about 15 million, are HIV positive; 52 000 persons died of AIDS in 1999 alone; 5 168 cases of new infection were recorded in 2000; and 91 000 AIDS orphans are on record.

While HIV/AIDS has the poise and posture of a global pandemic, there is no doubt that it is particularly an African problem.

The HIV/AIDS epidemic has overtaken every other disease as the top killer in Africa, where it has been responsible for an estimated 17 million deaths within a period of less than two decades. And, as Johanna McGeary has so aptly remarked, AIDS in Africa bears little resemblance to the epidemic elsewhere which is usually 'limited to specific high-risk groups and brought under control through intensive education, vigorous political action and expensive drug therapy' (McGeary 2001: 45). In Africa, by contrast, 'the disease has bred a Darwinian perversion. Society's fittest, not its frailest, are the ones who die – adults spirited away, leaving the old and the children behind. You cannot define risk groups: everyone who is sexually active is at risk' (Ibid.).

The HI virus probably found its way from still unknown origins into Cameroon in the late seventies or early eighties. By the late eighties, when the public health authorities first started timidly talking about it, most Cameroonians were still very sceptical about the existence of the virus, some claiming that it was a ploy to discourage sexual activity. Today, scarcely two decades afterwards, there is hardly a Cameroonian amongst 15 million inhabitants who can rightly claim not to have lost a close relative, neighbour, friend or colleague to the AIDS pandemic. And yet there has been little change in the sexual habits of Cameroonians, HIV/AIDS sensitisation campaigns notwithstanding.

VANHIVAV in Cameroon

In the field of research for an AIDS vaccine, one of the commonest current-day moral suspicions is the perception that the West is using Africa and other so-called 'developing world' regions as guinea pigs for research that will, eventually, only benefit Westerners (Benatar 2000, Greco 2000). This could well be alleviated if Africans could, on a much larger scale than is currently happening in South Africa for instance, become involved not only in assisting, but also conceptualising, initiating and executing this (often very costly) research. The problem is that African initiatives are mostly not taken seriously by the Western world and its large, wealthy, funding institutions, as well as by many African governmental authorities, some of them more preoccupied with personal political survival or with converting public resources into private property. Dictatorship, illegitimate power and corruption are, unfortunately, still the ailments bedevilling power, public authority and governance in many parts of Africa today (Tangwa 1998).

A local initiative in Cameroon, which unlike those of South Africa has not yet received any support, either from the Cameroon government or from any international or national sponsors, is that of Professor Victor Anomah Ngu, an oncologist and former laureate of the Lasker Award for cancer research. Professor Ngu, a former Minister of Health and former Vice-Chancellor of the University of Yaounde, started his research for a vaccine against the HIV/AIDS virus about a decade ago. His seminal hypothesis, published in *Medical Hypotheses* (Ngu 1994; Ngu 1997), is that, being an 'enveloped' virus, the HIV is 'perceived' by the host immune system as 'partly-self' because of the presence of the host cell wall membrane on the viral envelope and that this situation leads to an ineffective response by the body's immune system to the virus. He reasoned that viral core antigens *without the envelope* would be 'perceived' as 'non-self' by the host immune system, thereby eliciting an appropriate and effective immune response. In a normal uninfected person, therefore, such 'unenveloped' core antigens, he claims, would serve as an effective vaccine.

As a non-medical person with more than a passing interest in science and medicine, I found Professor Ngu's hypothesis simple and straightforwardly reasonable, coherent, interesting and well worth serious investigation in the face of the grave threat that is HIV/AIDS. But when he presented his hypothesis and preliminary investigative findings to his medical colleagues (many of them involved by government accreditation in 'the fight against HIV/AIDS') and to appropriate international agencies, with a view to obtaining assistance in systematically testing his hypothesis, he met with only scepticism and even derision. In a letter dated 15 January 1992 the 'Steering Committee on Clinical Research and Drug Development' of the WHO Global Programme on AIDS, in answer to Ngu's application for support, stated, *inter alia,* that they 'felt unable to recommend . . . financial support [because] the methods of antigen preparation and its standardisation were not fully described, and that the study did not have sufficient scientific basis'. But the deadly nature and apparent invincibility of the AIDS epidemic is surely an opportunity to take a hard, unbiased look at all serious efforts at finding a solution, including unconventional ones that may deliberately deviate from or otherwise fall outside of the dominant paradigm. Professor Ngu then proceeded, with meagre personal resources, to demonstrate his claims in sero-positive patients by preparing an *autologuous* vaccine for each of the patients. The results he obtained, even with his rudimentary facilities, clearly seemed to confirm his hypothesis (Ngu 1999).

In September 2000, Professor Ngu and I presented a joint paper at the Fifth World Congress of Bioethics, Imperial College, London, UK, under the title: 'Effective Vaccine against and Immunotherapy of the HIV: Scientific Report and Ethical Considerations from Cameroon' (Ngu and Tangwa 2000). The gist of our joint paper can be summarised in eight points, as follows:

- The HIV/AIDS is a terrifying and deadly disease, particularly for sub-Saharan Africa, where it has already claimed more than 17 million victims in less than two decades and is poised to wipe out the entire population.
- The central problem of the HIV infection is that immune responses by the body fail to kill the virus.
- The reason for this failure is that it is an enveloped virus. The envelope of the HIV is derived from host CD4 cell wall and killing the virus with its envelope will also kill host CD4 cells – leading to an auto-immune disease. The virus has used this threat to blackmail and to block, so to speak, effective immune responses that alone can kill the virus.
- The ideal solution for the body is to provoke immune responses to the HIV that are without an envelope. Such new immune responses will effectively kill only the virus, sparing the viral envelope and CD4.
- To obtain such new effective immune responses in an uninfected person, one starts with HIV antigens from which the envelope has been destroyed beforehand. Such antigens, which cannot infect, constitute an effective vaccine for the HIV. All HIV antigens, with only the envelope destroyed, constitute an effective HIV vaccine.
- Being unable to have such a vaccine tested on healthy persons, we tested it on patients, using their own auto-vaccine, under special conditions and have so far obtained results that confirm our hypothesis.
- This test showed that the auto-vaccine provoked immune responses that kill the virus, confirming its effectiveness as a vaccine. This procedure of using vaccines to induce the killing of the virus in patients constitutes a form of immuno-therapy for the HIV. A vaccine produced on the same basis as the auto-vaccine will be acceptable for trial on the public, because it has proved its worth in patients.
- Such a vaccine, in a world in which medicine and commerce seem to have become inseparable companions, holds the best hope of stopping the AIDS epidemic, especially in sub-Saharan Africa, because, *inter alia,* it is completely effective, simple and cheap to produce, using traditional as against modern high technology methods, and therefore affordable for the masses, who are highly vulnerable and most affected by the virus. (On the basis of the autologous vaccines he has been preparing for each of his patients, Professor Ngu estimates that, if produced on an industrial scale, a similar vaccine for healthy

persons would not cost more than an equivalent of about US$0.10 (ten cents) per shot).

Those who listened to our London presentation of what is in effect a candidate vaccine to which the name VANHIVAV has been given, seemed completely taken by surprise. First of all, no one seemed to have entertained the possibility of a 'home-grown' candidate vaccine proposal coming from Africa. What seemed to have been expected were proposals of how Western researchers could carry out ethical and acceptable HIV/AIDS vaccine research in Africa, with or without the collaboration of local scientists. Secondly, surprise was expressed as to why, with the interesting clinical results presented, no Western researchers or funding agencies had shown interest in VANHIVAV.

Since then Professor Ngu has obtained even more convincing results (Ngu 2001) from now being able to measure the viral load, but VANHIVAV has not yet aroused the sort of interest one would expect in the prevailing situation. There are those both at home and abroad who continue to dismiss his work as 'unscientific' without bothering to supply persuasive arguments for this sweeping judgement. (I was present at two recent conferences in Yaounde, given by Professor Ngu, at the Faculty of Medicine and Biomedical Sciences and the *Institut Goethe*, respectively, where some members of the audience still expressed their unsubstantiated scepticism about his optimism regarding his scientific proposals.) Others, while admitting that he may have discovered 'some sort of cure for AIDS, perhaps', seriously contest his claim to have a protocol for an HIV/AIDS candidate vaccine, on the grounds that a vaccine, by definition, is not something you give to a patient (which fulfils the definition of a drug) but rather something you give to a healthy person to prevent infection. This, of course, is trying to dismiss a claim on the basis of a stipulative definition. VANHIVAV is clearly a candidate vaccine with immuno-therapeutic effect, but why should this additional quality exclude it from the category of vaccines? Of course, a vaccine is not normally administered to a patient but rather to a healthy person. But Professor Ngu has not been *vaccinating* HIV/AIDS patients. He does not yet have a vaccine. What he does have is a proposal for making one. His involvement with patients was a way of proving that his hypothesis for a vaccine had scientific merit. The incidental immuno-therapeutic action of such an eventual vaccine, if it can be successfully manufactured, would in no way prevent it from being a vaccine. A boxer who also happens to be a sprinter cannot be said to be any less a boxer on the grounds that boxers are not usually sprinters.

VANHIVAV is clearly a candidate vaccine with immuno-therapeutic effect, but why should this additional quality exclude it from the category of vaccines?

Africa's unequal burden

While the prospect of the possible annihilation of the entire human race by the HIV/AIDS pandemic is indeed far-fetched, that of erasing the African continent of its human inhabitants is not too far from the realm of possibility. The reasons for this, which are mutually self-reinforcing, are many and varied and include, *inter alia*, the following:

- general paucity of modern health care facilities;
- acute and widespread poverty, exacerbated by war, refugee problems and unemployment;
- general lack of awareness of the pending AIDS disaster due to illiteracy and resultant difficulties in communication; and
- cultural attitudes and traditional practices that prevent or subvert recourse to or proper use of effective preventive methods, such as the condom or the bottle in place of breastfeeding.

The relationship between life expectancy and health, on the one hand, and economic growth on the other, indicates that with the AIDS epidemic Africa is caught within a vicious circle from which it will not be easy to bail out. To have the wherewithal to fight adequately against the epidemic, Africa needs to raise its level of production considerably; but those who could help do so – young adults or society's fittest – are the ones dying most from the epidemic.

If we look at global statistics for the distribution of the burden of disease generally in relation to population, the global economy, research resources and actual expenditure on health care, we realise that Africa with over ten percent of the world's population, controls less than one percent of the global economy and is saddled with over 66 percent of HIV/AIDS infections. Furthermore, over 90 percent of global research resources are devoted to diseases causing only 10 percent of the global burden of disease, while 87 percent of global health care expenditure is lavished on only 10 percent of the global population (Benatar 2000: 664 and Benatar and Singer 2000: 824). Above all else, industrialised world pharmaceutical companies, which control the manufacture of modern drugs, are demonstrably interested in making profits and maintaining monopolies and only secondarily in any other matter. As commercial enterprises, multinational corporations cannot be blamed for pursuing profit as such. The question, however, is whether the nature of the catastrophe in Africa does not require imaginative emergency measures, where such profit pursuit can be combined with more morally sensitive global co-operation aimed at helping those in dire need and towards discovering and manufacturing a cheap and affordable vaccine.

The situation of sub-Saharan Africa is indeed critical and such innovative emergency measures are urgently required. Among such putative measures, the search for an effective and affordable vaccine against AIDS occupies pride of place. What the experience of the last two decades in sub-Saharan Africa has demonstrated is that:

- education and sensitisation, while valuable and necessary in their own right, are of limited effect against the HIV/AIDS epidemic until such time as the general level of literacy in the African population is raised considerably; in the short term, given the levels of illiteracy in the adult population of even the most developed sub-Saharan African country (South Africa), viz. 41 percent, this does not seem very likely;

- therapies, such as AZT or Niverapine, which may prevent mother-to-child infection or palliate and prolong the life of AIDS patients, seem not to be generally accessible or affordable given the way they are currently priced. Imaginative measures, which necessitate global co-operation, as suggested in the previous paragraph, are required to make such drugs available and affordable, at least for the purpose of drastically reducing vertical transmission;
- it is not easy for people to suddenly change their behaviour, attitudes, customs or sexual habits.

Furthermore, it is instructive to note that all the major viral epidemics of the past – smallpox, poliomyelitis, yellow fever, cholera, measles etc. – were eliminated or controlled mainly by the use of vaccines. As the co-ordinator of South Africa's Aids Vaccine Initiative (SAAVI), Walter Prozesky is often quoted to have observed: 'Never in history has a viral disease been controlled by drugs. That's why a vaccine is the only possible way to fight HIV' (Galloway 1999: 10). In sub-Saharan Africa in particular, an effective cheap vaccine against HIV/AIDS clearly seems to be the only realistic and the most imperative of goals in the fight against the disease.

All the major viral epidemics of the past – smallpox, poliomyelitis, yellow fever, cholera, measles etc. – were eliminated or controlled mainly by the use of vaccines.

A possible strategy

From the African perspective, the Western approach to the AIDS pandemic, like many other things Western, is overly empirical, statistical and business-like. It is a question whether all problems that face us, including HIV/AIDS, can be solved by a purely analytical method where the base-line approach is to try to reduce complex systems to constituent parts, and where treatment of the parts of necessity implies salvage for the whole. This business-like statistical analyticity may, from some perspectives, appear like the epitome of rationality, but it ignores other perspectives and other aspects of being alive and being human. The analytic paradigm of knowledge is, without doubt, very important and is perhaps the most important kind of knowledge – prevalent to varying degrees in all human cultures – but it is not the only one. There are other types of human knowledge such as the intuitive, the metaphoric, the parabolic, the mythic, etc., which are, more or less, much better developed and more prominent in non-Western cultures.

In Africa a new movement is slowly emerging in which 'indigenous knowledge systems' are being researched, explored and, if possible, revitalised.

Research into indigenous knowledge systems, for instance, has recently been identified as one of the focal or preference areas for research that will be funded by the National Research Foundation, the officially government-sponsored endowment for scientific research in South Africa. In Camerooon, Professor Fabien Eboussi Boulaga and myself have lately been collaborating with Ulrich Loelke, a young German philosopher, in designing a research project based on a comparison of scientific knowledge and indigenous African knowledge systems. Many Africans see exciting possibilities in this reconstruction of traditional modes of knowledge and traditional approaches to problem-solving. Of course, the outcome of this research cannot be predicted and it can therefore not be said with any certainty in advance whether it will yield completely new knowledge systems or only elements that may complement and strengthen the existing dominant one.

The point is: globalisation should not be allowed to fix analytic knowledge as the sole paradigm of knowledge because there are aspects of reality and human life and existence with which that paradigm, important though it certainly is, cannot adequately deal. In any case, the HIV/AIDS epidemic in Africa is not one that will be easily solved by the present over-emphasis on study, statistical collection and analysis of data. It is not simply knowledge about how many people are being infected with HIV every second or how many children are dying from AIDS every minute that will turn the situation around. In African attitudes and expectations, when people are ill they want to be helped, not studied and analysed, and when people know that there is no cure for their illness, they quietly accept their fate with courage and hope.

The dilemmas confronting African countries and the international community in the face of the HIV/AIDS pandemic might be put in the following parable, whose interpretation, in accordance with African practice (Tangwa 1999: 218–219), I leave open for the reader. Suppose that you are very poor and almost starving. You are eating the last few rotting yams left in your barn. In this situation it would be highly morally commendable if you were to offer some of your rotting yams to a neighbour who is equally starving but whose barn is already completely empty. But, suppose that I, your third neighbour, have a barn full of yams from which I regularly select rotting yams to throw away. I now select my rotting yams and, instead of throwing them away, I offer them to you, cheaply or even freely. You will surely be very grateful and there is no doubt that my action is beneficial to you, in some sense. But is my action morally worthy or commendable?

We should be very careful not to confuse commerce or economic considerations in general, important as they may be in their appropriate context, with the ethics of health care or HIV/AIDS vaccine research in particular. Ethics is not about self-interest, not about bargaining, not about realism of the present moment but about what *ought* to be done in a given situation. It is also about sympathising and empathising with fellow humans *in need*, doing unto them as we ourselves would be done by if our respective situations were reversed, treating them as ends in themselves and never as mere means to any other end and, above all, doing them no harm (*primum non nocere!*). What ought to be done in the face of the AIDS pandemic evidently has not yet been done. An epidemic of the calibre of HIV/AIDS is not the ideal occasion for commercial bargaining, for calculation of profits and losses; it is not the ideal occasion for interminable wrangling, for scoring points or for opportunism of any sort; it is, first and foremost, the time to mobilise all available resources in the interest of those helplessly in need; it is the occasion to save lives without prior calculations or probing questions. Ethics is also about 'loving' one's neighbour and being unable to sleep with a quiet conscience should s/he happen to die of an ailment whose remedy or part thereof is locked up in one's cupboard.

References

Benatar, Solomon R. (2000). 'Avoiding Exploitation in Clinical Research'. *Cambridge Quarterly of Healthcare Ethics,* 9, 562–565.

Benatar, Solomon R. and Singer, Peter A. (2000). 'A New Look at International Research Ethics'. *BMJ,* Vol. 321, 824–565.

Galloway, Michelle (1999). 'Vaccine Initiative on Track as First Funding Allocations are Made: Four Projects to Receive Funding'. *AIDS Bulletin,* Vol. 8, No. 4, 10–11.

Greco, Dircue (2000). 'A Cure at any Cost?', *New Scientist,* 1st July 2000, 42–43.

McGeary, Johanna (2001). 'Death Stalks a Continent'. *TIME* Magazine, Vol. 157 (6), 12th February.

Ngu, V.A. (1994). 'Chronic Infections from the Perspective of Evolution: a Hypothesis'. *Medical Hypotheses,* 42: 81–88.

Ngu, V.A. (1997). 'The Viral Envelope in the Evolution of HIV: a Hypothetical Approach to Inducing an Effective Immune Response to the Virus'. *Medical Hypotheses,* 48: 517–521.

Ngu, V.A. (1999). 'Vaccines for the HIV: Past Efforts and Future Prospects', Paper presented to the Cameroon Academy of Sciences on 02/12/1999. [Unpublished.]

Ngu, V.A. and Tangwa, Godfrey B. (2000). 'Effective Vaccine Against and Immunotherapy of the HIV: Scientific Report and Ethical Considerations from Cameroon'. [Unpublished Manuscript], 1–8.

Ngu, V.A. (2001). 'Effective Vaccine Against and Immunotherapy of the HIV', forthcoming in the *Journal of the Cameroon Academy of Sciences,* Vol. 1, No. 1.

Tangwa, Godfrey B. (1998). *Road Companion to Democracy and Meritocracy (Further Essays from an African Perspective),* Bellingham, USA, Kola Tree Press, pp 2-15.

Tangwa, Godfrey B. (1998). Chapter 1: 'Democracy and Development in Africa: Putting the Horse Before the Cart', pp. 2–15).

Tangwa, Godfrey B. (1999a). 'GENETIC INFORMATION: Questions and Worries from an African Background', *Genetic Information: Acquisition, Access and Control,* edited by Alison K. Thompson and Ruth F. Chadwick, New York, Boston, Dordrecht, London, Moscow, Kluwer Academic/Plenum Publishers, pp. 275–281.

Tangwa, Godfrey B. (1999b). 'Globalisation or Westernisation? Ethical Concerns in the whole Bio-Business', *Bioethics,* Vol. 13, No. 3/4, 218–226.

Tangwa, Godfrey B. (2000). 'African Perspectives on Biomedical and Environmental Ethics', [forthcoming contribution to a book being edited by Kwasi Wiredu].

Tangwa, Godfrey B. (2001). 'Traditional African Perception of a Person: Some Implications for Health Research and Health Care Ethics', in J. B. Rugemalila and W. L. Kilama (Guest Editors) *ACTA TROPICA, Supplement Proceedings Seminar on Health Research Ethics in Africa,* Amsterdam - London - New York - Oxford - Paris - Shannon - Tokyo, ELSEVIER, pp. S32–S39.

Chapter 12

The dilemma of enrolling children in HIV vaccine research in South Africa: what is in 'the child's best interest'?

Should children be involved in the research for HIV vaccines? Children as a group would certainly benefit from an HIV vaccine, but as **Melissa Stobie, Ann Strode** *and* **Cathy Slack** *point out, the best interest standard for each child needs to be carefully interpreted in this ethical issue, and should broaden beyond individual interests to consider children as a class.*

In the fight to stem the HIV epidemic in South Africa, what would serve the best interests of children would be to vaccinate them against HIV infection before they become sexually active. This would require enrolling children (under the age of 18) in HIV vaccine trials, in order to gather scientific data on the effect of HIV vaccines in preventing infection or disease in this group. While the epidemiological and scientific necessity for enrolling children in HIV vaccine research seems clear, there are many ethical-legal complexities relating to the participation of children in HIV vaccine trials in South Africa. Children who are enrolled in these trials will be exposed to some significant risks, yet cannot be guaranteed direct health-related benefits. As such, it is difficult to claim that the research is in the individual child trial participant's 'best interest'. Such children will effectively be exposed to such risks for the greater good, to generate data that can be used to develop an efficacious paediatric HIV vaccine. This chapter explores the *best interests standard*, its application to research and the criteria that could be used when considering whether it is ethically and legally justifiable to enrol children in HIV vaccine research. We will not explicitly consider issues around who can consent, and when. Rather, we are interested in the tension between 'how to promote the best interests of children as a group through research while protecting the rights and welfare of individual research subjects' (Kopelman 2000: 745).

HIV vaccine trials

To understand the complexities attached to enrolling children in HIV vaccine trials, it would help to first understand the design of HIV vaccine trials, as well as the risks and benefits of participating in such trials. Phase I clinical trials include a small group of humans, to determine toxicity, safety and immunogenicity. Phase I trial participants do not have to be at high risk of HIV infection, as efficacy is not being tested. Phase II and III trials are conducted on larger scales, including trial participants who are at somewhat higher risk of HIV infection, to determine efficacy and ongoing safety. Phase II and III trial participants should be at somewhat higher risk of HIV infection, in order for efficacy to be tested. Results of the third phase are hoped to show that the vaccine has succeeded in stimulating an immune response to the HI virus that can prevent HIV infection or disease progression. In addition to these three phases, bridging trials can take place, to answer specific questions not asked in the previous three phases, building on from the knowledge gained in the previous trial. Children may well be involved in such bridging trials. Phase IV entails post-licensing monitoring of the efficacy and side effects of the drug.

Personal benefits of participating in HIV vaccine research include, amongst others: the knowledge that the child is contributing to the advancement of science and the attempt to halt the progression of a widespread, killer disease; access to high quality voluntary counselling and testing and psycho-social support networks, including risk-reduction counselling; physical examinations; treatment of some infections (such as STIs); guaranteed access to antiretrovirals if and when required; and modest reimbursement for time and travel expenses for each visit to the research site. The broader social benefits of such research would be great in a country such as South Africa, given our high HIV infection rates.

While risks differ for each phase, with Phase I facing greater uncertainties and thus greater risks, some generic risks directly related to the research include pain and discomfort from venipuncture and blood draws, fevers, malaise, skin reactions, stress, inconvenience, discomfort at having personal and invasive questions asked of one, discovery of one's HIV status, and suffering from social stigma. For child trial participants, conflicts of interest and problems with the principle of confidentiality may be encountered when children disclose underage sexual activity or sexual abuse. There is a theoretical risk of enhanced infection (where exposure to the vaccine candidate and hence the HI virus leads to a more rapid progression of disease), although this has not been experienced to date. There is also the theoretical risk that exposure to the candidate product may mean that one cannot participate in later vaccine trials, or even perhaps be a recipient of a different, successful vaccine once it has been developed. Furthermore, as a successful vaccine that elicits antibodies will result in a test of HIV positivity using standard methods of HIV testing (such as the commonly-used Elisa test), trial participants risk having a 'false positivity', and attending social complications (although they will be able to determine their true status using the sophisticated testing methods at the research site). Direct HIV infection from the candidate vaccine is not a risk for the HIV vaccines currently under development in South Africa, which do not use a live attenuated virus.

Exposing children to research-related risks: what is acceptable?

It is uncontroversial that to expose children to an unacceptable risk level is not in their best interests (Kennedy and Grubb 2000: 1729–1730). In order to evaluate them, research-related risks are classified in terms of probability and magnitude (MRC book 1, 9.12.4.1). The risks involved in HIV vaccine research meet the South African Medical Research Council (SAMRC)'s definition of minimal risk: a small chance of a trivial reaction, or a remote chance of a serious reaction. Leikin characterises HIV/AIDS epidemiologic research as minimal risk, yet he uses the more commonly accepted National Commission's definition of minimal risk, which is 'the probability and magnitude of physical or psychological harm that is normally encountered in the daily lives, or in the routine medical or psychological examination of, healthy children' (Leikin 1996: 203). The SAMRC refers to such risk as negligible.

For child trial participants, conflicts of interest and problems with the principle of confidentiality may be encountered when children disclose under-age sexual activity or sexual abuse.

While Leikin is probably correct that most AIDS/HIV epidemiologic research is of negligible risk, HIV *vaccine* research exposes children to risks that would surely be higher than those encountered in the daily lives of healthy children, especially those living in a 'stable society' (SA MRC Book 1). Indeed, the SAMRC holds that HIV testing (a necessary part of HIV vaccine research) entails a greater than minimal risk because of the potential social and psychological consequences of a positive test (9.12.4.3.3).

Against this background, one of the key ethical-legal complexities regarding the participation of children in HIV vaccine trials relates to a legal obligation for decision-making affecting children to take into account the child's best interests. The Constitution of the Republic of South Africa (Act 108 of 1996) provides in Section 28(2) that a child's best interests are of paramount importance in every matter concerning the child, and new health legislation provides more specifically that therapeutic research may only be conducted if it is in the 'best interests of the minor' [National Health Act, No. 61 of 2003, Section 71(2)(a)].

The ethical-legal complexities of the best interests standard in the context of research on children relate primarily to how to apply the principle in practice. It is not defined in the Constitution nor in legislation, and limited literature exists on how to apply it to research. Accordingly, this chapter has attempted to problematise the issue and it critically discusses the concept of the best interests of children in research by way of posing a dilemma: should the best interests standard apply to individual children, or to children as a group? That this is a dilemma is made obvious when one considers the case in the following light: it is in a child's best interest to not be exposed to risks, hence individual children should not be enrolled in HIV vaccine research. However, it is also in a child's best interest to have access to prophylaxis for HIV infection, and access to such medication requires that some children will have been used as trial participants.

How, then, do we interpret 'best interests'? On standard deontological grounds, 'best interests' would apparently be interpreted as applying to individual children whose rights are absolute, 'no matter what the anticipated social benefit' (Kopelman 2000: 746). On a crude account of utilitarianism, 'best interests' would apply to children as a group, legitimating individual child trial participant's exposure to risks for the 'greater good'. More sophisticated versions of both deontology and utilitarianism exist, and may be improved (Kopelman 2000). Nevertheless, the stark dilemma remains: do we attempt to save the future lives and well-being of many children by conducting research on a vaccine which will stem HIV infection rates at an epidemiologically appropriate point, or do we protect already vulnerable children from the risks attached to participating in HIV vaccine trials?

In order to explore this dilemma, this chapter outlines the background of the current legal and ethical regulation of research. Secondly, it describes the best interests standard and problematises the complexities of applying this to research. Thirdly, it makes recommendations for how the standard may be applied in a research context. It concludes that the best interests standard can apply to both the individual child and children as a class. While there are sound reasons for HIV vaccine research to proceed on the basis of its being in the best interests of children as a class, Research Ethics Committees (RECs) must carefully balance this public good with the best interests of individual child trial participants – ensuring, at the bare minimum, that the research is not against the child's interests. Finally, we explore some tools that RECs may employ when making a factual determination of the child's best interest.

Ethical-legal background

This section examines the diverse existing ethical-legal framework for regulating research involving children. It first describes international and South African ethical guidelines around the participation of children in HIV vaccine research. It then discusses the current and new South African legislation on child research participants. It ends with a critique of the existing ethical and legal frameworks, concluding that the ambivalences in these frameworks should be eradicated.

Current ethical guidelines and the involvement of children in HIV vaccine research

Current international research ethics guidelines differ regarding the inclusion of children in HIV vaccine trials. On the one hand, the UNAIDS 2000 guidelines recommend that children be involved in HIV vaccine research (guidance point

18), the CIOMS[1] guidelines could be interpreted to allow the inclusion of children in research (guidance point 14), and the 1998 National Institutes of Health research ethics guidelines (section III), which relies on the Code of Federal Regulations (especially, in this regard, 690.116), assumes a default 'inclusionary' position for children in research. On the other hand, the Nuremburg Code, with its emphasis on the necessity for informed first-person consent, would not allow for research with children.

South Africa's Medical Research Council's *Guidelines of Ethics for Medical Research: General Principles* (also known as 'MRC's Book One') adopts a protectionist stance arising from an interpretation of South Africa's constitutional provision that medical research cannot be conducted on a person 'without *their* ['first-person'] informed consent' (Section 12.2.c). While nominally respecting the autonomy of trial participants, this interpretation slips into paternalism by restricting the participation of vulnerable groups (such as children) to research that is 'therapeutic', or non-therapeutic but observation research with negligible risk[2] (MRC Book One), which would apparently exclude the involvement of children in HIV vaccine trials.

Current law on the participation of children in HIV vaccine research

There is currently no legislation dealing comprehensively with the participation of children in research. However, there are provisions in the Constitution, the Child Care Act (No. 74 of 1983) and the common law which could be applicable. Relevant provisions can be used to establish, for example, a child's right to participation with informed consent, privacy and compensation for research-related harm. The law does not directly regulate research on children by setting specific norms and standards. There is also no legal prohibition preventing children from participating in any form of research, provided that other prerequisites exist, such as: participation is in the child's best interests, the research is not contrary to public policy and consent or proxy consent is obtained (Strode, Slack, Grant and Mushariwa 2004). In this context where there is not a comprehensive legislative framework, most of the norm setting is done through ethical guidelines (Strode, Slack and Mushariwa 2004).

There is no legal prohibition preventing children from participating in any form of research, provided that other prerequisites exist.

This vacuum regarding research laws will to some extent be resolved when the National Health Act comes into operation, as section 71 of the Act specifically regulates research on children. Section 71 comprises three parts. Section 71(1) contains general provisions regulating consent on all research participants, including that: research or experimentation on a living person may only be conducted in accordance with regulations issued by the Minister of Health, with the written consent of the person and provided they have been advised of the objective of the research as well as any possible negative or positive consequences to their health. Sections 71(2) and (3) contain additional provisions for research with minors. These sections state:

> (2) Where research or experimentation is to be conducted on a minor for therapeutic purpose, the research or experimentation may only be conducted:
> (a) If it is in the best interests of the minor;
> (b) In such manner and on such conditions as may be prescribed;
> (c) With the consent of the parent or guardian of the child; and
> (d) If the minor is capable of understanding, with the consent of the minor.
> (3) (a) Where research or experimentation is to be conducted on a minor for a non-therapeutic purpose, the research or experimentation may only be conducted:
> (i) In such manner and on such conditions as may be prescribed;
> (ii) With the consent of the Minister;
> (iii) With the consent of the parent or guardian of the minor; and
> (iv) If the minor is capable of understanding, the consent of the minor.
> (b) The Minister may not give consent in circumstances where:
> (i) The objects of the research or experimentation can also be achieved if it is conducted on an adult;
> (ii) The reasons for the consent to the research or experimentation are not likely to significantly improve scientific understanding of the minor's condition, disease or disorder to such an extent that it will result in significant benefit to the minor or other minors;
> (iii) The reasons for the consent to the research or experimentation by the parent or guardian and, if applicable, the minor are contrary to public policy;
> (iv) The research or experimentation poses a significant risk to the health of the minor; or there is some risk to the health or well-being of the minor and the potential benefit of the research or experimentation does not significantly outweigh that risk.

The provisions within Section 71 of the National Health Act indicate a policy shift with greater emphasis now being placed on substantive and procedural protections for child research participants and less emphasis on child or parental autonomy. Examples of this shift in emphasis include:

- The Act does not allow children to consent independently to either 'therapeutic' or 'non-therapeutic research'. This is contrary to the way in which some commentators interpret the provisions in Section 39 of the Child Care Act (No. 74 of 1983) which allow a child from the age of 14 to consent independently to 'medical treatment' and accordingly allow children of this age to consent independently to therapeutic research (Van Wyk 2004: 8, 9).
- Both 'therapeutic' and 'non-therapeutic' research may only take place in a manner and on such conditions as may be prescribed in regulations that may be issued in terms of the Act.
- The Act places an additional procedural requirement on researchers undertaking 'non-therapeutic' research, as such research must be authorised by the Minister of Health.
- The Act only allows consent[3] by the child to research if they are 'capable of understanding'; in other words, children may only voice their opinion on

participation if they are able to demonstrate an understanding of the implications of participation.

In this context, it is argued by some that the role adopted by the Act is overly protective and does not facilitate research, particularly so-called non-therapeutic research on children (Slack, Strode, Milford & Grant 2004).

Disjunctive approaches in law and ethics towards the participation of children in research

The disjunction between the various laws and ethical guidelines on child participation in research is due in part to a tension between the paternalistic protection of specific children who might be involved in research, versus the anticipated, generic protection to be offered to children as a vulnerable population, who deserve special safeguards of their interests. The tension is thus not dissimilar to that between the deontological concern for the individual rights of specific humans, versus public health's primarily utilitarian stance which subordinates the good of individuals in favour of the good of the majority.

> *It might not be in the best interests of a child to have to report that she has tuberculosis, and it is a clear violation of her right to privacy; nevertheless, the reporting is justified on utilitarian grounds.*

To illustrate this point, we can take the example of notifiable diseases. It might not be in the best interests of an individual child to have to report that she has tuberculosis (she may suffer from social stigma, for instance), and it is a clear violation of her right to privacy; nevertheless, the reporting is justified on utilitarian grounds: other children deserve the protection which is made possible by the reporting procedures. Considering the case at hand, it might not be in the best interests of child trial participants to enrol in HIV vaccine research; nevertheless, it is in the best interests of children as a class to have the results of such a study.

Two approaches thus become evident in the law and ethical guidelines. The first approach gains its inspiration from the constitutional injunction to ensure that a child's best interests are of paramount importance in every matter concerning the child. This approach is protectionist – it attempts to protect individual children by, for example, not exposing them to research-related risks – and can be seen in MRC's Book One, which effectively precludes the enrolment of children in HIV vaccine trials. The second approach balances these concerns with a consideration of the broader social good generated by HIV vaccine research with children – as, for instance, Section 71 (3)(b)(iv) of the National Health Act does when it talks of the potential benefit of the research outweighing the risks to child trial participants. This chapter suggests that these two approaches need more exploring from the perspective of the best interests of the child, in an attempt to create a more coherent approach to the regulation of child participation in research.

Critique of the current and proposed ethical-legal framework

Slack et al. (2004) argue that there are three key problems with the current and proposed ethical-legal framework as it applies to children. Firstly, the framework is in a state of flux as the National Health Act has been passed by parliament but no date has been set for its implementation. The Children's Bill, which proposes considerable amendments to the health rights of children, is still being debated and again it is uncertain as to when this process will be completed. Furthermore, some key ethical guidelines such as the MRC's Book One are in the process of being revised and will only be available some time in the future. As a result there is uncertainty regarding many ethical-legal issues - for example, what implications the change in the consent law will have for trial protocols of ongoing studies.

Secondly, the emerging ethical-legal framework is ambiguous and inconsistent. There are a number of areas in which provisions in the National Health Act are not clear; for example, the Act retains the contested distinction between 'therapeutic' and 'non-therapeutic' research and does not define either term. As HIV vaccine trial participants are HIV negative when enrolled, they are considered to not have the condition under study. Hence, there are those who argue that such research is non-therapeutic and too risky to include children (Van Wyk 2004), with the implicit corollary that such research cannot be in the child's best interest. As forthcoming legislation relies on this distinction, researchers should think critically about the meaning of the terms 'therapeutic' and 'non-therapeutic'. Some scholars have cogently argued that instead of attempting to classify whole protocols as 'therapeutic' or 'non-therapeutic', one should ascertain whether the particular research intervention intends to confer direct health-related benefits or not (Levine 1988). Applied to HIV vaccine research, treatment for an STI, and the administration of risk reduction counselling is beneficial. In a context of frequently inadequate primary health care, these benefits of participating in HIV vaccine trials should not be underestimated, and are arguably in the 'best interests' of the child trial participant. On the other hand, assignment to placebo or blood draws for lab tests are non-beneficial. Hence, whole protocols are not evaluated as 'beneficial/therapeutic' or 'non-beneficial/non-therapeutic': their components are, and these beneficial components can be in the best interests of the child, even in previously so-called 'non-therapeutic' research.

Another ambiguity is that the South African ethical guidelines are not well harmonised on certain key issues, such as the level of risk children are permitted to be exposed to, or the nomenclature assigned to risk levels. A further inconsistency is that there are a number of instances in which the National

Health Act is in direct conflict with proposed sections in the Children's Bill: for example, the National Health Act requires dual consent from children and their parents for research while the Children's Bill proposes an age at which children may independently consent to 'medical treatment' and 'operations'. Furthermore, all four ethical guidelines that are relevant to HIV vaccine research have contradictory guidance regarding certain aspects of child participation (see Table 1).

Thirdly, the ethical-legal framework does not always protect children's welfare or promote critical research. For example, although the National Health Act is the first legislative attempt to expressly protect child research participants, it focuses on the right to informed consent without considering other issues such as children's right to preventive health care measures. The National Health Act also places additional procedural requirements on 'non-therapeutic' research which may delay the approval of such protocols (Slack, Strode, Milford and Grant 2004).

Applying the best interests of the child standard to research

This section describes the best interests standard in general terms, and discusses the complexities of applying it in a research context.

What is the best interests of the child standard?

The concept of the best interests of the child is well established in international law. Article 3 of the Convention on the Rights of the Child (1989) provides that in all actions concerning children, their best interests are of primary consideration. As such, the best interests of the child is a significant consideration in decision-making, but not the only consideration. However, this standard is considered so important within the framework of the Convention that it has been made into one of the four general principles that form the 'soul' of the Convention (Sloth-Nielsen 1995: 408).

In South Africa, the standard has been recognised within our common law for almost 100 years (Anderson and Spijker 2002: 365; *Cronje v Cronje* 1907 TS 871: 872). Section 28(2) of the Constitution of the Republic of South Africa (Act No. 108 of 1996) states that the child's best interests are of paramount importance in every matter concerning the child.

Although currently undefined in either the Constitution or other legislation, this principle has been well developed by the courts. Indeed, the principle may be undefined precisely because the courts have generally held that the principle requires a wide range of factors to be considered to promote a child's physical, moral, emotional and spiritual welfare during decision-making affecting the child (*McCall v McCall* 1994 (3) SA 201 (C): 204). The inquiry has both subjective and objective elements, as was articulated by Fogerty in the Australian case of *In the Marriage of Homan*:

> The test of the welfare of the child has to be determined having regard to contemporary social standards, that is, it cannot be a totally subjective test based upon the views or standards of the individual parent [or child or other interested party] but objective at least in the sense of falling within the wider range of existing social standards (1976 FLC 90–024 quoted in Heaton 1990: 97).

Although the principle has its roots in our divorce jurisprudence, it is increasingly being used in a broader context as a core principle in either legislation or the cases. For example, the South African Schools Act (No. 84 of 1996) provides in Section 4(1) that a school may exempt a learner from compulsory school attendance if it is in the 'best interests of the learner'.

This wider use of the standard is also reflected in the National Health Act where it provides that the conducting of so-called therapeutic research must be in the 'best interests of the minor'. The requirement of a best interests analysis in Section 71(2) of the National Health Act therefore introduces a novel concept into the considerations regarding the circumstances in which children should participate in so-called therapeutic research. A best interests analysis is not required in terms of the Act with so-called non-therapeutic research; however, this does not mean that researchers or research ethics committees cannot use it as a consideration in relation to such research, as the Constitution provides that a child's best interests are of paramount importance in every matter concerning the child.

The best interests standard is thus law's way of interpreting the deontological command to always treat others as ends-in-themselves.

The best interests standard is thus law's way of interpreting the deontological command to always treat others as ends-in-themselves, with the corollary that (due to their cognitive immaturity), children are incapable of always knowing what is indeed in their best interests. The law thus justifies its paternalistic stance, while leaving some flexibility in interpreting how we determine what truly is in any particular child's best interest.

Complexities of applying the best interests standard in courts

The Constitutional Court has stated that the standard should be flexible, as individual circumstances will determine which factors secure the best interests of a particular child (*Minister of Welfare and Population Development v Fitzpatrick and Others* 2000 (7) BCLR 713 (CC) at para 18). Although the standard does not have a fixed meaning, this does not mean that it is useless. An analogy has been drawn with the legal concept of the *boni mores* (legal convictions) of the community. This is also an indeterminate principle but has been successfully employed by the courts in a wide variety of circumstances to establish social standards of behaviour (Heaton 1990: 98).

However, others see this lack of legislative definition to be a weakness and argue that it fails to provide a reliable, determinate standard. Furthermore, lack of guidance on when it is applicable adds to the uncertainty about the standard (De Waal, Currie and Erasmus 2001: 415–416). For example, if it must apply in all circumstances, then could a child ever participate in non-therapeutic research, as it is unlikely that one could find that their participation was directly in their best interests? In addition, how does one apply this standard in a sentencing during the criminal trial of a child, as it would never be in a child's best interests to be sent to prison (ibid.)? In *S vs Howells* [1999 SACR (4) SA 675 (C)], the court held that the interests of society outweighed the best interests of the affected children when deciding to impose a custodial sentence on a single mother. These examples show that courts are continually faced with having to balance a range of competing interests when applying the best interests standard, and are prepared in certain circumstances to allow other factors – such as the best interests of society – to outweigh a child's best interests. The best interests standard thus is and should be applied both individually and socially. Some argue that it is for this type of reason that further legislative guidance is required (De Waal, Currie and Erasmus 2001).

Section 6 of the draft South African Children's Bill (B 70 of 2003) attempts to deal with these indeterminacies by codifying many of the factors established by the courts during a best interests analysis. These can include: the child's age; needs; gender; background; maturity and stage of development; physical and emotional security; intellectual, emotional, socio-cultural development; and the need to protect the child from physical and psychological harm.

Complexities of applying the best interests standard to research

Complexities arise when attempting to establish the most appropriate way in which to use the standard and the criteria that would be used in a research context. The key issues regarding the application of this standard to research include:

- Limited literature exists on what this legal obligation means in the context of research.
- Existing case law on the best interests standard applies primarily to the context of a divorce or custody hearing, and is based on a factual determination of what is in the best interests of individual children, not children as a class.
- The legislature has not established a set of general criteria that can be used to determine a child's best interests and although the Children's Bill in Section 6 does codify some factors to be taken into account in this analysis, these are not general principles that could be easily applied to research.
- There appear to be two competing interests – the best interests of individual child participants in research and the best interests of children generally as a class (Heaton 1990: 95), who may benefit from medical research. A potential

problem with this principle is that it fails to provide a mechanism for adjudicating between what might be in the best interests of children generally (e.g. the creation of an efficacious HIV vaccine), versus what would be in the best interests of a particular child (e.g. not being exposed to the physiological and psycho-social risks of HIV vaccine research participation).

In determining how to use the standard of the best interests of the child, the National Health Act is not clear on whether the principle must be used by Research Ethics Committees (RECs) to determine whether therapeutic research is in the best interests of a class of children, or whether it is going to apply at a more individual level when parents and children (if they have understanding) consent to the research protocol.

There appear to be two competing interests – the best interests of individual child participants in research and the best interests of children generally as a class.

It is possible that if the standard is narrowly applied as requiring a child's individual best interests to be of paramount importance that they would be excluded from so-called non-therapeutic research. Roscam-Abbing suggests that such research can never be in a child's best interests but rather such research should be 'not against the child's interests' (Roscam-Abbing 1994: 156).

Recommendations for applying the best interests standard to research with children

This section makes recommendations on the most appropriate way in which to interpret the best interests principle in a research context and outlines some of the key criteria that should be used in a best interests analysis.

The best interests standard should apply to both individual children and children as a class, and should be used as a mechanism to balance paternalism with empowerment

It is argued that the modern framework for children's rights is based on a careful balancing of protection and empowerment. Law is generally protective towards children as they are regarded as needing assistance due to their lack of experience (Kruger & Robinson in Robinson (ed.) 1997: 15). Accordingly, the South African law provides that children have limited legal capacity until they reach the age of 21 (Age of Majority Act, No. 57 of 1972). Furthermore, because children have limited capacity they need to be assisted by a parent or guardian when entering into transactions with legal implications (Kruger & Robinson in Robinson (ed.) 1997: 14).

This protection of children is accompanied by an increasing legislative recognition of the autonomy of children at an earlier age; for example, children may consent to 'medical treatment' from the age of 14 (Section 39, Child Care Act No.

74 of 1983), a termination of pregnancy at any age (Section 5, Choice of Termination of Pregnancy Act, No. 92 of 1996) and sexual intercourse at 16 (Section 14, Sexual Offences Act, No. 23 of 1957). There is also an increasing legal focus on child participation. Even if children do not have the capacity to act on their own, the law still requires their views to be taken into account. For example, Section 43 of the proposed Children's Bill provides that any major decisions involving a child must give due consideration to any views and wishes expressed by the child, bearing in mind the child's age, maturity and stage of development. This is in line with the Convention on the Rights of the Child.

The best interests standard is a useful mechanism to balance two considerations: firstly, the need to protect children must be balanced with an equal need to facilitate their participation in research. Secondly, the need to protect the child from research-related risks must be balanced against the potential health benefits of enrolment to child trial participants, as well as children in broader society who will benefit from receiving an efficacious vaccine. The criteria used in the best interests analysis are able to accommodate these diverse considerations when carefully balanced. It is not dissimilar to a risk-benefit analysis, as it requires a consideration of both what may be harmful to the child and what may benefit a child. What will be more difficult is weighing possible limited individual benefit against a wider benefit to all children, as there is no legal precedent for using the principle to determine the best interests of a class of children. In such circumstances, the courts and research ethics committees would have to weigh up the best interests of particular children versus other concerns, such as social interests or the need to promote public health.

There is an increasing legal focus on child participation. Even if children do not have the capacity to act on their own, the law still requires their views to be taken into account.

Proposed criteria for determining the best interests of children participating in research

Assuming, based on epidemiological evidence, that it is in the best interests of children as a class to have access to a safe and effective HIV vaccine, it remains to determine the best interests of individual children participating in research. Using as a basis the criteria established by the cases and those proposed in the Children's Bill, we suggest the following as criteria that can be used when applying the best interests principle to individual child participants. These are not different from those already established by the courts; rather, we have set out how these criteria could be usefully applied in a research context.

Age

It must be determined when a child has sufficient maturity to make decisions about what is in his or her best interests, with younger children being protected more carefully, while those over the age of 18 are treated as independent adults (Article 1, Convention on the Rights of the Child). However, under the age of 18 there are cognitive milestones which must be recognised. It will always be arbitrary to determine a specific age at which a milestone is reached, and children should always be regarded as unique individuals with evolving maturity. Nevertheless, children around the age of 14 are commonly regarded as being capable of making informed if not definitive decisions about what is in their best interests.

Needs

The needs of a child can be understood to fall into two camps: needs to maximise the benefits of life (beneficence) and the need to avoid harms (non-maleficence). As these are related considerations, they will be discussed together below.

In English law, subjecting a child to an unacceptable risk level is regarded as being contrary to a child's best interests (Kennedy & Grubb 2000: 1729–1730). The best interests standard is thus used as a risk standard to ensure that children are not unnecessarily harmed, physically or psychologically (for instance, by receiving frequent injections).

However, there is also the need to protect the child from future or potential harm. Knowing the incidence rates of HIV infection in South African youth, a legitimate way of doing so is to attempt to ensure that they run a reduced risk of becoming HIV infected. In this context, this can be achieved in two ways: firstly, by being the recipient of a potentially efficacious HIV vaccine; secondly, by participating in HIV vaccine trials to gain high quality VCT and an increased awareness of the disease.

Some may argue that a future harm could be HIV infection as a result of therapeutic misconception. This risk must be avoided at all costs, with every effort being made to educate the children appropriately about the study design.

An undeniable benefit to the child, which could satisfy a legitimate need to feel like a valuable member of society, is that the child will contribute to the production of generalisable knowledge about HIV and HIV vaccines.

View of the child

In *I v S* (2000 (2) SA 993 (C), p. 977 G–H) it was held that a child's views are not always indicative of their best interests but an informed, mature and intelligent opinion can carry substantial weight. In the spirit of treating children as ends-in-themselves, so that they do not feel exploited, either at the time or at a later date, it is imperative that children's voices are heard. The child's consent or assent should thus always be a necessary pre-requisite for participation in research.

Conclusions

Protecting individual children from potential harm is a complex process in the context of HIV infection rates in South Africa. Determining what is in an individual child's best interest can also be different from determining what is in children's best interests. It would clearly be in children's best interests to have an efficacious HIV vaccine, and this would seem to support the idea of including children in HIV vaccine trials. However, it is not immediately clear that participation in such trials is in the individual child's 'best interest', (despite the fact that components of the trial may be of direct benefit to the trial participant). It is for this underlying reason that there are tensions and ambivalences in South African legislation and guidelines.

In South Africa, Research Ethics Committees are only required to consider the best interests of the child in regard to 'therapeutic' research and accordingly they will have to undertake a factual investigation into what will be in the best interests of trial participants. However, the National Health Act does not require the best interests of children to be considered when establishing whether children should participate in 'non-therapeutic' research. Accordingly, if HIV vaccine research is classified as 'non-therapeutic' research, this debate may be moot in terms of current legislation. However, the Constitution, which is the supreme law of the land, deems that the best interests standard is of paramount importance in every matter concerning the child.

In conclusion, the best interests standard, as it applies to individual children, ensures that exploitation and abuse is minimised. But as useful as the mechanism is, it is not infallible, nor should it always override concerns for the best interests of society. It also has to be weighed against the best interests of children as a class, and it is up to Research Ethics Committees to carefully reflect on such a balance. In focusing on protecting the best interests of the child, we must not lose sight of the fact that we also wish to protect the best interests of children as a class.

Endnotes

[1] Council for the International Organisations of Medical Sciences.

[2] Negligible risk is here defined as risk that does not exceed everyday risk in a stable society.

[3] Although the Act uses the word 'consent' it is not independent consent by the child but consent alongside the consent of their parent or guardian.

References

Age of Majority Act: 1972, 57.

Anderson, A. & Sijker, A. (2002). Considering the views of the child when determining her best interest. *Obiter* Vol 24, No. 2, 365–372.

Child Care Act: 1983, 74.

Children's Bill, B70–2003, available from: http://web.uct.ac.za/depts/ci/plr/pdf/bills/bill27jan04.pdf. Accessed 30th November 2004.

Choice of Termination of Pregnancy Act: 1996, 92.

Constitution of the Republic of South Africa: 1996, 108, available: www.concourt.gov.za.

Convention on the Rights of the Child [online], available: http://www.unicef.org/crc/crc.htm.

Cronje v Cronje: 1907 TS 871 at 872.

De Waal, J., Currie, I. & Erasmus, G. (2001). *The Bill of Rights Handbook*. Kenwyn: Juta.

Heaton, J. (1990). Some general remarks on the concept 'best interests of the child'. *Tydskrif vir Hedendaagse Romeins-Hollandse Reg (THRHR), 53*, 95–99.

Kennedy, I. & Grubb, A. (2000). *Medical Law: Texts with Materials* (3rd ed). London: Butterworths.

Kopelman, L. (2000). Children as Research Subjects: A Dilemma. *Journal of Medicine and Philosophy, 25*, 745–764.

Kruger, J.M., & Robinson, J.A. (1997). The legal status of children and young persons. In: J.A. Robinson (ed.), *The Law of Children and Young Persons in South Africa.* (pp. 1–48). Durban: Butterworths.

Leikin, S. (1996). Ethical issues in epidemiological research with children. In: S.S. Coughlin, & T.L. Beauchamp. (Eds.). *Ethics and Epidemiology* (pp. 199–218). New York: Oxford University Press.

Levine, R.J. (1988). *Ethics and Regulation of Clinical Research (2nd ed.).* London: Yale University Press.

McCall v McCall: 1994 (3) SA 201 (C).

Minister of Welfare and Population Development v Fitzpatrick and Others 2000 (7) BCLR 13 (CC).

National Health Act: 2003, 61, available: www.doh.gov.za.

Roscam Abbing, H.D.C. (1994). Medical research involving incapacitated persons: what are the standards? *European Journal of Health Law, 1*, 147–160.

S v Howells: 1999 (4) SACLR 675 (C).

Sexual Offences Act: 1957, 23.

Slack, C., Strode, A., Grant, C., & Milford, C. (2004). Implications of the ethical-legal framework for adolescent HIV vaccine trials: Report of a consultative forum. To submit to *South African Medical Journal.*

Sloth-Nielsen, J. (1995). 'Ratification of the United Nations Convention on the Rights of the Child: Some implications for South African law'. *South African Journal on Human Rights, 11*, 401–420.

South African Schools Act, 1996, 84.

Strode, A., Slack, C., Grant, C., & Mushariwa, M. (2004). Pre-enrolment ethical legal complexities in adolescent participation in HIV vaccine trials. Submitted to *South African Journal of Science.*

Strode, A., Slack, C., & Mushariwa, M. (2004). An evaluation of South Africa's ethical-legal framework and its ability to promote the welfare of trial participants involved in HIV vaccine research. Submitted to *South African Medical Journal.*

Van Wyk, C. (2004). Clinical trials, medical research and cloning in South Africa. *Tydskrif vir Hedendaagse Romeins-Hollandse Reg (THRHR), 67*, 1–21.

Appendix

Table 1: Comparison of South African Ethical Guidance Regarding Inclusion of Children in Research.

	MRC BOOK 5	DOH GCP	MRC BOOK 1	INHREC
What approach is adopted to analysing risk?	Explicit approach is an analysis of interventions: • does the intervention confer direct health-related benefit or not? An 'intra-trial analysis'.	Spirit is an analysis of interventions: • does the intervention confer direct health-related benefit or not? An 'intra-trial analysis'. Refers to US CFR/IRB 96.	Approach to risk analysis rests on separating whole protocols into 'therapeutic' research or 'non-therapeutic' research. Disregards that most protocols include interventions not intended to confer benefit (e.g. randomization to placebo, extra tests).	Implicit approach is analysis of interventions.
How are risk standards in relation to children defined and named?	(Non-beneficial interventions): • risk of 'daily lives of pèople in a stable society' • risk of routine tests - medical or psychological. Termed 'negligible' risk.	Refers to IRB (1996): • risk of 'daily life' • risk of routine tests - physical or psychological. Termed 'minimal' risk.	('Non-therapeutic research'): • risk of daily lives of people in a stable society • risk of routine tests - psychological or physical. Termed 'negligible' risk.	Refers to: Risk of daily life or routine medical or psychological examinations. Termed minimal risk.
Who gives consent for child participation?	For HIV vaccine trials: • A 'parent or legal guardian' • Assent from the child according to his or her evolving capacity.	If research involves more than minimal (everyday) risk. and no direct benefit: • Both parents • Child assent. If research involves more than minimal (everyday) risk and direct benefit: • One parent • Child assent.	If research classified as 'non-therapeutic' research: • 'Parents' give consent. (Note: this is restricted to observation research; see below). If research is classified as 'therapeutic' research: • Independent consent from child 14 years and older is possible • Parental consent still 'desirable'.	The parents; and the minor where competent; If the minor is not competent then minor gives assent. Adolescents consent unassisted if: • The research is minimal risk and there is community endorsement.

What can be consented to by parents, in terms of kinds of studies or study designs?	Does not restrict parental consent to certain kinds of study designs.	Does not restrict parental consent to certain kinds of study designs.	Does restrict parental consent to certain kinds of studies. That is, if research is classified as 'non-therapeutic' then parental consent is restricted to 'observation' research only, and intervention research is precluded.	Does not restrict parental consent to certain kinds of study designs.
What can be consented to by parents, in terms of research risks when there is no direct benefit?	If intervention has no direct benefit: • Risk must be commensurate with daily lives of people in a stable society or routine medical or psychological examinations • Or minor increase over this, if justified by scientific or medical rationale (i.e. satisfactory risk-knowledge ratio). Note: Allows an increase over everyday risk.	Generally children should be exposed to minimal (everyday) risk in research. Research that involves greater than minimal (everyday) risk and no prospect of direct benefit: • Risks must be justified by generalisable knowledge. Note: Allows an increase over everyday risk.	Research that is classified as 'non-therapeutic': • Only if no or negligible (everyday) risk, i.e. daily life in stable society or routine tests. Note: Does not allow increase over everyday risk.	Refers to minimal risk or a minor increase over minimal risk. Note: Does allow an increase over everyday risk.
What can be consented to by parents, in terms of research risks when there is direct benefit?	If the intervention has direct benefit: • Risk must be justified by the potential benefit to participants. Note: No upper limit of risk.	Research that involves greater than minimal risk, but provides direct benefit to participants: • Risk must be justified by the benefit to participants. Note: No upper limit of risk.	Research that is classified as 'therapeutic research': • Only if risk of 'small chance of trivial reaction' or 'remote chance of serious injury or death'. Note: Does set an upper limit of risk. Note: Termed 'minimal'.	The risks must be justified by the potential benefit. Note: Does not set an upper limit of risk

Chapter 13

If HIV/AIDS is punishment, who is bad?

For centuries, a theory that **Loretta M. Kopelman** *calls 'the punishment theory of disease' has been used to explain epidemics and other catastrophes. In this chapter she identifies and analyses various forms of this ubiquitous theory, both secular and religious, arguing that all versions are irrational and thwart attempts to fight this pandemic and help those with HIV/AIDS.*

Sub-Saharan Africa is the epicentre of the HIV/AIDS pandemic. For compassionate as well as pragmatic reasons, we need to address the barriers to global efforts to find solutions in this impoverished region. Pragmatically, the security of the most stable countries could be threatened if AIDS continues to grow and eventually causes governments to fall, ethnic fighting to flair and economies to falter (Gellman 2000). Before the AIDS epidemic reaches such catastrophic proportions, we need a worldwide commitment to develop better public health, treatments, surveillance, preventive measures, education and nutrition; ultimately there must be a dedication to alleviate poverty and foster economic development in these regions (Folkers and Fauci 2001). Some obstacles to co-operation take the form of distrust, indifference and prejudice, especially by those in wealthy countries outside of sub-Saharan Africa to the misery of distant others.[1] One such impediment is an ancient prejudice about disease itself. As Secretary General Kofi Annan has said, addressing a special session of the United Nations (2001):

> We cannot deal with AIDS by . . . making out it is their fault [those who are sick] . . . Let no one imagine that we can protect ourselves by building barriers between them and us. For in the ruthless world of AIDS, there is no us and them.

From the earliest awareness of HIV/AIDS, people, including patients, have viewed this disease as punishment for sin. In 1986, when Charles Stanley was president of the Southern Baptist Convention, the largest Protestant group in the United States, he claimed that AIDS was sent by God to show displeasure that homosexuality was growing in social acceptance (New York Native 1986). Other members of the clergy agreed (Murphy 1988; Ross 1988), including such well-known figures as Jerry Falwell, leader of the moral majority, and Pat Buchanan, influential talk-show host, aide to Ronald Reagan and US presidential candidate in 2000. In Uganda, AIDS was thought to be divine punishment for the sin of adultery: Joseph Mayana, a local barrister, said that the Virgin Mary had revealed to him that '. . .no drug will be found for it. The only drug is repentance.' Groups sprang up there to seek divine absolution, protection or a cure from the Virgin Mary (Watson 1988: 1).

Even some health care professionals agreed HIV/AIDS was punishment for sin. At New York's Beth Israel Medical Center, a survey among clinicians who regularly dealt with AIDS patients revealed that of the 68 doctors and 172 nurses surveyed, almost 11 percent of the nurses and 4.5 percent of the physicians agreed with the statement 'AIDS is God's punishment to homosexuals' (Psychiatric News 1988). The following year another survey from the US reported that '40 percent to 70 percent of rural whites strongly endorsed the idea that acquired immune deficiency syndrome is the product of "divine intervention" or "divine retribution" . . . Two of five conservative clergy strongly agreed with the idea of divine intervention . . . [and] approximately one in ten physicians endorsed these propositions' (Francis 1989).

Today, one frequently hears comments about whether or not people are culpable for getting HIV/AIDS, such as, 'She is not to blame for having HIV/AIDS since she got it from her husband who is an intravenous drug user'. The implication is that while she is not blameworthy, he is. This explanation is deeply ingrained to account for why people get sick. For example, it is not unusual today to hear 'What did I do to deserve this?' when people are told that they or family members have any serious medical condition.

These comments reflect different versions of *the punishment theory of disease*[2] which I will identify and criticise. I define it herein as the view that being bad or doing bad things can directly cause disease, and when it does, blame should be placed on those who get sick. A modified version holds that one person might be blameworthy yet another person, somehow close to the culpable person, gets sick. Accordingly, I distinguish four forms of the punishment theory of disease, depending upon whether they are religious, secular, modified or non-modified (see Table 1).

Table 1: Four forms of the punishment theory of disease associating disease with moral blame

The punishment theory of disease	Non-modified	Modified
Religious	God or (a) transcendental being(s) inflicts punishment on the culpable person	God or (a) transcendental being(s) inflicts punishment on the culpable person or punishes someone close to the culpable person
Secular	People bring diseases on themselves by their bad lifestyles	People bring diseases on themselves by their bad lifestyles or bring about diseases in those close to the culpable person

A punishment theory of disease does not employ a causal concept of responsibility but a moral concept of blame or moral responsibility. A horse kicking over a kerosene lantern may be causally responsible for a fire, but not blameworthy or morally responsible. A person might be causally responsible for giving his disease to others, because he unknowingly donated blood that was infected, yet not blameworthy or morally responsible because he had no way of knowing that he might harm them. In contrast to the irrational association of disease with moral blame that I will be discussing, in some rare cases blame would be appropriate. For example, a person with HIV/AIDS would be morally responsible for infecting others if he could have done otherwise, intended the action done, and foresaw the potentially deadly consequences. In such rare cases, legal action might be appropriate. Unless indicated, I will be using a *moral concept of blame or moral responsibility* and not a *causal concept of responsibility* throughout this chapter.

In what follows, I will consider why the tendency to view disease as punishment is dangerous and irrational, and how such views thwart efforts to fight this pandemic and help those with HIV/AIDS. One of the greatest impediments to addressing the HIV/AIDS pandemic has been the tendency, especially among the affluent parts of the world, to dismiss the problem as belonging to others. With 70 percent of those infected with HIV/AIDS living in sub-Saharan Africa, we need to expose and criticise the assumptions that foster the disturbing tendency to regard this region as 'not our problem'. One source of this 'us' and 'them' thinking arises from the irrational and counterproductive tendency to view disease as a punishment (Kopelman 1988; Annan 2001).

Religious versions of the punishment theory

The association of disease and blame is ancient and ubiquitous, and divine punishment has been used in every epidemic throughout history to account for why some people get sick and some do not (Duffy 1979). According to religious versions of the punishment theory of disease, illness is divine punishment; it is inflicted on humans to punish them for an offence, to give them a chance for rehabilitation, to warn them to become more virtuous, to demonstrate that the bad perish or the good will thrive, or to show that some cosmic order requires the punishment of sin. For example, in Numbers 11: 31–33, the Israelites, who were trying to find their way to the promised land, had been instructed by God not to eat meat but they disobeyed:

> Then a wind from the Lord sprang up, it drove quails from the west, and they were flying around the camp for a day's journey, three feet above the ground. The people were busy gathering quails all that day, all night, and all the next day, and even the men who got the least gathered ten omers. They spread them out to dry all around the camp, but the meat was scarcely between their teeth and they had not so much as bitten it when the Lord's anger broke out against the people and He struck them with a deadly plague.

Scientific speculations exist about the causes of such a plague in this region (Amdur et al. 1991). The quail might have eaten hemlock berries containing coniine, a neurotoxin alkaloyd. Quails are resistant to this poison, but humans are not. By consuming the seemingly normal but contaminated quail containing the neurotoxin, the people could sicken or die. Another natural explanation is that the drying period might have permitted the outgrowth of pathogenic organisms.

While the religious version of the punishment theory of disease is ancient, so are its critics.

Yet, such scientific explanations do not necessarily dispel the power of the religious claims that illness is punishment for sin. Unless one can show that a scientific account is incompatible with, and not just different from, non-scientific and religious explanations, the former does not necessarily prove the latter wrong. Some believers may suppose that God used one of these means to warn or to test the Israelites, and the plague was nonetheless the consequence of their disobedience.

While the religious version of the punishment theory of disease is ancient, so are its critics. Job's friends tell him that God is punishing him with losses and illnesses for his evil ways, begging him to seek forgiveness. One of them states, 'Think now, who that was innocent has ever perished? Or where were the upright cut off? As I have seen, those who plough inequity and sow trouble reap the same. By the breath of God they perish, and by the blast of His anger they are consumed' (Job 4: 7–9). Job rejects this view, claiming that he has done nothing wrong. In the end, God answers from the whirlwind that Job's friends are ignorant: 'Who is this who darkens council by words without knowledge?' (Job 38: 2). Obviously, then, the punishment theory of disease and criticisms of it can exist side by side in sacred texts.

I will focus on three criticisms of the religious version of the punishment theory of disease. First, it fails as a general account; second, it is not clear that anything follows from it about how we should view or treat others; and third, it commits the fallacy of explaining the obscure by the still more obscure.

Fails as a general account

The religious version of the punishment theory of disease fails as a general account of why people get sick. One of the greatest tragedies of the AIDS epidemic is that millions of infants have been born with HIV. Yet they have done nothing wrong. Defenders may respond that these infants are being punished for the bad behaviour of parents who could have acted otherwise and thereby avoided the disease. Deity or deities sometimes are said to punish future generations instead of, or in addition to, the sinner. Consequently, sometimes innocent and blameless people suffer as a result of the sins of others, in this case the freely chosen behaviour of their parents.

This modification, however, acknowledges that the punishment theory of disease fails as a general account of why people get sick since it acknowledges that some innocent people get sick. Nonetheless it is implausible. If disease is sometimes but not always a punishment for sin and if this is to be a useful theory, then we should be given some way to distinguish the 'guilty-sick' from the 'innocent-sick'. That is, defenders of this modified version of the punishment theory of disease should offer a just and meaningful way to separate the sick who are innocent and the sick who are blameworthy. It seems unlikely that they could find criteria to do this reliably given the complex relation between the voluntary, non-voluntary and involuntary springs of human behaviour.

It seems unreasonable to conclude that the wicked perish while the good thrive in accordance with any understandable just system of punishment and rewards.

If we look at who thrives and who perishes in the world, it seems unreasonable to conclude that the wicked perish while the good thrive in accordance with any understandable just system of punishment and reward. Some good people die young and some wicked people have healthy lives into their old age. Currently, 26 million of the 36 million people infected with HIV/AIDS live in sub-Saharan Africa (UNAIDS 2000), and many of them are young children. The view linking disease and punishment suggests the offensive conclusion that people living in sub-Saharan Africa are morally worse than those in other areas or that a just God or gods regard a deadly disease as fitting punishment for whatever those living there are supposed to have done.

Nothing follows about how we should view or treat others

Assuming that this religious version of the punishment theory of disease is true, it is unclear that anything would follow about how humans should view and treat others. If someone has been or is being justly punished, then presumably it is wrong to give them additional punishment. If it is wrong to make people suffer intentionally and without cause, and if God or a divine being has already punished them, then it seems superfluous and wrong for humans to inflict additional blame or punishment. Moreover, if they – unlike the rest of us – have been warned or punished by a divine being, perhaps we should view them as blessed. Job suggests this in rebuking his friends: 'Behold, happy is the man whom God reproves; therefore despise not the chastening of the Almighty' (Job 5: 17).

Explains the obscure with the more obscure

This 'explanation' commits the fallacy of explaining the obscure by the still more obscure. We set out to explain why people get sick and end up by appealing to the intentions of a deity or supernatural beings. This appeal has been used for and against human rights, wars and every other human cause, so it is not surprising that it is used here as well. Lack of agreement about how to resolve disputes over the nature of God's intentions seriously undermines this view. Rather than clarify, this explanation creates more confusion and hardens people's hearts to rational inquiry. If disease is punishment, why should millions of innocent babies suffer and die? Why should 70 percent of the deaths occur in sub-Saharan Africa? Explanations of these differences in terms of who is sinful seem unsupportable.

Defenders might respond that these criticisms appeal to unreliable and finite notions of reason, compassion, consistency, proportionality and justice. Our untrustworthy notions of consistency and justice may require what seem to us to be similarly situated people to be treated in a similar way regarding proportional punishments, but a deity or deities transcend our imperfect notions. The problem with this response is that we have no others to use. Thus, as long as we disagree about what constitutes God's will or intentions and about how to resolve our disputes, such appeals are not likely to resolve our disagreements or be convincing.

Other defenders might disagree with my assumption that there are innocent beings who are punished by a merciful and just God, arguing that all members of the human race, even infants, are born sinners. On this view, all are sinners, no matter if the person is an infant or a mass murderer. (For example, the Calvinist doctrine, so far as I understand it, holds such a doctrine of original sin, a legacy of Adam's and Eve's sinful behaviour brought forward in the sex act.) Yet, this response also fails to support the cogency of the punishment theory of disease. There are few possibilities – either we are equally bad or not, but neither option supports the punishment theory of disease. First, if we are all equally bad and no real distinction can be made amongst us and if we should treat equals equally, then it is wrong to single out some for punishment. Punishments should be proportional, so if we are all equally bad and God cares to punish humans justly, then it is unfair to punish some but not all equally bad sinners. Second, if, on the other hand, we assume that we are not equally bad and some sinners are worse than others, then surely infants must be the best of the so-called sinners, and we return to the puzzle of why some of the most innocent beings amongst us should be punished more severely than others. Third, supposing that God or gods punish proportionally, then why are murderers in good health when infants are dying of HIV/AIDS?

Still other defenders of the punishment theory of disease might point to support within religious texts for assessments that some people should be treated or viewed differently when they get sick. They might cite the passage quoted above from Numbers stating that '. . . the Lord's anger broke out against the people and He struck them with a plague'. This passage, however, states that God can and does inflict punishment in the form of illness. It does not say that humans would necessarily know enough to judge when this occurs or how to pick out who is being punished for sin with diseases and who is not. This rebuttal, that humans do not know enough to judge, is also found in the previously cited passage from the book of Job where God comments from the whirlwind to show they speak in ignorance when associating blame and material misfortune with disease. In any case, support from religious texts will not convince those who do not believe that such divinities exist or that they care about humans enough to punish them, or do not believe the proffered interpretation.

Secular or moral versions of the punishment theory

According to secular or non-religious moral versions of the punishment theory of disease, illnesses are the result or punishing effects of irresponsible behaviour, bad habits or weakness of will. Because HIV/AIDS is an infectious disease, it is associated with behaviours such as having multiple sex partners, using intravenous drugs and engaging in prostitution. Defenders of this version of the punishment theory of disease, however, suggest that when people get sick after engaging in such behaviour it is 'their own fault'. Joseph Perloff, a professor of medicine at UCLA, asserts: 'It is not correct to say that nobody is to blame . . . Ninety percent of all AIDS cases are contracted by either specific sexual acts or specific drug abuse. The remaining ten percent – recipients of blood transfusions, children of female AIDS patients, haemophiliacs – may well be regarded as mere "victims"' (Ross 1988: 40–41)[3]. On this view, people who have multiple sex partners, engage in prostitution or pass around needles when they use drugs should know they are at greater risks for diseases, just as people who smoke or drink heavily should know they are more likely to get heart disease.[4] Yet this secular account is also problematic because, like the religious version, it fails as a general account of who gets diseases and does not establish blame reliably.

The millions of infants who get HIV/AIDS have not behaved badly, so they are not being punished for anything that they have done.

Fails as a general account

Like the religious version, this view also fails to offer a general account of why people get sick. The millions of infants who get HIV/AIDS have not behaved badly, so they are not being punished for anything that they have done. Defenders will either have to admit that this view in its unmodified form is wrong, or adopt the modified version that some people who get diseases such as HIV/AIDS have not engaged in bad behaviour. Such a modified secular view, however, has similar problems to those found in the modified religious version discussed earlier. That is, the view fails to explain cogently why good people and their relatives sometimes get sick and bad people and their relatives sometimes do not.

Perhaps defenders might want to say only those who *knowingly and intentionally* engage in risky behavior when they could have done otherwise, ought to be held blameworthy. Yet some people risk their health and well-being for higher goals, such as to save others, and do not deserve blame but praise. In the early days of the AIDS epidemic, clinicians were unsure how it was transmitted, and intentionally faced danger to care for others. They knowingly engaged in this 'risky behaviour,' but were serving higher goals or obligations including important professional duties. Even today, those who decide to work in areas with very high concentrations of HIV/AIDS to help others may be at greater risk than others who play it safe. Thus, the fact that people knowingly engage in risky behaviour may be heroic, not culpable.

Defenders would no doubt object that caring for sick people is not the sort of risky behaviour that they meant. But this example shows that the burden of proof would be on them to offer criteria for distinguishing which risky behaviour makes people morally blameworthy for their illnesses and which does not, bringing us to another problem with this position.

Cannot reliably ascribe blame

A second problem is that if a distinction between the blameworthy sick and blameless sick is to be useful and fair, we are owed some criteria for reliably separating these two groups. When do we know that someone is blameworthy for contracting HIV? *In the clearest case of ascribing blame, we would need to know that the person could have done otherwise, intended the action done, and foresaw the consequences.* As noted, in rare cases, someone might meet these conditions. More typically, however, it is often difficult to see if these conditions have been fulfilled. In some cases, socio-economic or cultural factors may make it very difficult for people to act otherwise. African women who have tried to prevent HIV/AIDS by bottle-feeding their babies, avoiding female genital cutting of their daughters or asking their husbands to wear condoms, for example, have been severely punished or held up to public ridicule. In addition, poverty, social norms, ignorance, temptation, compulsion, addiction and irrational views can create considerations of such complexity that untangling them to determine blame for illnesses seems hazardous, especially if the way people are treated hangs in the balance. For example, people may be trapped in a social structure where they acquired HIV/AIDS because the only means that they have for feeding their families is to engage in risky sexual practices.

It would be unjust and a case of 'blaming the victim' to encourage people who are sick to take moral responsibility for what was not within their control. By adding blame, shame or guilt to their problems, those who are sick suffer more. But those who inflict such harms are also diminished by their acts of injustice and inhumanity because they have hardened their hearts to the suffering of others. In addition, the decision to treat or view them differently has social risks. It would seem prudent to have a health care system that did not use resources to sort out who are responsible for their illnesses or do not deserve

Judgments about who are to blame for their illnesses would be mistaken in many cases and endanger important values encouraging a compassionate response to people.

care. To adopt this stance risks eroding the important moral norm of responding compassionately to people for no other reason than because they suffer. Ancient medical codes encourage clinicians to take care of patients just because they are in need and not to qualify their commitment. Allocation of health care resources on the basis of who we blame or excuse is not only unreliable, but also it endangers a compassionate response to people who need help. Thus, judgments about who are to blame for their illnesses would be mistaken in many cases and endanger important values encouraging a compassionate response to people. Charging sick people with moral weakness or blame is likely to increase their suffering and to undermine the duties of beneficence that are so important in the medical profession and in the society at large.

Dangers of the punishment theory

The world community must not turn away from the implications of sub-Saharan Africa having ten percent of the world's population, consuming one percent of the world's resources and yet containing 70 percent of those people living with HIV/AIDS.[5] With thousands of new infections each day, the worst is yet to come (Folkers and Fauci 2001; United Nations 2000). For both moral and pragmatic reasons, wealthy countries and persons should try to help stabilise this region and contain its epidemic. We need to address the obstacles to compassionate care and aid, including the prejudices that block people from responding as they should.[6] Some impediments are biases so ubiquitous and interwoven into our defence mechanisms that their power to endanger fair, rational and compassionate reactions to the people with HIV/AIDS may go unnoticed. One such prejudice is an ancient view associating punishment and disease, or what I have called the punishment theory of disease.

The punishment theory of disease is not only irrational, but also dangerous because it invites us to divide sick people into 'innocent' and 'guilty' at exactly the time when we need to unite, show compassion, cooperate and share resources. To combat this pandemic, we will need to stop thinking of the world as 'us' and 'them'. Labelling the sick as 'the other' fosters stigmatisation, prejudice, discrimination and abandonment. For those determined to place blame, insofar as cultural, social and economic forces make it difficult for people to act otherwise, then moral responsibility must fall on those responsible for such arrangements and on those who perpetuate them by such means as indifference, denial, intransigence or profiteering.[7] We need to aid and build alliances, not categorise, condemn or abandon.

Clinicians, investigators, politicians, and educators ought to work together in these emergency conditions to understand how best to fight this pandemic. Rich nations should work with poor nations to help them develop the resources, capacity and infrastructure to prevent, diagnose and treat this disease. This is not only the right thing to do, but also the prudent choice before governments and economies fail, and wars and famines follow (Folkers and Fauci 2001). It is in our mutual self-interest to help all countries fight and contain this illness. As partners, we can focus on the benefits of cooperating and developing reliable means of communication. Blaming victims of HIV/AIDS inhibits collaboration and abandons those in need.

The punishment theory of disease, however, is deeply ingrained. This powerful view has been used throughout history to rationalise why some get sick and some do not, so it is not surprising that it emerges today to 'explain' the HIV/AIDS pandemic. Psychiatrists Sigmund Freud (1917, 1959) and Eric Lindemann (1944) investigated the roots of the association of disease and sin. If they are right, its power may be related to understandable but irrational defence mechanisms that encourage the belief that 'we' will not get sick because 'we' have done nothing wrong; if 'others' get sick, they or those close to them must have done something bad. This could explain why this ancient view is well entrenched and has the power to shape policies affecting those who are suffering, especially distant others and to cause so much denial of the threat of HIV/AIDS.

The punishment theory of disease is an untenable and dangerous view in all its forms. Religious versions hold that disease is divine punishment and secular or moral versions hold we are punished for blameworthy lifestyles. Both fail as a general account of why people get sick and risk blaming people unjustly. Both also undermine compassionate care for people and can be an excuse to ignore or abandon people in need. Moreover, these views jeopardise the cooperation needed within and amongst nations to respond to this pandemic, the worst disease ever to sweep the world. HIV/AIDS is a worldwide crisis, and we need to cooperate and respond as befits this global public-health catastrophe, instead of engaging in the misguided and bad faith activity of dividing the world's peoples into the blameworthy and blameless.

Endnotes

[1] For example, there are concerns that public-private cooperation will not be for the common good but for the good of multi-national companies (WHO 2001).

[2] I dealt with it somewhat differently in Kopelman 1988. I discussed other diseases, and make less of the distinction between the non-modified and modified versions of the punishment theory (or as I say there 'concept') of disease.

[3] Ross (1988) cites *Los Angeles Times* 14th March 1986, Section 2, p. 4 for this quote.

[4] This view resonates with some writers in the holistic health movement who suggest that you will stay well if you live properly; this includes not only eating high-fibre cereals and exercising, but not smoking, drinking, overeating, abusing drugs, etc. (Kopelman 1988).

[5] See Benetar 2002; Van Niekerk 2002; United Nations 2000.

[6] A prejudice is different from a misconception or a mistake. Prejudice is a special form of unwarranted bias, having two components: (a) faulty or unwarranted beliefs such as over-generalisations, and (b) attitudes for or against certain persons or things based upon those unsubstantiated or faulty beliefs. What is distinctive about prejudices is that the negative attitudes persist after the faulty beliefs and reasons allegedly supporting them are exposed. As Gordon W. Allport has shown, prejudiced people resist having their rash reasoning exposed and shape 'reasons' to accommodate their attitudes. For further discussion see Kopelman, et al., 1998.

[7] Better arrangements are needed to address well-entrenched patterns of exploitation and discri-

mination. Legacies of privilege, sexism, imperialism, colonialism and other forms of exploitation are powerful forces shaping people's options.

References

Amdur, M., Doull, J., & Klassen, C. (1991). *Casaretti and Doull's toxicology, The Basic science of poisons* (4th ed., pp. 31–33/ London: Pergamon Press. [Original literature citation is Hall, R.L. (1979). *Proceedings of Marabou symposium on foods and cancer.* Stockholm: Castlan Press.].

Annan, K. (2001). 'Leadership, Partnership, Solidarity Needed in Fight Against AIDS', Address to the General Assembly by the Secretary-General on its special session of HIV/AIDS on 25th June 2001. http://www.un.org/News/Press/docs/2001/. Verified on 29th August 2001.

Benatar, S.R. (2002). 'The HIV/AIDS Pandemic: A Sign of Instability in a Complex Global System', *The Journal of Medicine and Philosophy*, 27(2), 163–177.

Duffy, J. (1979). *The Healers: A History of American Medicine.* Urbana: University of Illinois Press, 189–190.

Folkers, G.K. and Fauci, A.S. (2001). 'The AIDS Research Model: Implications for other Infectious Diseases of Global Health Importance', *The Journal of the American Medical Association* 286:4, 458–461.

Francis, R.A. (1989). 'Moral Beliefs of Physicians, Medical Students, Clergy, and Lay Public Concerning AIDS', *Journal of the National Medical Association* 81(11), 1141–1147.

Freud, S. (1917, 1957). 'Mourning and Melancholia', in *Collected Papers*, Vol. 4, tr. under supervision of J. Reviere, New York: Basic Books, 152–170.

Gellman, B. (2000, April 30). 'AIDS is Declared Threat to U.S. National Security', *The Washington Post*, A1.

Kopelman, L.M., Lannin, D.R., and Kopelman, A.E. (1998). 'Preventing and Managing Unwarranted Biases Against Patients', in *Surgical Ethics*, (ed.) Laurence B. McCullough, James W. Jones, and Baruch A. Brody (eds), Oxford University Press, 242–254.

Kopelman, L. M. (1988). 'The Punishment Concept of Disease', in *AIDS: Ethics and Public Policy* by C. Pierce and D. VanDeVeer, (eds.), Wadsworth Publishing Company, Belmont, California, 49–55.

Lindemann, E. (1944). Symptomatology and management of acute grief. *American Journal of Psychiatry* 101:141–148.

Murphy, T. F. (1988). 'Is AIDS a just punishment?' *Journal of Medical Ethics* 14, 154–160.

New York Native. (1986). 'Baptist Leader Links AIDS to Tolerance of Gays', February 10–16,7.

Psychiatric News. (1988). 'Ignorance About Aids, Homophobia Still Strong Among Health Professionals', *Psychiatric News*, 17th June, pp. 11, 25.

Ross, J.W. (1988). 'Ethics and the Language of AIDS', in *AIDS: Ethics and Public Policy* by C. Pierce and D. VanDeVeer (eds.), Wadsworth Publishing Company, Belmont, California, 39–48.

Sigerist, H.E. (1955). *History of Medicine.* New York: Oxford University Press, Vol. 1, pp. 180ff, 442ff; and Vol. II, 298ff.

The World Health Organisation (WHO). (2001). 'Public-private health partnerships can bring improved health', Home page (20th August 2001) http://www.who.int/bulletin.-pressrelease/BULLETIN.2001.5.htm. Verified 28th August 2001.

United Nations: UNAIDS 2000 Report, December. http://www.unaids.org/epidemic_update/report. Verified 29th August 2001.

Van Niekerk, A.A. (2002). 'Moral and Social Complexities of AIDS in Africa', *The Journal of Medicine and Philosophy*, 27(2), 143–162.

Watson, C. (1988). 'Virgin invoked as Aids strikes', *The Independent*, 7th June, p. 1.

Index